Mette Fossberg
HRAI

MEDICAL RECORD MANAGEMENT

EDNA K. HUFFMAN, RRA

Eighth Edition, Revised by the
American Medical Record Association
RITA FINNEGAN, MA, RRA, and
ELIZABETH PRICE, RRA, Editors

1985
PHYSICIANS' RECORD COMPANY
BERWYN, ILLINOIS

PREFACE

The eighth edition of *Medical Record Management* continues in the style of its previous versions by presenting a basic approach to medical record science. With each new edition, some practices, once important but grown obsolete over time, are replaced by newer concepts, approaches and technology. These all reflect the medical record manager as a health information specialist who occupies a unique position in health care. Where once the major role and responsibility for records were custodial, today's medical record manager occupies an ever-widening sphere of expertise in data management, usage and quality.

Accurate, timely and pertinent data are often a deciding or critical factor in claims payment and fiscal solvency. The present day medical record manager must be a compiler, provider, and coordinator of health information that justifies the payment of patients' bills, allows for the purchase of goods and services, and helps in planning the operations and activities of the health care facility.

It may seem odd to say that a health professional belonging to an organization that has been in existence for almost 60 years is a member of an "emerging profession" but that is where medical record professionals stand today. The world of prospective payment and the trend toward corporate health care involving all states of disease/health/severity of illness have created a need for better oriented, more informed individuals who can manage all kinds of data and prepare them for their ultimate usage as a management tool for patient care.

AMRA is grateful to many of its members for assisting with this edition – not only to those who made valuable suggestions for inclusion in various chapters, but also to those who wrote new chapters or updated others. A list of these includes Kathryn Piazza, RRA, for chapters on "The Medical Record – Value and Uses," and "Development and Content of the Hospital Medical Record"; Susan C. Miller, MBA, RRA, for "Medical Records in Ambulatory Care, Home Care, and Hospice Programs"; Joan

C. Liebler, MPA, RRA, for "Health Records in Long Term Care Facilities"; Mary Strosser, RRA and D. Jon Green, ART, for "Mental Health Records"; Juanita Sevilla Pursel, MSW, RRA, for "Hospital Organization – An Overview"; Margret Amatayakul, MBA, RRA, for chapters on "The Medical Record – Management of Content," and "Medical Record Department Management"; Evelyn Whitlock, RRA, for chapters on "Forms Design and Control" and "Filing Methods, Storage, and Retention"; Carol E. Osborn, MS, RRA, for "Microfilming"; Rita Finnegan, MA, RRA, for "Nomenclature and Classification Systems"; Laura Feste, RRA, for "Indexes and Registers"; Patricia Pierce, MS, RRA, for "Health Care Statistics"; Kathryn Sheehy, RRA, for "Word Processing Management in Transcription and Medical Record Services"; Leslie Blide, MA, RRA, for "Computer Applications for Medical Records"; Jennifer Cofer, RRA, for "The Legal Aspects of Medical Records"; and Patrice L. Spath, ART, for "Quality Assurance."

The Editors

TABLE OF CONTENTS

Chapter   *Page*

chapter *1*

INTRODUCTION TO
MEDICAL RECORD ADMINISTRATION

EVOLUTION OF HEALTH CARE
IN THE UNITED STATES

EARLY AMERICA

The science of medical record administration is relatively new in the health care field. When America was discovered almost 500 years ago, medical care was almost nonexistent; and the physicians of that day, all European educated, were few in number. There were no organizations or hospitals to assist them; and, of course, there were no medical records except for the few individual efforts made by doctors or townspeople to keep them for various reasons. Records have only become important because medicine and health care have achieved very high standards. But to appreciate just how far these standards have come, one need only to look back at America's beginnings.

History books abound which tell us of how medicine has evolved through the centuries. Plagues were common and often followed the routes of travelers. Lepers were isolated, and monks practiced medicine and attended nearly all the hospitals that existed. In the New World, the arriving colonist was subjected to epidemic diseases, hostile savages, and such severe winters that some early settlements were completely obliterated. Smallpox, measles, yellow fever, influenza, scarlet fever, and diphtheria were just a few of the contagious diseases that threatened their existence.

RENAISSANCE PERIOD

The Renaissance in Europe in the 16th and 17th centuries brought about not only a revival of interest in the arts, literature, and philosophy, but the beginning of a new concept of society which was based on economic growth and care for its citizens. In England there was a growing awareness that a healthy population was a positive factor in economic growth. A Hospital Council for London was planned to provide care for plague patients, maternity care, and some general care. At the same time in America, settlements began to appoint commissions to control the spread of disease, although their chief functions at first were to care for the sick, provide for orphans, and bury the dead. Little was done to prevent disease except through isolation and quarantine. But in general, in both Europe and America, some improvements were being made.

18th AND 19th CENTURIES

Health care improved slowly during the early decades of the 18th century, and it wasn't until after the American Revolution that there was evidence of real progress made. Benjamin Franklin was one of the leaders in a movement to establish the first incorporated hospital; and this institution, now known as Pennsylvania Hospital, was established in Philadelphia in 1752. Franklin served as secretary of the hospital, and many of its earliest records are in his handwriting. For the first 50 years of its existence, medical records were kept in a register in which the patient's name, address, disorder, and dates of admission and discharge were recorded. This information has been preserved from the first admission to the present time. In 1803 it was ordered that a detailed record be kept of the interesting cases, and many of these are found to be illustrated with pen-and-ink sketches. In 1873 the hospital began to keep histories and has an unbroken file to the present day.

The New York Hospital opened in 1771 and started its first register of patients in 1791. This register gives interesting notes concerning the patients; and many of the histories follow a definite routine similar to that which is used today: stating diagnosis, age, date of admission, occupation, illness, treatment, and progress notes.

Massachusetts General Hospital in Boston opened in 1821

and has the distinction of having a complete file of clinic records for every patient admitted. From these records all diseases and operative procedures were cataloged; and the findings were used for patient care, research, and statistical purposes.

As the population of the United States increased and moved westward, the demand for medical practitioners far exceeded the supply. By this time there were a few medical schools scattered about the country; but with the opening of hospitals and the increasing population, many private proprietary schools sprang up almost overnight. Called "diploma mills," they graduated students of medicine in as little as six months. By 1869 there were 72 such medical schools in the United States. Reform came slowly; but during the next two decades, there was a growing awareness that something needed to be done.

TWENTIETH CENTURY

In 1909-1911 Abraham Flexner, financed by the Carnegie Foundation, made a comprehensive study of the status of medical education in the United States. Flexner laid bare the sad picture that there were many inferior schools incapable of providing an acceptable level of medical education. After the appearance of this report, many of the inferior schools closed their doors.

Improvement of Records Through Hospital Standardization

In 1913 the American College of Surgeons was founded under the leadership of Dr. Franklin H. Martin. One of the objectives of this new group was to raise the standards of surgery. In order to accomplish this aim, they felt that a sound standard of surgical training would have to be adopted; and this would require data on the training of the surgeon in the hospital as well as in the medical school. Because every procedure in the hospital is designed for the welfare of the patient and is for this reason inseparable from the training of the surgeon, the College felt that it could best elevate the standards of surgery by a continent-wide standardization of hospitals.

In order to properly evaluate the surgical work of their candidates for fellowship, the College required the submission of 50 complete copies and 50 abstracts of case records of patients upon whom the candidate had performed major surgery. It soon became apparent that neither the hospital records of the patients nor the surgeon's office records were adequate for proper appraisal of the work of the surgeons. The College thus realized that some method would have to be devised in their Hospital Standardization Program to provide better medical records for use not only by candidates for fellowship, but also for something much more important – for efficient care of the patient in present and future illnesses; for the medicolegal needs of the hospital, physician, and the patient; and for use in medical research. They, therefore, adopted as one of the minimum requirements for hospital standardization "that accurate and complete case records be written for all patients and filed in an accessible manner in the hospital." It is interesting, and even shocking, to note that in 1918 only 89 hospitals met the standards of the first survey. Thus, only 1.6 percent of the hospitals registered in the United States (5,323) were approved. Numerous others were not even registered. During one of the early years, the results of the survey were so shocking that in the best interests of the general public the records were burned.

Steady improvement, both in the quantity and quality of medical records, began with the advent of hospital standardization. Each year on the initiative of Dr. Franklin H. Martin and Dr. Malcolm T. MacEachern, Director of Hospital Activities of the American College of Surgeons, subjects pertaining to medical records were put on the hospital standardization programs. The subjects ranged from discussions regarding the medical record itself and its care to the qualifications necessary for the persons responsible for the records. Later, round-table conferences were devoted exclusively to the subject of medical records.

Improvement of Records Through Organization

As these conferences had been successful in creating greater interest in the improvement of the quality of medical records, Dr. Malcolm T. MacEachern issued a special invitation to the medical record workers of the United States and Canada to attend a meeting in Boston during the Clinical Congress of the American College of Surgeons. The meeting was to be devoted exclusively to medical records and medical record keeping. He appointed Mrs. Grace Whiting Myers, librarian emeritus of Massachusetts General Hospital, as general chairman to organize committees, direct the preparation of a program, and plan exhibits. This was the first meeting lasting more than a day where medical records and problems concerned with their content, availability, and preservation were exclusively discussed. It was also the first meeting where exhibits of exclusive interest to medical record workers were shown.

As this meeting was drawing to a close on October 11, 1928, Mathew W. Foley, editor of *Hospital Management* and father of National Hospital Day, who was interested in elevating the standards of medical records, spoke briefly and pointed out that organization had brought about improvements in many fields and would undoubtedly accomplish the same in this one. He concluded by saying, "If you do not organize now, perhaps you never will." That brought on the motion to organize, and Mrs. Myers was elected first president; Florence G. Babcock of University Hospitals, Ann Arbor, Michigan, treasurer; and Frances Benson of Bryn Mawr Hospital, Bryn Mawr, Pennsylvania, secretary. The new group called itself the Association of Record Librarians of North America and took as its main objective: "To elevate the standards of clinical records in hospitals, dispensaries, and other distinctly medical institutions."

Not only those registered at this meeting but any other medical record workers interested in the objectives of this new group were permitted to submit applications for charter membership until the following April (1929). Thirty-five of the group in attendance at this first meeting availed themselves of this opportunity before leaving for home; and when charter membership was closed, there were 58 charter members. During the first year, members were admitted from 25 of the 48 states, the District of Columbia, and Canada.

The years proved that Mr. Foley's advice was sound, for organization has brought about great progress toward the objectives established. It has been of great individual benefit to the workers themselves as they have risen from the status of medical record clerks to a professional level. More important are the better medical care given the patient through greater interest on the part of the medical profession and the unceasing vigilance of well-trained medical record practitioners for accurate and adequate medical records. Thus, through the cooperation of the hospital and medical associations with medical record personnel working toward the same goal – the proper care of the sick and injured – the quantity and quality of medical records steadily improved.

Accreditation Replaces Standardization

The era in which the American College of Surgeons carried the primary responsibility for the establishment of standards for the hospitals of the United States and Canada came to an end on December 6, 1952, after thirty-four years of outstanding progress in the improvement of medical care. On that date the Joint Commission on Accreditation of Hospitals assumed the responsibility not only of carrying on but also of furthering this great work consistent with the patient-centered type of medical care necessary in our hospitals in this last half of the twentieth century.

The Joint Commission on Accreditation of Hospitals (JCAH) is composed of five member organizations: The American Medical Association, the American Hospital Association, the American College of Surgeons, the American College of Physicians, and the American Dental Association, the latter added in 1979. Upon receipt of an invitation by a hospital, a survey team is dispatched by the Hospital Accreditation Program to determine the compliance of the facility with the minimum requirements for quality patient care, published in the JCAH *Accreditation Manual for Hospitals*. All final decisions concerning accreditation of hospitals and the administration of the Commission itself rest with the JCAH Board of Commissioners.

Over the years, changes have been made in accreditation requirements which have raised the previous minimum standards for all areas, including medical records. Since the patients' records reflect the care given by the hospital, the accuracy and completeness of medical record documents are an important factor in determining a hospital's accreditation status. In the *1985 Accreditation Manual for Hospitals*, the Joint Commission on Accreditation of Hospitals states:

> "Substantial serious or sustained medical record deficiencies or delinquency may be the basis for a hospital's receiving less than the maximum accreditation status."

As of this writing, more than 90 percent of the eligible acute general hospitals in the United States are accredited by the Joint Commission on Accreditation of Hospitals. While both the accreditation program and its predecessor, hospital standardization, have always been voluntary in nature, accreditation today has come to signify that a hospital is operating under a high set of standards and good patient care is being rendered. Because of widespread knowledge regarding this fact, public pressure is brought to bear on hospitals which are not accredited.

Medicare and Licensure

In 1965 Congress enacted a health care program to provide hospitalization and medical insurance for the aged. Title XVIII of the Social Security Act contains the provisions for the Medicare program, officially titled "Health Insurance for the Aged and Disabled." At the same time, Title XIX, "Grants to States for Medical Assistance Programs," was enacted to form the basis for states' medical programs.

On July 1, 1966, Public Law 89-97 became effective. Known as Medicare, it had a profound effect on all health institutions. At the outset, this law, administered by the Social Security Administration (SSA), gave financial assistance under certain conditions to most of the nation's population 65 years of age and over. Since then other federal laws have been enacted to admit groups such as the handicapped; and at this writing, approximately 25 million people in our over 200 million population are covered with some kind of national insurance.

In adjudicating payment of federal funds for health care, the SSA accepted the basic premise that accreditation by the Joint Commission on Accreditation of Hospitals would also fulfill their requirements for funding medical care. Therefore, most accredited hospitals became licensed for Medicare. Most Medicare funds are handled on an area-wide basis by a fiscal intermediary, often the Blue Cross Association or other health insurance carriers.

Requirements for health facilities' reimbursement under the Medicare program are contained in the reference *Regulation Number 5, Federal Health Insurance for the Aged.* Within this publication are subparts entitled "Conditions of Participation" for each of the various types of health care facilities. Regulations relative to the compilation and maintenance of patients' medical records are found throughout the regulations, emphasizing the concept that good medical records reflect good quality patient care rendered by a health care institution.

State Licensure

Federal legislation serves as a guideline for those states who wish to promulgate individual regulations for health care programs. Modifications are made by each state on the basis of their own particular needs. As long as the states do not conflict with federal requirements, they are free to enact their own laws, considering those areas which are important to that state.

To complement federal requirements for Medicare patients, most states have legislation for hospital licensure, which includes specific mention of medical record requirements. Laws frequently have been enacted in response to controversial areas relating to the medical record field, such as computerization of medical record data and confidentiality.

HEALTH CARE TODAY

Until the 20th century the emphasis was on the care of the sick and mainly involved physicians, nurses, and hospitals. Today the health care delivery system includes many different kinds of practitioners, facilities, and organizations working together to serve their consumers or clients. Services run the gamut from providing acute care treatment to convalescent care, from preventive care and guarding against communicable diseases to giving annual checkups and conducting classes on family planning and health education. Although published in 1975, Figure 1 shows very graphically the evolution in the treatment of patients – from one concerned only with disease – to a concept of total health and well-being.

One of the major factors that has contributed to this broadening of health care has been the advancement in medical research. In the last century significant progress has been made in learning about the disease process and all the factors that predispose one to disease and illness. Where once health was defined simply as the absence of disease, health now is defined as the state of complete physical, mental, and social well-being. In this more comprehensive definition, consideration is given to health care which includes the prevention of disease and health maintenance, in addition to medical care which is curative or palliative.

With these changing attitudes toward health, the public now considers health care to be a right to which everyone is entitled regardless of financial status.

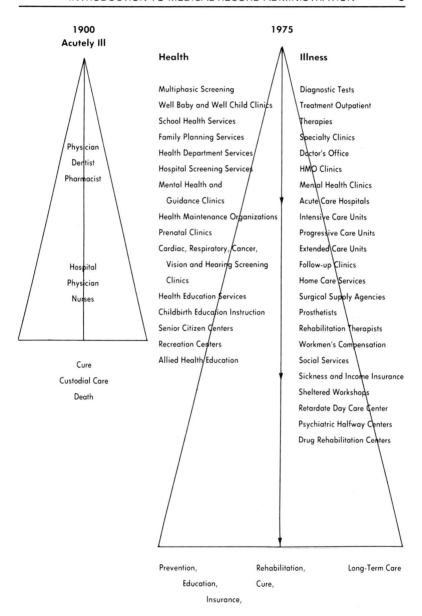

FIG. 1 – THE EVOLUTION OF HEALTH CARE IN THE U.S.

Reprinted with permission from Lee, Ruth M., *Orientation to the Health Sciences.* Bobbs Merrill Company, Inc., Indianapolis, IN, 1978.

HEALTH CARE FACILITIES

HOSPITAL CARE

As can be gathered from reading the chart in Figure 1, the multitude of services available today are provided by many kinds and types of health care facilities. The primary one is the hospital, which is an establishment that provides inpatient

---

Essential Characteristics of Hospitals*

1. The primary function of the institution is to provide diagnosis and treatment, both surgical and nonsurgical, for patients who have any of a variety of medical conditions.

2. Inpatient beds are maintained in the institution.

3. There is governing authority legally responsible for the conduct of the institution.

4. There is an administrator to whom the governing authority delegates the full-time responsibility for the operation of the institution in accordance with established policy.

5. There is an organized medical staff to which the governing authority delegates responsibility for maintaining proper standards of medical care.

6. Each patient is admitted on the medical authority of, and his care is under the direction of, a member of the medical staff.

7. The nursing services are under the direction of a full-time registered professional nurse.

8. Registered professional nurse supervision and other nursing services are continuous.

9. A medical record is maintained for each patient.

10. Pharmacy services are maintained in or by the institution and supervised by a licensed pharmacist.

11. Diagnostic x-ray services, with facilities and staff able to conduct a variety of procedures, are maintained in the institution.

12. Clinical laboratory services, with facilities and staff able to conduct a variety of tests and procedures, are maintained in or by the institution, and anatomical pathology services are regularly and conveniently available.

13. Operating room services, with facilities and staff, are maintained in the institution.

14. Food served to patients meets their nutritional requirements, and modified diets are regularly available.

FIG. 2 – ESSENTIAL CHARACTERISTICS OF HOSPITALS

*Classification of Health Care Institutions, American Hospital Association, Chicago, 1974.

beds, medical services, and continuous nursing services for diagnosis and treatment by an organized medical staff. Hospitals have certain basic characteristics but are controlled by different types of ownership or sponsorship (Figures 2 and 3).

U.S. HOSPITALS BY TYPE OF CONTROL

I. Government Owned

    A. Federal   Army/Air Force/Navy/

                       Veterans Administration

    B. State   Psychiatric/Chronic Disease/State

                       University/Medical School

    C. Local   Hospital District/County/City

II. Non-Government Owned

    A. Voluntary   Church Owned or Affiliated

                       Other, i.e., Community/Regional/

                       Kaiser/Union

    B. Proprietary   Individual Ownership

                       Corporation Owned/Single/

                       Chain (multi)

FIG. 3 – U.S. HOSPITALS BY TYPE OF CONTROL

Hospitals may also be classified as to length of stay. This term refers to the average length of time patients stay in a facility. If the average is less than 30 days, the hospital is classified as short-term. If over 30 days, it is referred to as a long-term care facility.

AMBULATORY CARE

When ambulatory care was first provided by hospitals, its purpose was to give medical care to the poor who could not afford a private physician. This concept is no longer true today, mainly because most outpatient clinics are open around the clock and patients, regardless of their financial status, can receive care whenever the need arises.

There are many types of ambulatory care facilities available, either free-standing and not affiliated with a hospital, or hospital-related. Some examples of free-standing ambulatory care facilities are health maintenance organizations, neighborhood health centers, community mental health care centers, physicians' offices, and private group practices. Examples of those that are hospital-related are hospital outpatient clinics or departments, emergicenters, surgicenters, as well as some health maintenance organizations and neighborhood health centers.

Health Maintenance Organizations

The Health Maintenance Organization (HMO) Act of 1973, amended several times since, describes an organized health care delivery system that provides a wide range of health services to a voluntarily enrolled population in exchange for a fixed periodic fee.

A health maintenance organization can be organized and sponsored by a medical foundation (usually organized by physicians), by community groups, by labor unions, by a government unit, by a profit or nonprofit group allied with an insurance company or some other financing institution, or by various other arrangements. The health maintenance organization also may be hospital or medical-school based, a free-standing outpatient facility, or a group of such outpatient facilities.

Community Health Centers

Another alternative health care facility is the community health center. With the enactment of the Economic Opportunity Act of 1964 and subsequent legislation, federally funded health centers were established in response to unmet health needs. A series of four types of health care programs is currently under the direction of the Bureau of Community Health Services within the Department of Health and Human Services: neighborhood health centers, family health centers, community health networks, and the rural health initiative.

Community Mental Health Centers

Development of mental health programs has been encouraged with the passage of several laws by Congress. The basic goals of the community mental health center are: (1) to provide comprehensive treatment to all who need it; (2) to provide this treatment within the community; and (3) to have the patient's family physician continue to see the patient and participate in his or her treatment. Federal regulations have also defined adequate services for the mentally retarded. Appropriate facilities to serve the mentally retarded would include clinics, day facilities (i.e., for treatment, education, training, custodial care, sheltered workshop), and residential facilities.

LONG TERM CARE

In the long term care field, there are three major types of facilities. These are *skilled nursing, intermediate care,* and *resident care* facilities. The brief descriptions here can be supplemented by reading Chapter 5 of this textbook.

Skilled Nursing Facility – A facility that provides nursing care on a 24-hour basis for as long a time as is necessary. The nursing care and skilled services must meet the standards as outlined in the *Conditions of Participation: Skilled Nursing Facilities* to receive federal funding.

Intermediate Care Facility – A facility that provides continuous nursing care on a 24-hour basis but not to the high degree of difficulty or sophistication as that given for skilled nursing care. Compliance with the standards as outlined in the *Conditions of Participation: Intermediate Care Facilities* will provide federal funding.

Resident Care Facility – A facility that provides residents with living arrangements, meals, and social and personal programs.

HOME CARE PROGRAMS

Home care programs are not facilities themselves but describe the location in which health care is provided – in patients' own homes. Federal regulations for home care programs are published under several forms. Public Law 89-97, previously mentioned, sets forth the *Conditions of Participation for Home Health Agencies.* Agencies eligible for participation in this program to provide health care services to patients in their own homes include the following:

1. Visiting Nurse Association.
2. Subdivision of a local or state health department.
3. Subdivision of a local or state welfare department offering home health services.
4. Combination of Visiting Nurse Association and a health department agency.
5. Department of a hospital, medical school, medical clinic, extended care facility, or rehabilitation facility offering home health services.

Other providers include companies that furnish meals, medical equipment, companions, homemakers, or therapists to the homebound.

HOSPICE CARE

The hospice is another alternative to routine institutional care. It provides palliative and supportive care for terminally ill patients and their families. Emphasis is placed on the control of symptoms and preparation for and support before and after death. The hospice can be free-standing, hospital based, or home based. A hospice is really not a type of facility but a new concept of providing health care services where they are necessary. See Chapter 4 for a more detailed discussion of hospice care.

HEALTH CARE PRACTITIONERS

Providing health care is no longer the sole responsibility of the physician. The physician relies on a great number of health care professionals whose contributions to patient care fulfill and complement the physician's orders. These individuals who contribute to both direct and indirect patient care comprise the *health care team*.

PHYSICIANS

A *physician* is a person skilled in the art of healing. There are two accepted types of physicians today: the Doctor of Medicine (MD) and the Doctor of Osteopathy (DO).

An MD is a graduate who received a doctor of medicine degree from an accredited medical school. Upon obtaining the degree and obtaining state licensure, a physician may practice general medicine. Most physicians, however, wish to practice a specialty, such as internal medicine or surgery, and continue study in that chosen specialty by completing a residency in the specialty area.

Osteopathic physicians are physicians who obtain a doctor of osteopathy degree from an approved school of osteopathy. The literal meaning of osteopathy is "disease of the bone." The osteopath believes that disease is related to the structure of the body. The osteopath prefers treatments restoring the integrity of the musculoskeletal system to interventions such as drug therapy and surgery.

Other doctoral practitioners include podiatrists (DPM), dentists (DDS or DMD), chiropractors (DC) and optometrists (OD). Practice, treatments, and drug prescriptions are limited to their particular field of preparation. Hospitals may grant admitting privileges to dentists and podiatrists with the provision that a physician prepares the patient's history and physical examination. The physician is also responsible for the overall medical supervision of the patient.

Traditionally, diagnosis and treatment have been the physician's tasks. However, today's health care scene has grown more complex; and greater demands are placed on physicians. As a result, physicians are forced to delegate more and more tasks to nonphysicians.

Among the types of physician extenders are *physician's assistants*. The function of a physician's assistant is to perform diagnostic and therapeutic tasks under the responsibility and supervision of a physician. By performing these functions, the physician's assistant allows the physician to extend his or her services through more effective use of the physician's knowledge, skills, and abilities. The physician's assistant, however, does not supplant the physician in the decision-making required when establishing diagnoses and planning therapies.

The majority of physician's assistants are classified in a category designated as Type A. Their training and education is broad enough to prepare them to manage the more common problems that occur in most primary care settings. In contrast, the physician's assistant categorized in the Type B group has specialized training in one particular area. The surgeon's assistant, the orthopedic physician's assistant, and urological assistant are examples of Type B physician's assistants. The final classification, Type C, includes those practitioners who act only as technical aides to physicians.

NURSES

Nursing is one of the oldest, most well-established health care professions. The history of nursing shows a continually expanding role for its practitioners.

The *registered nurse* (RN) is a health care practitioner whose major task is coordinating the factors that influence the patient's health, such as observing symptoms and reactions, accurate recording of facts, carrying out treatments, and administering medications. In the inpatient setting the nurse carries out physician's orders, helps the patient adjust to hospitalization, assists with discharge planning, and provides health care information and counseling to the patient. In the outpatient setting the nurse interfaces with physicians, hospitals and clinics, as well as school authorities, social agencies, housing authorities, and the state health department.

RNs are graduates of approved schools of nursing and have passed a state licensure examination. Nursing programs may be in two-year junior colleges, three-year diploma schools, or in four-year baccalaureate institutions. Three groups of nurses, nurse anesthetists, nurse midwives, and nurse practitioners, have special training in addition to a nursing degree. The *nurse anesthetist* has special training in anesthesia to assist the anesthesiologist (a physician who specializes in anesthesiology) and to administer anesthesia without direct supervision in certain predefined situations. The *nurse midwife* specializes in obstetrical care and has sufficient training to manage routine pregnancies and deliveries. The *nurse practitioner's* role is similar to that of the physician's assistant. Because of the nurse practitioner's background in nursing skills, however, the nurse practitioner's approach to patient care is believed to be more comprehensive than that of the physician's assistant. Nurse practitioners may also work more independently of physicians than physician's assistants.

A *licensed practical nurse* (LPN) is an individual who has received a formal course of instruction (usually nine months to a year) in practical nursing and who has taken a state examination to become a licensed practical nurse. Practical nursing is the performance of nursing duties which do not require the professional knowledge and skills of a registered nurse, including the care of convalescent, chronically ill, aged or infirm patients, and the carrying out of medical and nursing orders under the supervision of registered nurses or as directed by a licensed physician.

PHARMACISTS

A *pharmacist* is an individual who prepares, preserves, compounds, and dispenses drugs. Pharmacists are engaged in various aspects of pharmacy in many different settings, both within health care facilities and in health-related organizations. Pharmacists may own and manage pharmacies, they may hold positions in governmental regulatory agencies – for instance the Food and Drug Administration – and they may be involved in research, development, manufacturing, and distribution of drugs in a pharmaceutical company. Pharmacists play an important role in patient health care settings, educating physicians and nurses to recent developments in pharmacy, developing drug policies and control systems, upgrading distribution procedures, and counseling patients.

ALLIED HEALTH PRACTITIONERS

Allied health is a concept that is much newer than medicine and nursing. Although some of the occupations within allied health existed before the term allied health was used, such as medical social work, many are the result of very recent technological advances. For example, the electron microscopist came into existence only after the electron microscope became commonly used in health care. The term allied health is generally applied to occupations whose primary function is to provide health services or promote health. Preparation for such occupations ranges from on-the-job training to postgraduate education. The occupations include those who have direct patient care responsibilities, such as physical therapists and occupational therapists, and those with little or no direct patient contact, such as medical laboratory technologists, community health educators, and medical record practitioners. Figure 4 is a table of allied health occupations arranged by educational preparation and orientation.

HEALTH CARE ADMINISTRATORS

The health care delivery system also includes individuals who are often not referred to as health care practitioners because they have no medical background but who play a significant role in the health care delivery system and have special training in areas of health care administration. These are individuals who manage health care facilities and perform administrative services in health care organizations.

A *hospital (or other health care facility) administrator* is responsible for providing the environment in which direct health care services are provided. The terms chief executive officer or president are also used to describe these individuals. Administrators coordinate intrahospital resources, make decisions about expanding available facilities, incorporate new health care services, and maintain established programs for health care. The administrator works with agencies and regulatory bodies external to the hospital for purposes of quality assurance, cost containment, accreditation, and licensure.

Administrators usually have a master's-level preparation in hospital or business administration. Licensure requirements vary according to the type of facility and state in which the administrator works. Several organizations, including the American College of Hospital Administrators and the American Health Care Association (for long-term care administrators), provide a form of certification and encourage standards of excellence among their members. Continuing education activities play a prominent role in the ongoing career development of administrators.

EDUCATIONAL REQUIREMENT	PATIENT ORIENTED	LABORATORY ORIENTED	ADMINISTRATION ORIENTED	COMMUNITY ORIENTED	OTHER
Postbaccalaureate	Audiologist Clinical Psychologist Medical Social Worker Rehabilitation Counselor Speech Pathologist Psychiatric Social Worker Corrective Therapist Music Therapist Art Therapist		Hospital Administrator Biostatistician	Public Health Administrator Health Educator Nutritionist Engineering Specialties	Biomedical Engineer Health Physicist
Baccalaureate (Some with Postbaccalaureate Clinical Training)	Dietitian Occupational Therapist Physical Therapist Dental Hygienist Orthoptic Technologist Prosthetist	Medical Technologist	Medical Record Administrator	Sanitarian	Medical Illustrator Medical Writer Medical Librarian Nuclear Medical Technologist
Associate Degree and Other Prebaccalaureate	Dental Assistant Dispensing Optician Food Service Supervisor Occupational Therapy Assistant Orthoptic Technician Emergency Medical Technician Dietary Technician Recreation Technician Therapeutic Recreation Technician Speech and Communication Aide Physical Therapist Assistant	Cytotechnologist Dental Laboratory Technician Medical Laboratory Technician Radiologic Technician	Medical Record Technician Medical Secretary Ward Manager		Environmental Technologist Biomedical Instrument Technician
1-Year	Respiratory Technician Dietary Aide	Certified Laboratory Assistant	Medical Assistant Medical Office Assistant Nursing Unit Clerk		

FIG. 4 – ALLIED HEALTH PRACTITIONERS

A *chief hospital financial manager*, or chief financial officer, of a health care facility is responsible for overseeing all accounting and financial affairs of the health care facility. The background of the financial manager is often that of a certified public accountant but may also be that of master's preparation in business or finance. The Hospital Financial Management Association offers a certifying examination which addresses the special issues of financial management in health care facilities.

Public health administrators are most commonly found in health care organizations which do not provide direct patient care, especially governmental. Public health administrators set policy and develop procedures for health care programs apart from individual health care facilities, such as those administered by state health departments, etc. A master's in Public Health is the preparation most of these individuals have for their jobs.

HEALTH-RELATED ASSOCIATIONS, ORGANIZATIONS, AND AGENCIES

Much of the progress in achieving high standards of health care in the United States must be credited to the efforts of health-related associations, organizations, and agencies. Some of the major groups will be described here.

AMERICAN MEDICAL ASSOCIATION

This is the oldest of the medical associations. It was founded in 1847 and has its headquarters in Chicago, Illinois. Its components are state, county, and territorial groups of physicians.

The organizational structure is made up of several officers, a Board of Trustees, a House of Delegates, and several councils. Each council has its own purposes, projects, and responsibilities. The Council on Medical Education, for example, approves internship and residency programs for physicians and sets standards for medical schools throughout the country.

AMERICAN COLLEGE OF SURGEONS

The American College of Surgeons (ACS) was founded in 1913. This is a professional association for surgeons and was formed to establish standards of surgical education and practice.

As mentioned earlier in this chapter, the American College of Surgeons was the first association to become aware of the great need to improve the quality of medical care. Its Hospital Standardization Program, begun in 1918, was a major influence in improving this care over the next few decades. In 1952 an accreditation program replaced standardization, adding additional medical groups to its base and becoming known as the Joint Commission on Accreditation of Hospitals.

Today the primary purpose of the ACS, which is headquartered in Chicago, is to improve the quality of care for surgical patients by elevating the standards of surgical education and practice.

AMERICAN COLLEGE OF PHYSICIANS

Founded in 1936, the American College of Physicians (ACP) has its headquarters in Philadelphia, Pennsylvania. The ACP certifies specialists in internal medicine through its certification board. The board determines the qualifications of candidates and administers examinations to physicians who meet its standards. These physicians must be doctors of medicine (MDs).

AMERICAN OSTEOPATHIC ASSOCIATION

The American Osteopathic Association (AOA) was founded in 1897 and is headquartered in Chicago. Members include osteopathic physicians (DOs), surgeons, and graduates of osteopathic medicine. The purposes of the AOA include the promotion of public health, the encouragement of scientific research, and the maintenance and improvement of high standards of medical education in osteopathic colleges.

AMERICAN HOSPITAL ASSOCIATION

The American Hospital Association was founded in 1898 and is headquartered in Chicago. Its major purpose is to promote public welfare through its leadership and to provide better health services.

The AHA conducts research and educational projects in a wide variety of areas such as health care administration, hospital economics, hospital facilities and design, and community relations. It represents hospitals by speaking on their behalf on national legislative issues. It conducts many educational programs and seminars, maintains an excellent library, and publishes an annual survey of hospitals.

JOINT COMMISSION ON ACCREDITATION OF HOSPITALS

The Joint Commission on Accreditation of Hospitals was founded in 1952 to take over the accreditation program for hospitals from the American College of Surgeons. Its five-member organization included the Canadian Medical Association, but in 1959 Canada withdrew to form its own accreditation program. Today the JCAH includes the American Medical Association, the American College of Physicians, the American College of Surgeons, the American Hospital Association, and the American Dental Association.

The accreditation of hospitals has expanded into other health care facilities; and the JCAH now establishes standards for and conducts surveys of psychiatric facilities, long-term care, ambulatory care, and services for the mentally retarded and developmentally disabled.

GOVERNMENT HEALTH AGENCIES

The major health responsibilities and activities of the United States Government are centered in the Department of Health and Human Services (HHS). This department, formed in 1953, was originally known as the Department of Health, Education, and Welfare (HEW). In 1980 it was redesignated as the Department of Health and Human Services.

The department is responsible for more than 300 programs that promote good health among Americans and places special emphasis on those individuals who are least able to provide for themselves.

State and local health departments coordinate and carry out health programs at the local level. A state health department, for example, coordinates efforts with local groups to enforce sanitary regulations, control waste disposal, and maintain the quality of water. Other programs range from collecting and analyzing vital statistics to providing laboratory services to its citizens.

WORLD HEALTH ORGANIZATION

The World Health Organization (WHO) was founded in 1948 and maintains its headquarters in Geneva, Switzerland. It functions through six regional offices which are located as follows:

- Africa – Brazzaville
- Americas – Washington, DC
- Southeast Asia – New Delhi
- Europe – Copenhagen
- Eastern Mediterranean – Alexandria
- Western Pacific – Manila

Membership is open to any country. The WHO collaborates with the United Nations and assists governments in strengthening their health services wherever possible.

THE HEALTH CARE CONSUMER

As the concept of health has changed from the treatment and care of acute conditions to that of maintaining a state of well-being, the concept of the patient has changed as well. Once patients were merely recipients of direct services for the treatment of diseases. In its changing view, the public is increasingly concerned with prevention of disease, improved health conditions, safety of the work place, and safety of foods and products. In this role all Americans become consumers of health care, whether direct or indirect.

Not only have the expectations of the health care consumers changed, but also the level of participation in that care. Consumers want to have a voice in selecting their health care services. They want explanations of their problems and knowledge of what is going to take place in their care plans. Health care services are finding it necessary to reorient themselves to this more open and informed attitude.

THE MEDICAL RECORD PROFESSION

THE PROFESSIONAL ASSOCIATION

Mission

As discussed earlier in this chapter, the American Medical Record Association was founded in 1928. It is the national organization of professional medical record administrators and technicians. Its mission is to

- achieve and maintain the highest attainable levels of professional competence in those who manage health records and health information systems;
- be the nation's authoritative body on health records and health information systems, and to be an advocate for the profession on governmental, academic, and social or business issues that affect the management of health records or health information systems;
- advance the professional standing of those who manage health records and health information systems; and
- contribute, within the scope of the profession, to quality and efficiency in health care.

Membership

Membership is open to anyone who is interested in promoting the purposes of the Association. Accredited record technicians and registered record administrators are eligible for active membership. Other persons working in the medical record field or working in a related field may join as associate members. Student membership is available for those enrolled in a program for medical record administrators or technicians. Corporate membership is open to interested agencies or associations.

State Organizations

State associations are organized as integral components of the national association. National bylaws provide for one such association to be organized in each state, the District of Columbia, and the territorial possessions of the United States. An AMRA member belongs concurrently to the national and component state association in the same membership category.

House of Delegates

The Association's legislative body is the House of Delegates. Delegates from each component association comprise its membership, and at each annual meeting advise the Board of Directors in the development and modification of Association plans.

Board of Directors

Members of the Board of Directors are elected from the active membership. Each year a president-elect and two directors are elected. The board consists of the president, president-elect, and seven directors, one of whom is the immediate past-president. Each term of office is for three years, and members serve their terms while continuing their regular employment.

The Board of Directors takes its direction and derives its authority from the AMRA membership through bylaws and policies established by the House of Delegates. It acts for the Association between annual meetings and is responsible for the management of the business and professional affairs of the Association. It fulfills these responsibilities by direct action; through the Association's councils, subcouncils and committees; through the Executive Director whom it employs; and the staff positions which it authorizes.

Councils/Subcouncils/Committees

The Board of Directors is responsible for meeting the constantly changing needs of the Association through council/committee action. It may establish, oversee, and act on the recommendations of all councils and committees, except as otherwise stated in the bylaws. It also has the responsibility to make all council and committee appointments.

Councils and committees report and make recommendations to the Board of Directors. At present there are six councils:

- *Council on Certification* – oversees the certification process to ensure that it promotes competence in the delivery of medical record services.

- *Council on Organization and Communication* – responsible for the continuing development of the Association and its members by addressing new issues as they arise and communicating those issues or policies derived from them through available media or by advocate leadership.
- *Council on Professional Practices* – concerned with the development of medical record practitioners and assuring that their roles, functions, and qualifications meet current needs of health care systems.
- *Council on Education* – oversees the maintenance of educational standards through accreditation of educational programs for the medical record technician and the medical record administrator.
- *Council on Research* – explores research possibilities and encourages practitioners to test theories using research criteria and methods.
- *Council on Public Affairs* – monitors legislative affairs as well as other public issues, which have an impact on the health care delivery system.

THE EXECUTIVE OFFICE

The Board of Directors employs an Executive Director to conduct the day-to-day business of the Association, whose headquarters are located in Chicago. Through the Executive Director and staff, the various programs are carried out, an important one of which is that of maintaining a registry of credentialed medical record practitioners.

Registry – The process through which applicants who write the credentialing examinations are screened and scheduled for testing. Official results are maintained in a registry.

Divisions – The *Academic Division* works closely with the Council on Education in defining standards and in developing and recommending educational policies and accreditation procedures. It provides information and materials for colleges and universities interested in establishing medical record administration and medical record technician curricula, and it conducts workshops for faculty development.

The *Communications and Professional Practice Division* is responsible for publishing a monthly *Journal of AMRA*, monitors activities pertaining to professional practice including giving members assistance where needed, and assisting with Ethics Committee matters.

The *Continuing Education and Member Information Division* maintains records of all members including records for all practitioners who participate in the continuing education program.

The *Independent Study Division* administers and provides materials for persons who enroll in the independent study program in medical record technology. Graduates of this program with 30 semester hours of appropriate academic credits are eligible to write the examination for certification as an accredited record technician.

FOUNDATION OF RECORD EDUCATION

The Foundation of Record Education of AMRA, a nonprofit corporation affiliated with AMRA, was founded in 1962. Its purposes are threefold: to "Promote the education of students in medical record science and related areas by providing financial assistance through loans"; "Engage in research and other programs designed to organize, develop and disseminate useful information pertaining to the science of medical records to and for the benefit of the interested public"; and "Engage in other exclusively charitable, scientific, or educational activities in the field of medical records and related areas."

To accomplish these goals, the Foundation maintains the Grace Whiting Myers-Malcolm T. MacEachern Student Loan Fund, the FORE Resource Center, the Sally Mount Memorial Fund, the Research Council, and a Program Development Center.

The loan fund provides low-interest loans to students enrolled in medical record education programs. The Resource Center maintains a specialized library of medical record materials which are available on loan to members and the public. They also perform literature searches on selected topics, compile bibliographies for publication in the *Journal*, and distribute course outlines and videotapes upon request. The Resource Center also administers the Sally Mount Memorial Fund, established in 1984, which offers audiovisual materials to the membership for a handling fee. The Program Development Center sponsors continuing education seminars throughout the country on subjects of interest to today's health care practitioners. The Research Council explores research possibilities and encourages members to conduct research.

PUBLICATIONS

The *Journal of the American Medical Record Association* (JAMRA) is the official publication of the Association. It began in 1930 as the *Bulletin of the Association of Record Librarians of North America* and served members in both Canada and the United States. When the Canadian medical record practitioners formed their own association, the publication title was changed to *Journal of the American Medical Record Association*, although during the period from 1962 to 1980, it was known as *Medical Record News.*

Formerly a bimonthly publication, supplemented in the alternate months with a newsletter called "Counterpoint," the two were merged in 1983 to become a monthly publication.

Other publications include Independent Study Modules, Professional Practice Standards, position statements, bibliographies and workbooks on various topics as the needs arise.

AMRA CODE OF ETHICS

The medical record profession has its own code of ethics which applies to all medical record practitioners. It must be understood that while there are many special phases of ethics, each is a part of general ethics. A knowledge of general ethics, the science of proper conduct, is necessary because it guides individuals in differentiating between right and wrong in their daily lives. Medical record practitioners are concerned, not only with general ethics, but also with the special code of ethics which governs their conduct in the performance of their duties.

The Oath of Hippocrates is the oath upon which all medical ethics is based. In part, it states:

> Whatever, in connection with my professional practice or not in connection with it, I see or hear, in the life of men, which might not be spoken of abroad, I will not divulge, as reckoning all should be kept secret.

The American Hospital Association and the American College of Hospital Administrators also adhere to ethical codes for all hospital employees which are based in part on the Hippocratic Oath. An example of the ethical principles outlined in the American Hospital Association's *Guidelines on Ethical Conduct and Relationships for Health Care Institutions* is included here:

Health care institutions should, wherever possible and consistent with ethical commitments of the institution, ensure respect and consideration for the dignity and individuality of patients, employees, physicians, and others.

Health care institutions should establish and maintain internal policies, practices, standards of performances, and systematic methods of evaluation that emphasize high quality, safety, and effectiveness of care.

Like the American Medical Association, the American Hospital Association, and many allied associations, the American Medical Record Association, in 1957, adopted a code of ethics which defines basic principles for the conduct of its members. In 1977 the Code of Ethics was reexamined and redefined to provide those in the medical record field with definitive and binding guidelines of conduct. Because of the trust placed in every person who works in a medical record department, all, whether members of the Association or not, should observe this code which follows:

AMERICAN MEDICAL RECORD ASSOCIATION CODE OF ETHICS*

PREAMBLE

The medical record professional abides by a set of ethical principles developed to safeguard the public and to contribute within the scope of the profession to quality and efficiency in health care. This code of ethics, adopted by the members of the American Medical Record Association, defines the standards of behavior which promote ethical conduct.

PRINCIPLES

1. The medical record professional demonstrates behavior that reflects integrity, supports objectivity, and fosters trust in professional activities.

2. The medical record professional respects the dignity of each human being.

3. The medical record professional strives to improve personal competence and quality of services.

---

*Draft version subject to confirmation by 1985 House of Delegates.

4. The medical record professional represents truthfully and accurately professional credentials, education, and experience.

5. The medical record professional refuses to participate in illegal or unethical acts and also refuses to conceal the illegal, incompetent, or unethical acts of others.

6. The medical record professional protects the confidentiality of primary and secondary health records as mandated by law, professional standards, and the employer's policies.

7. The medical record professional promotes to others the tenets of confidentiality.

8. The medical record professional adheres to pertinent laws and regulations while advocating changes which serve the best interest of the public.

9. The medical record professional encourages appropriate use of health record information and advocates policies and systems that advance the management of health records and health information.

10. The medical record professional recognizes and supports the Association's mission.

PLEDGE AND EMBLEM OF AMRA

The pledge for the members of the American Medical Record Association was written and first read by Grace Whiting Myers, founder of the Association, at the annual convention in Boston in 1934. It is in part the Oath of Hippocrates and states:

> I pledge myself to give out no information from any clinical record placed in my charge, or from any other source, to any person whatsoever, except upon order from the chief executive officer of the institution which I may be serving.

The position of the medical record practitioner is, therefore, one

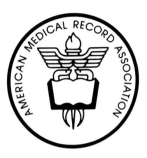

RECOGNIZING that the AMERICAN MEDICAL RECORD ASSOCIATION seeks to develop and enforce the highest standards of work among its members, I hereby pledge myself, as a condition of membership, to conduct myself in accordance with all its principles and regulations.

IN PARTICULAR I pledge myself to pursue the practice of my profession in a spirit of unselfishness, and of loyalty to the Association and to the institution which I am called to serve; to bear always in mind a keen realization of my responsibility; to seek constantly a wider knowledge of my profession through serious study, through instruction by competent approved teachers, through interchange of opinion among associates, and by attendance at meetings of this and of allied associations; to regard scrupulously the interests and rights of my fellow-members, and to seek counsel among them when in doubt of my own judgment.

MOREOVER, I pledge myself to give out no information concerning a patient from any clinical record placed in my charge, or from any other source, to any person whatsoever, except upon order from the chief executive officer of the institution which I may be serving; and to avoid all commercialization of my work.

FINALLY, I pledge myself to co-operate in advancing and extending by every lawful means within my power, the influence of the AMERICAN MEDICAL RECORD ASSOCIATION.

FIG. 5 – PLEDGE AND EMBLEM OF THE AMRA

of trust. The patient has a legal right to privacy and it is the ethical obligation of all who handle patient information to uphold this right.

When the pledge was adopted, it became evident that an official emblem was needed for use on papers and documents, as well as for jewelry signifying membership in the Association. An emblem was adopted in 1935. It bears the name of the Association, the date of organization (1928) and a design symbolizing a medical record superimposed upon an adaptation of the caduceus (Figure 5). It is usually printed in the official colors of the Association – green, gold, and white – which were officially adopted in 1942.

Just how the winged caduceus, which has no legendary association with medicine, came to represent the medical profession in a great part of the world is not known. The word caduceus is a Latin adaptation from the Greek meaning herald's wand, and the Greek god Hermes, referred to as Mercury by the Romans, was believed to have been the messenger who originally carried the wand. He is believed to have been a progression from the old Babylonian snake god, the awakener of life and vegetation and the master of the healing art. The snake has been a symbol of medicine from antiquity. Some say the snake was selected because of its long life; others think that the renewal of its skin suggests the renewal of youth and health; and still others think it was selected because of its keen sight. The caduceus incorporates a winged staff with two snakes entwined around it in opposite directions, their heads confronting each other. One legend states that Hermes found the two fighting each other and that when he separated them with his wand, they entwined themselves around it in appreciation.

Since Hermes was the messenger of the gods, two wings were added to the staff; and it became the emblem of commerce and of peace as he also brought armistice messages to fighting armies. This is thought to be the reason that the caduceus was selected as an administrative symbol by the Medical Corps, the noncombatant branch of the United States Army, while the Aesculapian staff, with one snake entwined was used as the medical symbol incorporated in the coat of arms of the United States Army. The caduceus is universally the symbol of the medical profession except in the British Commonwealth, France, Germany, and the United States. In these countries the knotty staff of Aesculapius with one snake entwined around it is the symbol of the medical profession, and it is the emblem of the American Medical Association as well.

As the caduceus is a medical administrative symbol, it, with the medical record and the flame signifying the light of knowledge, constitutes a very appropriate design for the emblem of the American Medical Record Association.

THE MEDICAL RECORD PROFESSIONAL

EDUCATIONAL GROWTH

For the first few years after organization of the Association of the Record Librarians of North America, the founding members were busy bringing about needed changes in their own departments. As time went on, they realized that those trained by the apprenticeship method, which had until then been the only method available, could no longer cope with the problems of their work. They could not adequately meet the objectives which they had established when the Association was organized; they could not be expected to go out and organize departments that would meet the newer, more stringent requirements for medical record services. This led to the appointment of a committee to plan for the training of medical record practitioners.

Under the leadership of Je Harned Bufkin, a curriculum was drawn up for the use of hospitals desiring to establish schools. The prerequisites for application, the content and length of the courses, and the procedures to be followed for approval of the schools were also established.

By 1935 the educational program was ready to function, and the following schools and instructors were approved in the order listed:

(1) Massachusetts General Hospital, Boston; Genevieve Chase, instructor;

(2) Rochester General Hospital, Rochester, New York; Je Harned Bufkin, instructor;

(3) St. Mary's Hospital, Duluth, Minnesota; Sister M. Patricia, O.S.B., instructor; and

(4) St. Joseph Hospital, Chicago; Edna K. Huffman, instructor.

St. Mary's Hospital in Duluth was affiliated with the College of St. Scholastica from the very beginning, and its program was the first to grant a baccalaureate degree in medical records. Other programs gradually made the transition from the hospital setting to academic affiliation.

Presently there are approximately fifty accredited educational programs in medical record administration, all of which either grant degrees or require them for entrance. Accredited educational programs for medical record technology number about seventy-five throughout the United States.

Until 1942 the Association inspected and approved its own schools, but by this time it was felt that the educational experience of the Council on Medical Education and Hospitals of the American Medical Association would be of great benefit to the educational programs for medical record personnel. Accordingly, in that year, a formal resolution was presented to the House of Delegates of the American Medical Association, requesting them to assume responsibility for the approval of the schools for medical record administration. This received favorable action, and the Council on Medical Education and Hospitals was authorized to establish standards, inspect training programs, and publish lists of approved schools.

Today the Committee on Allied Health Education and Accreditation (CAHEA) of the American Medical Association and the American Medical Record Association jointly share responsibility as accrediting agencies for these educational programs. Educational standards for medical record programs are approved by the Council on Medical Education of the American Medical Association and the AMRA House of Delegates. These standards have been elevated to meet today's prerequisites for competent medical record administrators and technicians.

The AMRA educational committee for these schools, now the Council on Education, was for many years composed of representatives from the American College of Surgeons, the American Medical Association, the American Hospital Association, and the American Medical Record Association. In 1952 representatives from the American College of Physicians and the American Public Health Association were added. Thus the Council, concerned with the education of medical record personnel, always had the advantage of the broad experience of groups with allied interests to guide in preparing workers to help in raising the standards of clinical records.

MEDICAL RECORD ADMINISTRATOR

An approved educational program for individuals preparing to become medical record administrators must grant a bachelor's degree in medical record science or accept only candidates who already have a baccalaureate degree. The curriculum includes courses in anatomy and physiology, medical record science, medical terminology and medical science, organization and management, statistics, data processing, and directed practice in medical record departments. Students also gain background in the natural sciences including chemistry and biology, in humanities, in social science, in languages, and in philosophy. Upon successful completion of the medical record administration program, the graduate is eligible to take the national registration examination to become a registered record administrator.

MEDICAL RECORD TECHNICIAN

Because of the great shortage of properly trained medical record administrators, it became evident by 1951 that there was a need for trained ancillary workers who would have less training and experience than the medical record administrator, but who would be qualified to work under the supervision of a qualified medical record supervisor or medical record committee in a small hospital, or under the supervision of a registered record administrator in a large hospital. Accordingly a curriculum was drawn up, and prerequisites for entrance (high school graduation) established for schools to train an additional level of medical record personnel.

In 1953 the first schools for the education of medical record technicians were approved. These were largely hospital-based programs. By the end of the 1960s, most hospital-based schools had been phased out due to increased demands on the full-time RRAs who were required to administer both the hospital's educational program and the medical record department. At the present time most programs are two years in length and are found in colleges and universities which grant an associate degree. A sampling of the curriculum for technician's programs includes courses in anatomy and physiology, medical record science, medical terminology, basic pathology of disease process, and directed practice in a medical record department. Successful completion of a technician's training program provides eligibility to take the national accreditation examination given by the AMRA each year to become an accredited record technician.

Independent Study Program

While the medical record profession underwent its growing pains, the demand for qualified medical record personnel far exceeded the supply. In order to provide some measure of balance, the 1957 AMRA House of Delegates approved the development of a correspondence course for medical record personnel. Enrollment began in 1962, and by 1979 over 15,000 students had availed themselves of this educational opportunity. Open to individuals with a high school diploma who worked in a medical record department, the correspondence course consisted of twenty-five lessons in basic medical record science and medical terminology. The course was designed to cover a period of eighteen to twenty-four months, and satisfactory completion entitled the student to sit for the accreditation examination to become an accredited record technician.

In 1979 the AMRA introduced a new, more comprehensive home study program entitled "Independent Study Program in Medical Record Technology" (ISP/MRT) to replace the original correspondence course for medical record personnel. A total of seventeen modules with ninety-seven lessons must be completed in the enrollment period of thirty-six months. Course content includes such subjects as medical terminology, medical transcription, medical record science, health care delivery trends, supervisory concepts, and directed clinical practice. In order to enroll in the ISP/MRT, a candidate must be a high school graduate. Although enrollment is open to qualified applicants, students who satisfactorily complete the program must also have 30 semester hours of college credit to sit for the accreditation examination to become an accredited record technician.

REGISTRATION AND ACCREDITATION

As medical record work began to take on a professional status, it was felt that a yardstick for measuring the ability of the workers was needed. In 1932 the American Medical Record Association set up qualifications, including a written examination, to establish recognition of highly qualified medical record practitioners as professionals. These qualifications were raised

American Medical Record Association

no. _____

This Certifies that

has satisfactorily complied with the requirements
of this Association and is therefore qualified as a

Registered Record Administrator

In Witness Whereof we have hereby ascribed our names
this   day of   19

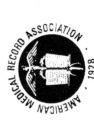

President
American Medical Record Association

Executive Director
American Medical Record Association

FIG. 6 – CERTIFICATION OF REGISTERED RECORD ADMINISTRATOR

American Medical Record Association

no. ____

This Certifies that

has met the qualifications of Accreditation of this Association and is thereby awarded the title of

Accredited Record Technician

In Witness Whereof we have hereby ascribed our names

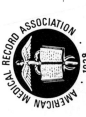

Executive Director

President

FIG. 7 – CERTIFICATION OF ACCREDITED RECORD TECHNICIAN

as prerequisites for all allied health professionals in the field advanced.

Prior to 1965 many experienced medical record practitioners were credentialed under this "grandfather clause." As of January 1965, applicants for registration were required to be graduates of a school approved for education of medical record administrators. This stipulation was further defined in 1970 to specify possession of a baccalaureate degree for all MRAs who wished to write the registration examination.

Upon successful completion of the examination, the individual receives a Certificate of Registration (Figure 6), and is entitled to use the letters RRA (Registered Record Administrator) after his name.

The American Medical Record Association also provides a written examination to establish recognition for accredited record technicians, awarding a Certificate of Accreditation to successful candidates (Figure 7).

CONTINUING EDUCATION

Just because the medical record professional receives his credentials (RRA or ART) does not mean his education has ended. The American Medical Record Association, recognizing that the true professional is never finished with learning, began to plan a continuing education program in the early 1970s. In January 1975 the Association launched its first five-year cycle of Continuing Education, requiring 15 hours per year or 75 hours total for registered record administrators, and 10 hours per year or 50 hours total for accredited record technicians to retain their credentials. At present the cycles are only two years in length, although yearly hours required remain the same. Failure to complete the required education hours results in revocation of the individual's registration or accreditation status, and the person is no longer eligible to use his designated credentials. Appropriate completion of the requirements at a later date may result in the individual's reinstatement as a qualified medical record professional.

ROLES

Medical record practitioners have traditionally been employed in hospitals and other health care facilities. In recent years, however, many other areas of employment opportunity have opened up. Some of these are in insurance companies, accounting firms as consultants, law firms, as sales representatives for computer or office equipment companies, or any business organization where data storage and retrieval – whether health or not – is of great importance.

Many medical record practitioners have obtained advanced degrees in Business Administration, Education, or Public Administration so that they could pursue higher level jobs in special settings. Some of these include educational institutions; governmental settings; and administrative posts of various kinds, both at home and abroad.

Those who have studied the job-market opportunities and trends predict that over the next ten years there will be a healthy upward movement for many allied health professionals. Medical record professionals, because of the widening of their job opportunities to include more and more nonhospital settings, will probably continue to be in short supply for some time.

INTERNATIONAL FEDERATION OF HEALTH RECORD ORGANIZATIONS

The American Medical Record Association, organized in 1928, was the first national association. While the original membership included many Canadian medical record librarians, they (the Canadians) soon realized the advantages of having their own organization with common national goals; and in 1942 they organized the Canadian Association of Medical Record Librarians.

Prior to World War II, the medical record personnel of Great Britain were preparing for organization but had to delay until after the war. They organized in 1948 as the Association of Medical Records Officers of Great Britain.

By 1949 the Australian Hospital Association recognized the value of trained medical record personnel and sparked the impetus that brought about the organization of two state groups, the New South Wales and Victorian Associations of Medical Record Librarians. In 1952 the Australian Federation of Medical Record Librarians was organized. The responsibilities of the Australian medical record librarians are very similar to those of their counterparts in Canada and the United States. This addition to the medical scene brought about added interest in research from medical records and thus a great improvement in the quality of the medical record per se, just as had occurred in other countries.

Channels of communication were soon established between the members of the organized associations as well as with isolated workers in other countries around the world. It was believed that worldwide participation of medical record personnel would bring about greater and more rapid advances in the establishment of international standards, the compilation of statistics that could be used for international comparisons, as well as disease classifications that could be adopted on an international basis. Therefore, the First International Congress on Medical Records was held in London in 1952 with representatives from nine countries participating. Additional Congresses were held every few years until the Fifth International Congress in Stockholm, where the International Federation of Health Record Organizations was established. The Sixth Congress, and first meeting of the Federation, was held in 1972 in Sydney, Australia. It is evident that international interest in medical records has spread rapidly and that the enthusiasm of the original sponsoring group, including the American Medical Record Association, has been amply rewarded.

The International Federation of Health Record Organizations meets every four years at various locations around the world. The purposes of the Federation are similar to those adopted by the national organizations. The Federation attempts to serve as a means of communication among medical record practitioners in various countries and thus advance the standards of medical record science worldwide. The Federation promotes the development of techniques to improve the quality of medical record services. This is done partly by educational programs and other media developed for the exchange of ideas and experiences by medical record personnel on an international level.

SUMMARY

The medical record professional plays a major role in the ever-expanding health care field. To provide competent assistance to health professionals involved in the complex process of quality patient care, he is called upon to advance daily by continuing his own education and maintaining a thorough knowledge of his specialty. With the dedication of a true professional, the medical record practitioner often donates valuable time and assistance to medical record association activities and other health-related organizations and agencies to advance the art and science of medical record administration. The medical record professional realizes the importance of membership in his state and national associations. Such membership provides him with a unified voice to influence legislative bodies and governmental and nongovernmental regulatory agencies. In return for his contributions to his professional associations, the medical record professional benefits from the vast amount of information disseminated to members on new techniques and requirements for the sound practice of medical record science. In a world whose climate is often tense with conflict, it is encouraging to note that medical record professionals are dedicating themselves internationally to the improvement of medical record services and quality patient care in all areas of the world.

STUDY QUESTIONS

1. Identify the following persons or organizations:
   a. the first medical record librarian
   b. the first hospital to establish a medical record department
   c. the "Father of Medicine"
2. Summarize the reasons for the development of the Hospital Standardization Program by the American College of Surgeons.
3. In 1952, which organization assumed responsibility for the Hospital Standardization Program?
4. Summarize the efforts toward professionalism by medical record practitioners which eventually led to formation of the American Medical Record Association in 1970.
5. Distinguish between the medical record administrator and medical record technician in each of the following areas:
   a. educational requirements
   b. credentialing examination

    c. continuing education requirements

    d. roles of each

6. Name the organization which shares responsibility with the AMRA for accrediting medical record education programs.

7. Explain the reasons why it is important for all medical record department employees to abide by the AMRA Code of Ethics.

8. Identify the composition and functions of the AMRA House of Delegates, Board of Directors, and Councils.

9. Describe the activities of the Foundation of Record Education.

10. Identify the advantages to AMRA of participating in the International Federation of Health Record Organizations.

REFERENCES

Accreditation Manual for Hospitals. Joint Commission on Accreditation of Hospitals. Chicago, Illinois, 1985.

BURDA, DAVID. "More Positions Available Than Wanted in Medical Record Job Market." *Journal of the American Medical Record Association,* October, 1984.

Classification of Health Care Institutions. American Hospital Association, 1974.

Conditions of Participation – Subpart K: Skilled Nursing Facilities, Social Security Administration.

Conditions of Participation for Hospitals. HIR-10, Social Security Administration.

Dynamics of Health Care. 3rd Ed. RUTH M. FRENCH. McGraw Hill, 1979.

Editorial on Hospital Standardization. *Hospital Management,* May, 1919.

MARTIN, FRANKLIN H. "Hospital Standardization – Its Inception, Development and Progress in Five Years." *Surgery, Gynecology and Obstetrics,* 34:135-160, 1922.

Mustard's Introduction to Public Health. 5th Ed. LENOR S. GOERKE and ERNEST L. STEBBINS. Macmillan Company, 1968.

MYERS, GRACE W. *Autobiography.* Berwyn, Illinois: Physicians' Record Company, 1949.

————. *History of Massachusetts General Hospital.* Boston, Massachusetts: *Griffith-Stillings Press, 1929.*

————. *"Presidential Address."* Bulletin of the Association of Record Librarians of North America, January, 1930.

Orientation to Health Services. RUTH M. LEE. Bobbs Merrill, 1978.

Public Health and Community Medicine. 3rd Ed. LLOYD E. BURTON and HUGH H. SMITH. Williams Wilkins, 1980.

chapter *2*

THE MEDICAL RECORD —
VALUE AND USES

THE MEDICAL RECORD

The medical record is a compilation of pertinent facts of a patient's life and health history, including past and present illness(es) and treatment(s), written by the health professionals contributing to that patient's care. The medical record must be compiled in a timely manner and contain sufficient data to identify the patient, support the diagnosis, justify the treatment, and accurately document the results. The medical record practitioner must ensure that the medical record contains all of the pertinent information needed by health personnel to treat the patient now and in the future; information needed by approving agencies to license, certify, and accredit health care facilities; information needed by third-party payers (insurance companies and government agencies) to pay for health care; information needed by educators, researchers, and public health officials to improve health care practices; and information needed by the patient. The process of ensuring that the medical record is complete and useful is a challenging and complex task for the medical record practitioner. This task entails a thorough knowledge not only of the medical record and its content, but also ancillary information concerning purpose, ownership, value, uses of and responsibility for the medical record.

PURPOSE

The main purpose of the medical record is to accurately and adequately document a patient's life and health history, including past and present illness(es) and treatment(s), with emphasis on the events affecting the patient during the current episode of care.

OWNERSHIP

The medical record developed in the hospital, clinic, other health care facility or under its auspices is considered to be the physical property of that facility. The information contained therein, however, is the property of the patient and thus must be available to the patient and/or his legally designated representative upon appropriate request. Regulations regarding access to the medical record may vary depending on state law. The fact that the facility owns the pieces of paper upon which the record is written does not prevent others from submitting legitimate claims to see and copy the information therein. Discussion of the release of medical record information is presented in Chapter 17.

USES

The document compiled as the medical record contains a wealth of information and has many uses, both personal and impersonal. Personal use refers to usage in which the identity of the patient is retained and is necessary. A request for copies of portions of a patient's record by the insurance company which provides hospitalization coverage for the patient is an example of personal use. The copies are needed for the company to process the patient's claim and thus provide a service to the particular patient.

Impersonal use refers to the usage in which the identity of the patient is not retained and is not necessary. Use of the data in the record for a research project involving 1,000 medical records is an example of impersonal use. The major reason the medical record department concerns itself with these differences is that a proper authorization by the patient or his legal representative for release of information is required before information can be released for personal use.

The medical record is used in a number of ways:

Patient Care Management –
   a. to document the course of the patient's illness and treatment during each episode of care;

b. to communicate between the physician and other health professionals providing care to the patient; and

c. to inform health professionals providing subsequent care.

Quality Review – as a basis for evaluating the adequacy and appropriateness of care.

Financial Reimbursement – to substantiate insurance claims of the health facility and patient.

Legal Affairs – to provide data to assist in protecting the legal interest of the patient, the physician, and the health care facility.

Education – provides actual case studies for the education of health professionals.

Research – provides data to expand the body of medical knowledge.

Public Health – identifies disease incidence so plans can be formulated to improve the overall health of the nation and world.

VALUE

The data within the medical record are valuable to many users:

To the Patient

A medical record contains data regarding a patient's past and present health and presents documentation by health professionals of the patient's current condition in the form of: physical findings, results of diagnostic and therapeutic procedures, and the patient's responses.

Because health professionals provide care to a number of people during a given time period, they are not expected to remember the details of each patient's illness and response to treatment. The patient also may not remember the significant details of his illness and treatment. Thus the record serves as a reference for both the patient and health professional. It provides substantiation of care given, which is needed for the processing of the patient's health insurance claims. The record also serves the patient by providing data to health professionals who treat the patient on subsequent episodes of care, so continuity of care is provided to the patient. The record can provide data which may protect the legal interests of the patient in workers' compensation, personal injury, or malpractice cases.

To the Health Care Facility

The medical record is of value to the health care facility in that it provides data to evaluate the performance of health professionals working in the health care facility and to evaluate use of the facility's resources, such as special diagnostic equipment and services offered by the facility. The record is used in surveys by licensing, certifying, and accrediting agencies in evaluating care which the facility provides and in determining compliance with the standards of the respective agency.

The record is relied upon more and more to substantiate claims submitted to third-party payers. Hospitals extract data from throughout the medical record to determine all the diagnoses and procedures related to a given patient in order to correctly file a payment claim. Because the record documents the care given, it can be used, if necessary, to protect the legal interest of the facility in lawsuits.

To Health Care Providers

The medical record provides information to assist all professionals in caring for a patient during the current episode of care and during subsequent visits to a facility. The record documents the care given by each professional, thus protecting their legal interests.

The record assists physicians, in particular, in providing continuity of care when the patient is discharged from a hospital and is followed in the clinic or private office setting. For their own education, all professionals can review records of patients for whom they have provided care.

To Educators, Researchers, and Public Health Officials

The medical record contains data which assist the health professional and the student in health professions in the educational process when they review the record for study purposes. The record is indispensable in furthering medical research by supplying a data base for evaluating the effectiveness of treatments for specific diseases.

The medical record also provides data for reporting vital events such as births and deaths to the public health agency in each state. Requirements for reporting certain diseases, for example, venereal diseases and gunshot wounds, also exist in each state to protect the health of the individual and the public. Statistics developed from data gathered in this manner may document the need for state, national, and world health programs.

To Organizations Responsible for Health Care Claim Payments

Insurance companies and federal/state program reviewers scrutinize medical records to determine if documentation exists to substantiate the facility's claim for insurance benefits. For continued participation in federal/state health insurance programs, the medical records maintained by a facility are reviewed to determine compliance with standards regarding medical record content.

RESPONSIBILITY FOR THE MEDICAL RECORD

The medical record is the property of the health care facility and is maintained for the benefit of the patient, the physician, and the facility. It is the responsibility of the facility to provide a record for each patient and safeguard the record and its content against loss, damage, tampering, and unauthorized use. Responsibility for providing, directly or indirectly, an adequate medical record is shared by many members of the hospital and medical staff.

Governing Body

Because of the corporate nature of hospitals, the final responsibility in all matters pertaining to hospital management is vested in the governing body. In almost all states, the governing body is held responsible for the proper care of the patient as well as for the proper selection of a qualified medical staff and hospital administrator or chief executive officer. As the final authority, it is legally and morally responsible for determining that each patient receives high quality medical care, documented by a complete and accurate medical record. The governing body fulfills this responsibility by delegation to the chief executive officer as its representative and usually takes

no active part in hospital operations except in evaluating recommendations made by the chief executive officer or the medical staff.

Hospital Administration

The authority to manage a hospital is delegated to the chief
executive officer by the governing body. Medical records generated by a facility are the property of that facility and thus are
rightfully the concern of the chief executive officer. The administration is responsible for ensuring that the medical staff adopts
rules and regulations providing for the maintenance of complete
medical records in a timely manner. Further, the administration
must see that such policies are consistently enforced. The administration delegates to the staff of the medical record department
responsibility for processing, storing, and retrieving the medical
record. However, the administration is responsible for providing
to this department adequate direction, space, equipment, and personnel to perform these tasks effectively.

Medical Record Department

The director of the medical record department works with
physicians and the directors of all hospital departments to educate the hospital and medical staff in proper documentation
practices and to assist them in designing medical record forms
which facilitate documentation.

The staff of the medical record department reviews the record
for completeness and compliance with established rules and regulations regarding the record. It is most often in the medical record
department that errors or deficiencies in documentation are discovered and notification given to the responsible parties. Another
responsibility of the medical record department is providing accurate and efficient medical transcription services to assist physicians and other health professionals in documenting patient care.
The medical record department is also responsible for storing the
record in a secure manner, retrieving the record efficiently, and
providing access to the record by those so authorized.

Attending Physician and Other Health Care Professionals

The major responsibility for an adequate medical record rests with the patient's physician. Other physicians and health care professionals are responsible for correctly documenting the care they provide.

As a group, the medical staff is responsible for determining bylaws and rules and regulations by which it is governed. Licensure, certification, and accreditation agencies all have standards requiring that the medical staff rules and regulations address certain issues regarding the medical record. Generally, these issues include:

- provisions for the keeping of accurate and complete clinical records

- delineation of individuals authorized to make entries in the medical record

- time limit following admission of the patient in which a history and physical examination must be entered in the patient's record

- time limit following discharge for completion of the record

The JCAH requires the medical staff to review the quality of medical records at least quarterly for clinical pertinence and timely completion. Further, the JCAH specifies that individuals who perform the medical record review function should determine or recommend the format of the medical record, the forms used in the medical record, and the use of electronic data processing and storage systems for medical record purposes.

It is evident, from the many perspectives discussed in this chapter, that concise, complete, and accurate medical records are of utmost importance. To support this idea, various agencies and organizations involved in health care have established requirements or standards that address the medical record and its content. In the next section, the most prominent organizations and the roles they play in evaluating and improving health care and the health record will be discussed.

DESIGNATIONS OF APPROVAL
FOR HEALTH CARE FACILITIES

"Health care is a right, not a privilege" is a principle commonly expressed by the public today. To accommodate demands for increased health services, a multitude of local, state, and federal programs are available to offer health care services. As a result, hospitals and other types of health care facilities are subject to regulations set by multiple government agencies which provide reimbursement for health care. Voluntary accreditation organizations also have requirements or "standards" which must be met by facilities seeking accreditation from these organizations. Broad concepts involving licensure, certification, and accreditation of health care facilities will be discussed in this section and detailed requirements specific to the medical record will be discussed in Chapter 3.

LICENSURE

Licensure of health care facilities is a governmental activity which gives legal approval for a facility to offer the services for which it is licensed. In order to obtain a license, the facility must meet certain specified requirements for physical aspects of the facility, services provided, and personnel employed to provide these services. These standards are generally considered to be the very minimum and may vary from locale to locale.

Government Agencies

Licensure is a designation provided by local or state governments. Each licensing body develops the regulations used to evaluate facilities in that area. Because most hospitals are licensed by the state, regulations for licensure reflect the law in that state. Federal facilities, such as Veterans Administration and Public Health Service hospitals, are established by law and do not require licensing. They do, of course, seek accreditation and certification as appropriate to their functions. Each medical record practitioner should be familiar with and have access to the licensure regulations in the state in which he works.

CERTIFICATION

Certification of health care facilities is also a governmental activity. This designation allows a facility to be reimbursed by the government for providing services to patients enrolled in certain government programs (Medicare and Medicaid). Participation of the facility is voluntary, but to be certified, the facility must adhere to certain regulations. The requirements have been developed by the federal government and are considered to be minimum acceptable standards. Compliance with these regulations is monitored by each state through an agreement with the Secretary of the Department of Health and Human Services.

Department of Health and Human Services

The Department of Health and Human Services (DHHS) – prior to 1980 Department of Health, Education and Welfare – is the Cabinet level department of the federal executive branch most often concerned with people and most involved with the nation's human concerns, including health. It has among its major subdivisions the: Social Security Administration (SSA); Health Care Financing Administration (HCFA); the U.S. Public Health Service (USPHS); which includes among others the National Center for Health Statistics, National Center for Health Services Research, Center for Disease Control (CDC), Food and Drug Administration (FDA), and National Institutes of Health (NIH). The Secretary of DHHS advises the President of the United States on health, welfare, income security plans, and other policies and programs of this department and directs the department staff to carry out programs approved by Congress.

The Department of Health and Human Services oversees the certification process which is administered through HCFA. The concept of certification came about as a result of these amendments to the Social Security Act: Title XVIII (Medicare) and Title XIX (Medicaid). These amendments provide federal funds to qualifying hospitals, skilled and intermediate nursing homes, and home health agencies for treating patients enrolled in the above-named federal programs. To qualify, a hospital must follow the regulations set forth in the *Conditions of Participation– Hospitals*. There are also individual *Conditions of Participation* for nursing homes and for home health agencies.

ACCREDITATION

Accreditation is a completely voluntary activity of a facility and is not designed to affect the right of a facility to offer services or to participate in the governmental programs mentioned above. Accreditation implies that there is voluntary conformance to high standards which are more rigorous than the minimum licensing or certification standards.

Some of the common goals of the accrediting agencies described in this chapter are to: develop and maintain standards by which health care facilities may measure and strengthen their programs; improve the quality of services offered by these facilities; and offer to the facility, community, and the consumer a mechanism of accountability and assurance of high quality care. The standards used in the survey process are developed by the respective accrediting agencies with the aid of experts in that particular field. These standards are revised as changes in the state of the art, government regulations, demand, or need of the public occur.

In the following section the most widely recognized accrediting organizations for health care facilities will be discussed.

Joint Commission on Accreditation of Hospitals

The Joint Commission on Accreditation of Hospitals has as its mission to help improve the quality of care and services and the quality of the environment of care provided in health care settings through the voluntary accreditation process.

The American Hospital Association, the American Medical Association, the American College of Surgeons, the American College of Physicians, and the American Dental Association sponsor the JCAH, and each provide representatives who comprise the JCAH Board of Commissioners. These commissioners write and publish the standards developed by JCAH and determine the accreditation status of various types of health care facilities.

JCAH surveys and has developed standards manuals for: acute care hospitals (*Accreditation Manual for Hospitals*); psychiatric, substance abuse, and mental retardation facilities (*Consolidated Standards Manual for Child, Adolescent, and Adult Psychiatric, Alcoholism, and Drug Abuse Facilities and Facilities Serving the Mentally Retarded/Developmentally Disabled*); long-term care facilities (*Long-Term Care Standards Manual*); nonhospital ambulatory care health organizations (*Ambulatory Health Care Standards Manual*); community mental health programs (*Principles for Accreditation of Community Mental Health Services Programs*); and hospices (*Hospice Standards Manual*). JCAH also published various guides, a newsletter (*JCAH Perspectives*), and a periodical (*Quality Review Bulletin*).

Presently JCAH grants a maximum of three-year's accreditation (with or without contingencies) if a hospital is in substantial compliance with the standards. Approximately 18 months from the date of its survey, each accredited hospital is asked to conduct an interim self-survey using procedures and submitting reports as required by JCAH. When a hospital is accredited, subject to one or more contingencies, JCAH monitors the hospital's efforts to improve an area of concern identified during an accreditation survey. Usually these hospitals are required to either submit a written progress report or to undergo a focused on-site survey. Accreditation may be denied or withdrawn. Because accreditation is not automatically renewable, a hospital must undergo the full accreditation process each time its accreditation status approaches expiration.

The JCAH accreditation survey may serve purposes other than the accreditation process. The District of Columbia and thirty-nine of the states have legislation, regulation, and/or administrative arrangements enabling their hospital licensure agencies to recognize JCAH hospital accreditation in whole or in part for licensure purposes. Each of these licensure agencies requires the hospital to submit evidence of accreditation in connection with their application for relicensure. Over half of these licensure agencies require the hospital seeking relicensure to send a copy of the recommendations made by JCAH in connection with its most recent accreditation survey as a condition for using the accreditation survey in lieu of the licensure inspection.

In a few states, representatives of the state hospital licensure agency join in the JCAH survey process to review licensure requirements not covered under JCAH requirements. In all cases the licensure and accreditation decisions are made independently by the respective organizations. Many agencies perform periodic validation inspections of a sample of hospitals using accreditation status as a method to replace state licensure inspection.

These state-specific arrangements have resulted from initiatives by state hospital associations in order to reduce the number of redundant surveys/inspections which member hospitals must undergo. The reason for providing these arrangements is that survey/inspection preparations and performance divert hospital resources from patient care activities.

Hospitals accredited by JCAH (and AOA) are recognized as meeting the *Conditions of Participation*. The state certifying agency conducts random validation surveys of a sample of hospitals certified by virtue of accreditation and complaint investigations in such hospitals. The results of these surveys and investigations are reported annually by HCFA to Congress.

American Osteopathic Association

Osteopathic hospitals voluntarily obtain accreditation from the American Osteopathic Association (AOA). To qualify for accreditation by the AOA, hospitals with only doctors of osteopathy (DOs) on their medical staffs must use the term "osteopathic" in their titles and on hospital stationery. Hospitals in which the medical staff is composed of both osteopaths and medical doctors (MDs) are eligible for AOA accreditation but need not use the "osteopathic" designation in the hospital title.

The accreditation manual, *Accreditation Requirements of the American Osteopathic Association*, includes specific requirements for compliance along with interpretive remarks. The accreditation process itself is similar to that of the JCAH. The AOA may grant a hospital accreditation for either one, two, or three years. If a hospital receives accreditation for only one year, the AOA may mandate a consultation for deficient areas. The AOA may also withdraw or deny accreditation. A hospital must apply for accreditation annually. Hospitals applying for accreditation for the first time must have consultation.

American College of Surgeons

The American College of Surgeons (ACS) is the only agency in the United States which surveys and approves cancer programs and cancer registries. This approval, like accreditation by JCAH and AOA, is a voluntary effort on the part of the facility and indicates high quality care. The two ACS publications used to provide guidelines for approval of cancer programs and registries are the *Cancer Program Manual* and its companion publication *Supplement on the Tumor Registry.*

Commission on Accreditation of Rehabilitation Facilities

Commission on Accreditation of Rehabilitation Facilities (CARF), founded in 1966, was established by and for the fields of rehabilitation and habilitation to adopt and apply standards in these types of facilities throughout the United States.

Sponsoring members of CARF are the: American Hospital Association; American Occupational Therapy Association; Goodwill Industries of America, Incorporated; National Association of Jewish Vocational Services; National Easter Seal Society; and United Cerebral Palsy Association, Incorporated.

Some of the goals of CARF, as outlined in its bylaws, are to: develop and maintain standards for rehabilitation facilities; improve the quality of services provided to the disabled and disadvantaged; and offer to the facility, community, and the consumer a mechanism of program accountability and assurance of continuing high level of performance.

To be eligible for a survey by CARF, the facility's major purpose must be rehabilitation of individuals requiring restorative and adjustive or employment services in an integrated and coordinated individualized program. In carrying out its program, the facility may place emphasis on one or more of the following: physical restoration, personal and social development, vocational development, sheltered employment, speech pathology, audiology, or work activity. The standards are published by CARF in the *Standards Manual for Rehabilitation Facilities.*

Accreditation Association for Ambulatory Health Care

The Accreditation Association for Ambulatory Health Care (AAAHC) was incorporated in 1979. This organization is continuing a program of voluntary accreditation for ambulatory care facilities originally developed in 1969 by the American Group Practice Association and expanded in 1975 by the Joint Commission on Accreditation of Hospitals. In 1978, however, the JCAH was reorganized but still maintained a mechanism for accrediting ambulatory care facilities. However, several ambulatory care groups believed the Joint Commission's new organizational structure would not allow them full participation in the accreditation process; and as a result, six organizations, whose primary interests were ambulatory care, created AAAHC. The charter members of the AAAHC are the American College Health Association (ACHA); the American Group Practice Association (AGPA); the Free Standing Ambulatory Surgical Association (FSASA); the Group Health Association of America, Inc. (GHAA), the Medical Group Management Association (MGMA); and the National Association of Community Health Centers, Inc. (NACHC).

The purpose of the AAAHC is to assist ambulatory health care professionals in improving the quality of care provided in their organizations, to compare their performance with recognized standards, and to provide for sharing of expertise through consultation among members.

A health care facility must be formally organized and must provide primarily ambulatory care services to be eligible for an AAAHC accreditation survey. AAAHC has accredited single and multispecialty group practices, ambulatory surgery centers, health maintenance organizations, college and university health services, and community and neighborhood health centers. The AAAHC standards are very similar to those of JCAH and are contained in the *Accreditation Handbook for Ambulatory Health Care.*

THE SURVEY PROCESS

The method by which the licensing, certifying, and accrediting agencies determine compliance with their regulations or standards is generally the same. To be considered, the interested facility must submit an application and complete a comprehensive questionnaire. These are reviewed to determine if the facility meets the basic accreditation requirements. If it appears the facility is in compliance, an on-site survey is scheduled. The survey team consists of professionals in various health care disciplines. Accreditation-survey teams usually include at least a practicing physician and hospital administrator. The surveyors review the survey documents and then provide on-site observation. At the end of their visit, these professionals provide a summation conference with representatives of the facility's governing body, administration, medical staff, and other staff members as appropriate. In this conference the surveyors report their findings, discuss major deviations from the regulations or standards, and make recommendations for correcting them. The representatives of the facility are given an opportunity to comment on any adverse findings.

The surveyors file their findings in a report to the licensing, certifying, or accrediting agency for whom they conducted the survey. The report may also include information submitted by the public, state or federal agencies, or associations. The facility receives a copy of the report and is allowed to respond in writing regarding the findings. The appropriate bodies in these organizations, on written recommendations of the surveyors, make the decision on licensure, certification, or accreditation, as appropriate for that particular organization. If a decision is contrary to what the facility believes to be appropriate, the facility may appeal the decision by submitting additional information supporting its view. The surveying organization will review this information along with all other pertinent information and make a final decision. Surveys for determining continued compliance with the standards for licensure, certification, and accreditation are conducted at specified intervals, according to the regulations of the various agencies.

SUMMARY

The medical record contains pertinent information about each patient provided care at a health facility. The medical record must be written in a timely manner and contain sufficient information to identify the patient, support the diagnosis, justify the treatment, and accurately document the results. The medical record generated by a facility is owned by that facility, but the patient has a legitimate claim on the information within the record. The medical record has many uses: patient care management, quality review, financial reimbursement, legal, education, research, and public health. It is valuable to the patient, the health care facility, all health care providers, educators, researchers, and public health officials.

In the hospital setting, the responsibility for a complete and useful record is shared by: the governing body, the administration, the medical record department, the attending physician, and other health care professionals.

Health care facilities seek designations of approval for the purpose of licensure, certification, and accreditation. Agencies which provide these designations have developed requirements or standards, including some concerning the medical record, which health care facilities must meet in order to earn the designation of approval of the respective agency. In order to determine compliance with its standards, the respective approving agency requires the health care facility to submit documentation and submit to an on-site survey. The approving agency then makes its determination of approval or nonapproval.

It is the role of the medical record practitioner to be knowledgeable of the many aspects of the medical record, including requirements of the approving agencies. In this way the medical record practitioner provides valuable assistance to the health professionals employed therein in developing an adequate medical record for quality patient care.

STUDY QUESTIONS

1. Define the terms licensure, certification, and accreditation in regard to health care facilities.

2. Through what two federal programs may health care facilities receive reimbursement by virtue of being "certified"?

3. Describe the general survey process by which facilities are evaluated to determine compliance with standards for licensure, certification, or accreditation.

4. What is the significance of JCAH accreditation to a hospital which is seeking "certification"?

5. Name the six general types of health care facilities/services which JCAH accredits.

6. What organization(s) specifically accredits/approves: rehabilitation facilities, cancer programs, and ambulatory care facilities?

REFERENCES

A Discursive Dictionary of Health Care. Subcommittee on Health and the Environment, Committee on Interstate and Foreign Commerce, U.S. House of Representatives. Washington, D.C.: U.S. Government Printing Office, 1976.

Accreditation Handbook for Ambulatory Health Care. Accreditation Association for Ambulatory Health Care, Inc. Skokie, Illinois, 1985.

1985 Accreditation Manual for Hospitals. Joint Commission on Accreditation of Hospitals. Chicago, Illinois, 1984.

Accreditation Manual for Long Term Care Facilities. Joint Commission on Accreditation of Hospitals. Chicago, Illinois, 1980.

Accreditation Requirements of the American Osteopathic Association. American Osteopathic Association. Chicago, Illinois, 1979.

Ambulatory Health Care Standards Manual. Joint Commission on Accreditation of Hospitals. Chicago, Illinois, 1985.

Cancer Program Manual. American College of Surgeons, 1981.

Cancer Program Manual: A Supplement on the Tumor Registry. American College of Surgeons, 1981.

Consolidated Standards Manual for Child, Adolescent, and Adult Psychiatric, Alcoholism, and Drug Abuse Facilities and Facilities Serving the Mentally Retarded/Developmentally Disabled. Joint Commission on Accreditation of Hospitals. Chicago, Illinois, 1985.

Hospice Standards Manual. Joint Commission on Accreditation of Hospitals. Chicago, Illinois, 1983.

Principles for Accreditation of Community Mental Health Service Programs. Joint Commission on Accreditation of Hospitals. Chicago, Illinois, 1979.

Privacy and Confidentiality of Health Care Information. Jo ANNE CZECOWSKI BRUCE. Chicago, Illinois: American Hospital Publishing, Inc., 1984.

Standards Manual for Facilities Serving People With Disabilities. Commission on Accreditation of Rehabilitation Facilities, Tucson, Arizona, 1984.

The United States Government Manual. Office of the Federal Register, National Archives and Records Service, General Services Administration. Washington, D.C., 1984.

United States Department of Health, Education, and Welfare, Social Security Administration, "Subpart I: Conditions of Participation – Home Health Agencies" of Regulations No. 5. Federal Health Insurance for the Aged, 1972.

United States Department of Health, Education, and Welfare, Social Security Administration. "Subpart J: Conditions of Participation – Hospital" of Regulations No. 5. Federal Health Insurance for the Aged, 1972.

United States Department of Health, Education, and Welfare, Social Security Administration, "Subpart K: Conditions of Participation – Skilled Nursing Facilities" of Regulations No. 5. Federal Health, Insurance for the Aged. Federal Register, Volume 39, Number 12, January 17, 1974.

chapter *3*

DEVELOPMENT AND CONTENT OF THE HOSPITAL MEDICAL RECORD

The medical record is the who, what, why, where, when, and how of patient care. Medical records are the visible evidence of what the hospital is accomplishing. This chapter will explain how the medical record evolves to protect the interests of all parties who are involved in the care of a patient and have legitimate uses for the record. It is imperative that accurate, timely documentation be provided for each patient on each contact with a health care provider and facility. Reinforcing the importance of documentation in hospital medical records, the Department of Health and Human Services (DHHS) in the document *Conditions of Participation for Hospitals* and the Joint Commission on Accreditation of Hospitals (JCAH) in its *Accreditation Manual for Hospitals* state that an adequate medical record shall be maintained for every individual who is evaluated or treated at the hospital through inpatient, ambulatory, home health, or emergency services.

In order to clarify the term "adequate medical record," this chapter will discuss requirements of the *Conditions of Participation*, JCAH standards, and generally accepted guidelines for hospital medical record content. The medical record practitioner should consult the most current editions of the aforementioned documents and also the licensure requirements of the applicable state.

FLOW OF THE MEDICAL RECORD

The medical record for the inpatient usually originates in the admitting department of the hospital. In this office, the patient or his representative provides identifying and financial data and signs consent forms for treatment and for release of information. This office, in cooperation with the medical record department, assigns the patient a hospital number which is used on all medical record forms for the patient throughout each episode of care. The admission department sends relevant portions of this information to other departments in the hospital to inform them the patient is being admitted. The departments usually receiving data are the business office, data processing, medical records, and nursing service.

The next department to generate data on the patient is the nursing service via the nursing station to which the patient is assigned. Here a medical record of basic forms is compiled for the patient. When orders for various tests, treatments, and consultation are provided by the patient's physician, nursing service generates and routes the requests to the appropriate department. Nursing service is usually responsible for filing test results and making entries regarding nursing care on certain forms within the record.

The attending physician who admits the patient is primarily responsible for the patient's care. He generates data by compiling a history of the patient, performing a physical examination, and recording the results. The physician also generates data regarding the patient when he orders diagnostic and therapeutic services, when he assesses the patient's condition and response to treatment through progress notes, and when he summarizes the patient's course at the end of the episode of care. During hospitalization, data may be generated by other physicians who give care to the patient, such as in providing consultation, surgery, or other specialized evaluations or treatments. Data dictated by various physicians may be transcribed and entered in the medical record. Usually pathology and radiology departments employ transcriptionists who type these reports. The medical record department employs transcriptionists who type patient histories, physical exams, consultation and operative reports, and discharge summaries. The physician who generates each of these reports must review and sign his reports.

Ancillary services provide additional support in the care of the patient. Departments most frequently referred to as ancillary are dietary, medical laboratory, physical therapy, occupational therapy, respiratory therapy, and social service. These departments receive requests for services, evaluations, and/or

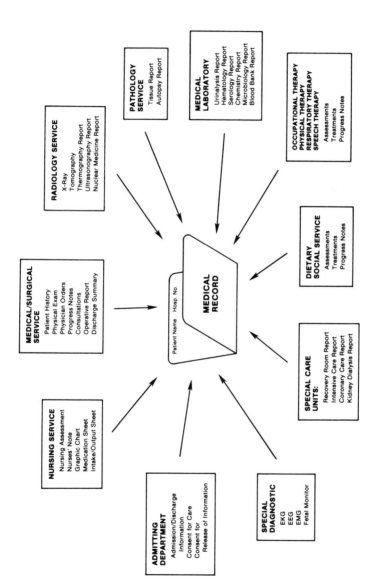

Fig. 1 – Routing of the Medical Record Data Within the Hospital

treatments for individual patients. The data thus generated become part of the medical record, either by being placed in the record at the nursing station or, in the case of a patient who has been discharged, in the record while it is being analyzed in the medical record department. (See Figure 1.)

After the patient is discharged, the medical record department receives the medical record and is responsible for performing certain procedures involving the record and the data therein. These may be performed in varying order, depending on the needs of a particular department. The tasks are mentioned briefly here and discussed in greater detail in other chapters.

Although unit clerks sometimes place the medical record in permanent order according to the hospital's prescribed order, this procedure is often completed in the medical record department. The record is reviewed for completeness, with the major emphasis on determining that all necessary forms are included; that the forms are properly completed; and that the entries are dated and signed. Notation is made of incomplete content areas and of the health professionals responsible for their completion. This procedure is usually referred to as "quantitative" analysis and is discussed in Chapter 8. At this time the record may be placed in the area designated as the "incomplete record area," where the responsible professionals complete it; or it may continue to be processed. Coding (applying code numbers to the diagnoses and procedures) and abstracting data from the record are usually performed next. These tasks are discussed in Chapters 12 and 14 respectively. When the record is determined to be complete, it is then filed in the area reserved for completed records of discharged patients (permanent files) for use at a later date if necessary. (See Figure 2.)

FORMAT TYPES

Medical record format refers to the organization of the forms within the medical record. There are three types of format: source-oriented, problem-oriented, and integrated.

SOURCE-ORIENTED MEDICAL RECORD

Traditionally, the hospital medical record is organized in sections according to the patient care departments which provide

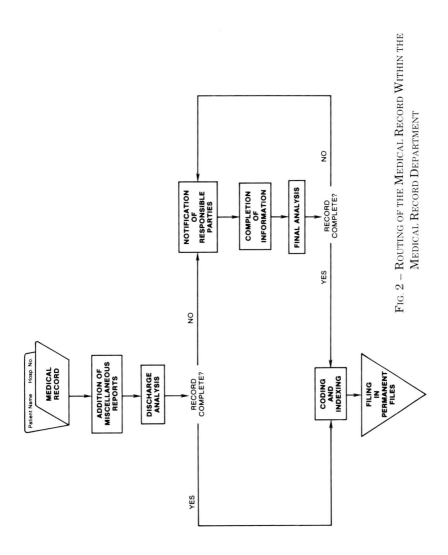

FIG. 2 – ROUTING OF THE MEDICAL RECORD WITHIN THE MEDICAL RECORD DEPARTMENT

the care and the data; thus the term "source-oriented" medical record. The sections may be separated by dividers with the source name. Within each section the forms are arranged according to date. Usually the record is arranged in "reverse" chronological order at the nurses' stations, so the most recent information is at the front and the oldest information is at the back of each section. Upon discharge of the patient, the record is rearranged in chronological order.

The major advantage to the source-oriented format is that it organizes reports from each source together, thus making it easy to determine the assessment, treatments, and observations a particular department has provided. Most health care professionals are accustomed to this arrangement because it is the traditional format.

Critics of the source-oriented medical record state it is not possible to quickly determine all of the patient's problems with this format. It is also difficult to determine all the treatments being provided for the patient at a given time, since the data from the various departments are organized in sections and not according to the problems of the patient.

PROBLEM-ORIENTED MEDICAL RECORD

The problem-oriented medical record, commonly referred to as POMR, was introduced by Lawrence L. Weed, MD, in the 1960s. The POMR provides a systemic method of documentation to reflect logical thinking on the part of the physician directing the care of the patient. The physician defines and follows each clinical problem individually and organizes them for solution. Proponents of the POMR state that its structure facilitates this process. The POMR must contain four basic components: (1) the data base, (2) the complete problem list, (3) initial plans, and (4) progress notes.

The data base is described as being "defined," that is, there are specific data to be obtained on every patient treated in a particular facility. The elements of the data base include: the chief complaint, present illness(es), patient profile (how he spends his day) and related social data, past history and review of systems, physical examinations of defined content, and baseline laboratory data.

The problem list is contained on a sheet which is placed in the front of the chart. This list has as "problems" anything that requires management or diagnostic workup, including medical, social, economic, and demographic problems, past and present. The problems are titled and numbered and serve as a table of contents. The list should state the problems at the level of the physician's understanding of a particular problem.

Thus, the problem list may contain a statement of a symptom, an abnormal finding, a physiologic finding, or a specific diagnosis. Conditions suspected or to be ruled out are not listed as problems but are noted in the initial plan. Additions or changes are made in the list as new problems are identified and active problems resolved. Problems are not erased; they are marked "dropped" or "resolved" and the date of the change recorded.

The initial plans describe what will be done to learn more about the patient's condition, treat the condition, and educate the patient about his condition. Specific plans for each problem are delineated and fall into three categories: more information for diagnosis ("rule out" statements may be made here) and management; therapy (including statements of drugs, procedures, goals, and contingency plans); and patient education. The plans are numbered corresponding to the problem which they address.

Progress notes are the follow-up for each problem. Each note is preceded by the number and title of the appropriate problem and may consist of any or all of the following elements: subjective (symptomatic); objective (measurable, observable); assessment (interpretation or impression of the current condition); and plan statements. The acronym for this process is SOAP, and the writing of progress notes in the POMR format is often referred to as "soaping." The emphasis is on unresolved problems. A slightly different way to describe the patient's progress other than the narrative method mentioned above is with the use of flow sheets. Flow sheets are recommended in situations in which there are several factors being monitored or when the patient's condition is changing rapidly. The discharge summary and transfer note are also included in the "progress note" category. These should address all the numbered problems on the patient's list. It may be necessary for the physician to write an overall summary and use flow sheets to clarify the patient's progress.

Weed recommended that certain other forms, such as physicians' orders, consultant reports, and nurses' notes, be in the problem-oriented style, with reference to titled and numbered problems. Other data in the record may be in the conventional format, such as laboratory and operative reports.

Proponents of the POMR identify many advantages to this format: the physician is required to consider all the patient's problems in total context; the record clearly indicates the goals and methods of the physician in treating the patient; medical education is facilitated by the documentation of logical thought processes of the attending physician; and the quality assurance process is easier because the data are organized.

The major disadvantage of POMR is that the format usually requires additional training of the medical and professional staffs. Also, for the POMR to be effective in a facility, a significant number of physicians must be convinced of the system's worth or at least be willing to try it. Few acute care facilities maintain problem-oriented medical records.

INTEGRATED MEDICAL RECORDS

In the integrated format, the information is organized in strict chronological order with the most current entries at the beginning of the record. The forms from various sources are intermingled. Thus the history and physical examination may be followed by a progress note, a nurses' note, an x-ray report, a consultation, and so on. The forms for each episode of care are organized in separate sections of the record.

The advantage of the integrated format is that all information on a particular episode of care is together, thus providing a clear picture of the patient's illness and response to treatment.

The disadvantage of the integrated format is that it is difficult to compare similar information, for example, fasting blood sugar levels, over a series of admissions because the reports are not in the same section of the record.

There may be varying degrees of integration of information. The most common variation allows for integrated progress notes, with all providers recording on the same form(s), in sequence. All other reports are maintained in sections.

Some of the advantages to using integrated progress notes are: a patient's progress can be determined quickly because the current notes of all disciplines are together; the number of specialized forms is reduced, thus reducing the bulk of the record; and the team concept of health care is encouraged.

Some of the disadvantages of integrated progress notes are: only one individual can document at a time; it may be difficult to identify the profession of the individual making a particular entry unless notes are always followed by the title of the recorder; and physicians often feel their documentation requires highlighting in some manner to differentiate it from that of other professionals caring for the patient.

The decision regarding the format of the medical record is usually made by the medical staff with recommendations from the medical record committee. The JCAH recommends a standardized format for hospital-wide use. This facilitates use of the record by those so authorized for purposes of clinical, administrative, statistical, and quality assessment activities.

REQUIRED CHARACTERISTICS OF ENTRIES IN MEDICAL RECORDS

It has often been said that an adequate medical record indicates adequate care, and conversely, a poor medical record indicates poor care. It may be possible for a complete and thorough record to exist for a patient who received poor care, but the reverse is more likely to be true. A patient may have received adequate care which is poorly documented. For continuity of care it may be necessary to refer to the original record. If it lacks information, the patient may receive less than optimal follow-up care. Characteristics of adequate medical record documentation are discussed in the following two sections.

APPROPRIATE DOCUMENTATION

The quality of the medical record depends, in part, on information entered by those professionals authorized to provide care and responsible for documenting that care. Hospital and medical staff policies should determine who has this right and responsibility. The Conditions of Participation require that the medical staff have bylaws, rules, and regulations which include a provision for the medical staff to keep accurate and complete clinical records. It is further required that the record contain the originals of all reports.

The JCAH makes approximately the same statement adding that the record must contain information to identify the patient. The JCAH specifically states that entries may be made only by individuals given that right in hospital and medical staff policies. They describe the content of the record by stating that it must incorporate all significant clinical information pertaining to a given patient. Further, the record shall be sufficient to enable the attending physician to provide effective continuing care and to determine the patient's condition at any given time. The record shall also enable a consultant to review the patient and his record and render an opinion, and another physician to assume the patient's care at any time. Additionally the record shall provide pertinent information for utilization review and quality assessment purposes.

SIGNATURES

Those professionals providing care to a patient and authorized to make entries in the record must document the care they provide and date the entry. They also verify that this care was given by signing the entry. The *Conditions of Participation* state that every physician is to sign the entries he makes; and a single signature by the physician on the admission/discharge record, where diagnosis(es) and procedure(s) are listed, is not sufficient to authenticate the entire record. In hospitals with house staff, the attending physician must countersign at least the history, physical examination, and discharge summary written by the house staff.

The JCAH requires that medical records be dated and authenticated, and that there be a method established for identifying the authors of entries. The identification may be a written signature, initials, or computer key. When rubber stamps of signatures are allowed as a means of authentication (most commonly for pathologists and radiologists), the individual whose signature is represented by the stamp must place in the hospital's administrative offices a signed statement that he has the stamp and is the only one who will use it. There is no delegation of the use of the stamp according to JCAH.

The parts of the record that are the responsibility of the attending physician are to be authenticated (signed) by him. If, for example, a physician assistant conducts and records the medical history and physical examination, the attending physician is required to sign these reports. Any entry which requires countersignature of the attending physician must be defined in the medical staff rules and regulations.

ABBREVIATIONS

The JCAH specifically states that abbreviations and symbols are to be used only when they have been approved by the medical staff and when there is an explanatory legend available to those authorized to make entries in the record and to those who must interpret them. Each abbreviation and symbol should have only one meaning.

TIMELINESS

Because human memory can easily fail, it is imperative that entries regarding patient care be made as close as possible to the time of occurrence of the event(s) being documented. The *Conditions of Participation* address this issue by requiring that current and discharged patient records be completed promptly. Current records (the history, physical examination, and pertinent laboratory and x-ray data) are those which are completed within 24-48 hours after admission. Upon discharge of the patient, the record is to be completed within 15 days.

The JCAH requires that each clinical event shall be documented as soon as possible after its occurrence. In general, the records of discharged patients are to be complete within 30 days, the period of time being specified in the medical staff rules and regulations. Completeness implies that the required forms are assembled and authenticated; all final diagnoses are recorded without use of abbreviations; and transcription of any dictated information is completed and inserted in the record. The JCAH also has specific requirements on the timeliness of certain data which will be described when these data elements are discussed in the section on content in this chapter.

LEGIBILITY

The usefulness of the record depends in part on the legibility of the entries. The JCAH requires that records be legible and recommends that, when it is economically feasible and appropriate, medical entries be typed. They state that special consideration should be given to the typing of certain forms: radiology, pathology, operative reports, and discharge summaries. The JCAH further notes that when the typing and filing of these reports cannot be accomplished in a timely fashion, entries providing sufficient information for continuity of care are to be made in the record.

CORRECTION OF ERRORS OR OMISSIONS

Errors are properly corrected by drawing a single line through the mistake, writing the word "error" near it, and recording the correct information. The individual who writes the error corrects, dates, and signs the entry. The error should not be erased or painted out with correction fluid. If an entry is accidently omitted, the entry is made after the last entry on that day, with an explanation of the omission and the reason for its being out of sequence. If the entry is made at a later date, it is added between the lines on the proper day and in the correct time sequence with an explanation of the reason for the late entry, and date of the entry. The entry, of course, is signed by the individual recording it.

FORMS IN THE MEDICAL RECORD

This section will discuss the content of all basic medical record forms. These forms are called basic because they are necessary in the majority of hospital medical records.

Unless specified by requirements of approving agencies, the organization of data within the individual forms is determined by each health care facility. Sample forms are included in this chapter to demonstrate arrangements of data. Inclusion of a form is not to be construed as meaning the form is required or approved by licensing, certifying, or accrediting agencies. Individual health facilities should organize data to allow for efficient gathering and dispersing within its data system. Before adopting any form, it is imperative that a health facility critique the form to be certain it meets the individual needs of that facility.

Because of the reduced size of the forms, they have been left blank so the data items can be more easily read. In actual practice each item should have an entry. Items not pertinent to a

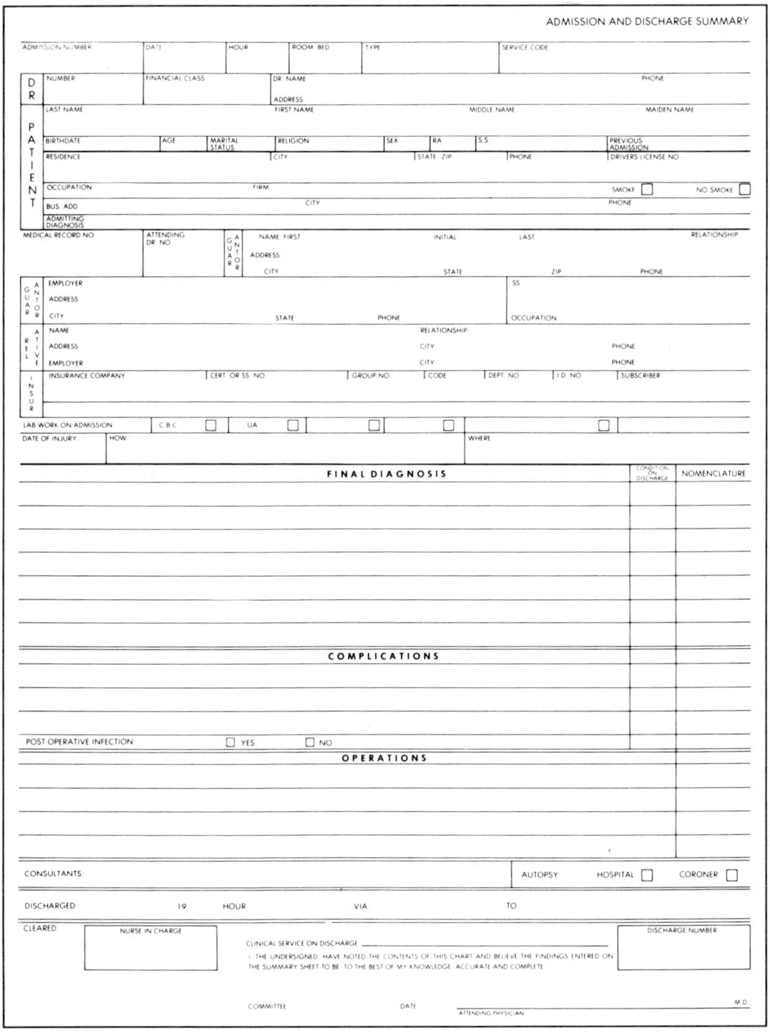
ADMISSION AND DISCHARGE SUMMARY

ADMISSION NUMBER | DATE | HOUR | ROOM BED | TYPE | SERVICE CODE

DR: NUMBER | FINANCIAL CLASS | DR NAME | ADDRESS | PHONE

PATIENT: LAST NAME | FIRST NAME | MIDDLE NAME | MAIDEN NAME
BIRTHDATE | AGE | MARITAL STATUS | RELIGION | SEX | RA | S.S | PREVIOUS ADMISSION
RESIDENCE | CITY | STATE ZIP | PHONE | DRIVERS LICENSE NO
OCCUPATION | FIRM | SMOKE ☐ | NO SMOKE ☐
BUS. ADD. | CITY | PHONE
ADMITTING DIAGNOSIS

MEDICAL RECORD NO | ATTENDING DR NO | GUARANTOR: NAME FIRST | INITIAL | LAST | RELATIONSHIP | ADDRESS | CITY | STATE | ZIP | PHONE

GUARANTOR: EMPLOYER | ADDRESS | CITY | STATE | PHONE | SS | OCCUPATION

RELATIVE: NAME | RELATIONSHIP | ADDRESS | CITY | PHONE | EMPLOYER | CITY | PHONE

INSUR: INSURANCE COMPANY | CERT OR SS NO | GROUP NO | CODE | DEPT NO | I D NO | SUBSCRIBER

LAB WORK ON ADMISSION | C B C ☐ | UA ☐ | ☐ | ☐ | ☐

DATE OF INJURY | HOW | WHERE

FINAL DIAGNOSIS | CONDITION ON DISCHARGE | NOMENCLATURE

COMPLICATIONS

POST OPERATIVE INFECTION ☐ YES ☐ NO

OPERATIONS

CONSULTANTS: | AUTOPSY | HOSPITAL ☐ | CORONER ☐

DISCHARGED 19 | HOUR | VIA | TO

CLEARED | NURSE IN CHARGE | DISCHARGE NUMBER

CLINICAL SERVICE ON DISCHARGE ____

I, THE UNDERSIGNED, HAVE NOTED THE CONTENTS OF THIS CHART AND BELIEVE THE FINDINGS ENTERED ON THE SUMMARY SHEET TO BE, TO THE BEST OF MY KNOWLEDGE, ACCURATE AND COMPLETE

COMMITTEE | DATE | M D | ATTENDING PHYSICIAN

Form courtesy of Physicians' Record Company

FIG. 3 – ADMISSION/DISCHARGE FORM

particular patient are indicated by some type of entry, such as "not applicable" (NA). This indicates the item was not accidentally overlooked, which might be inferred from the presence of a blank item. In actual practice each form would include the hospital name and address, a form number, and the date the form was approved.

The medical record contains data compiled by different entities. There are two broad classifications of hospital medical record data: administrative and clinical. Clinical data are usually subdivided into medical, nursing, and ancillary data. There are specific considerations for clinical data present in "special" types of hospital records such as obstetric, newborn, and short-stay records.

ADMINISTRATIVE DATA

Admission/Discharge Form

Basic identification and financial data are routinely collected on every patient except where not available. The data are collected at admission or prior to admission if preadmission processing is done. These data are found on a form referred to as the identification/summary sheet, admission/discharge record, and summary sheet or face sheet (Figure 3). It is usually the first form in the permanent record. Usually the upper portion contains sociological information, while the lower section contains clinical data.

Enough information is contained in the sociological section to positively identify the patient. This usually includes:

1. the full name of the patient, address, phone number, place and date of birth, age, sex, race, marital status, religion, occupation, social security number, and possibly father's name or mother's maiden name and birthplace;

2. name, address, and telephone number of nearest relative or friend;

3. name and address of patient's employer and/or spouse's employer;

4. date and time of admission, hospital number, room number and service to which patient is assigned, and date and time of discharge;

5. attending and referring physician; and

6. insurance carrier(s), policy number(s), and guarantor.

Except for date and time of admission, hospital and room number, the sociological information is obtained from the patient or from the nearest relative or friend at the time of admis-

CONDITIONS OF ADMISSION

TO

1. **General Duty Nursing:** The hospital provides only general duty nursing care. Under this system nurses are called to the bedside of the patient by a signal system. If the patient is in such condition as to need continuous or special-duty nursing care, it is agreed that such must be arranged by the patient, or his legal representative, or his physicians, and the hospital shall in no way be responsible for failure to provide the same and is hereby released from any and all liability arising from the fact that said patient is not provided with such additional care.

2. **Medical and Surgical Consent:** The patient is under the control of his attending physicians and the hospital is not liable for any act or omission in following the instructions of said physicians, and the undersigned consents to any x-ray examination, laboratory procedures, anesthesia, medical or surgical treatment or hospital services rendered the patient under the general and special instructions of the physician. The undersigned recognizes that all doctors of medicine furnishing services to the patient, including the radiologist, pathologist, anesthetist and the like, are independent contractors and are not employees or agents of the hospital.

3. **Release of Information:** The hospital may disclose all or any part of the patient's record to any person or corporation which is or may be liable under a contract to the hospital or to the patient or to a family member or employer of the patient for all or part of the hospital's charge, including, but not limited to, hospital or medical service companies, insurance companies, workmen's compensation carriers, welfare funds, or the patient's employer.

4. **Personal Valuables:** It is understood and agreed that the hospital maintains a safe for the safekeeping of money and valuables and the hospital shall not be liable for the loss of or damage to any money, jewelry, glasses, dentures, documents, furs, fur coats and fur garments, or other articles of unusual value and small compass, unless placed therein, and shall not be liable for loss of or damage to any other personal property, unless deposited with the hospital for safekeeping.

5. **Financial Agreement:** The undersigned agrees, whether he signs as agent or as patient, that in consideration of the services to be rendered to the patient, he hereby individually obligates himself to pay the account of the hospital in accordance with the regular rates and terms of the hospital. Should the account be referred to an attorney for collection, the undersigned shall pay reasonable attorney's fees and collection expense. All delinquent accounts bear interest at the legal rate.

The undersigned certifies that he has read the foregoing, receiving a copy thereof, and is the patient, or is duly authorized by the patient as patient's general agent to execute the above and accept its terms.

_____
PATIENT

_____
PATIENT'S AGENT OR REPRESENTATIVE

_____
RELATIONSHIP TO PATIENT

A copy of this Document is to be delivered to the patient.

Time of signing_____ 19____, Hour _____.M.

Witness: _____

FORM A-144　　　　PHYSICIANS RECORD CO. BERWYN, ILLINOIS　PRINTED IN U.S.A.　　　CONDITIONS OF ADMISSION

Form courtesy of Physicians' Record Company

FIG. 4 – CONDITIONS OF ADMISSION

sion. When this information is not obtainable, the reason should be stated in the record. It is extremely important that the admitting clerk securing this information be accurate. For a married woman, her legal name is entered, i.e., her given, maiden, and married (family) names. It is most helpful to enter the last name first, then first name, and middle or maiden name. The date and time of discharge are often entered on this form by medical record personnel.

The clinical portion of this form will be discussed briefly under the clinical section of the medical record.

Conditions of Admission

The back of the admission/discharge form is often used for the conditions of admission (admission consent or authorization for admission form). The form provides a statement indicating that the patient agrees to receive basic, routine care. There usually is a statement to the effect that the hospital cannot guarantee the outcome. This form (Figure 4), when signed by the patient or his guardian at admission, provides a record of consent to routine services, diagnostic procedures, and medical treatment. It is the responsibility of the admitting clerk to explain to the patient the contents of this form and its purpose.

AUTHORIZATION FOR RELEASE OF INFORMATION

To_____ Hospital Number_____
(NAME OF HOSPITAL)

You are hereby authorized to furnish such professional information, in accordance with the policy of your hospital, as may be

necessary for the completion of my hospitalization claims by_____
(NAME OF THIRD PARTY)

_____ from the medical records compiled during my hospitalization
(NAME OF THIRD PARTY)

from_____ 19____ to _____ 19____ and are

hereby released from all legal liability that may arise from the release of the information requested.

Date _____ Signed _____
(PATIENT OR NEAREST OF KIN)

Signed_____ _____
(PARTY INSPECTING RECORD) (RELATIONSHIP IF SIGNED BY OTHER THAN PATIENT)

Date of inspection of record_____ 19____ Signed _____
(ATTENDING PHYSICIAN)

Authorization must be signed by the patient, or by the nearest relative in the case of a minor or when patient is physically or mentally incompetent.

FORM C-409   PHYSICIANS RECORD CO., BERWYN, ILLINOIS   PRINTED IN U.S.A.

Form courtesy of Physicians' Record Company

FIG. 5 – CONSENT FOR RELEASE OF INFORMATION

Consent for Release of Information

The consent or authorization for release of information (Figure 5) allows the hospital to send to specifically named organizations copies of the patient's medical record. The patient's signature on this form authorizes the hospital to release medical information compiled during the current episode of care. The organizations which may receive this information are those which provide hospitalization insurance coverage including Medicare/Medicaid, workers' compensation, Blue Cross-Blue Shield, and private carriers. This form is often found on the back of the admission/discharge form. Again, it is the responsibility of the admitting clerk to explain to the patient the content of the consent and its purpose.

AUTHORIZATION FOR MEDICAL AND/OR SURGICAL TREATMENT

Date_____ 19____ Time_____ a.m. p.m.

I, the undersigned, a patient in_____Hospital, hereby authorize

Dr._____(and whomever he may designate as his assistants) to administer

such treatment as is necessary, and to perform the following operation_____
(NAME OF OPERATION AND/OR PROCEDURES)
_____and such additional operations or procedures as are considered
therapeutically necessary on the basis of findings during the course of said operation. I also consent to the administration of such

anesthetics as are necessary, with the exception of_____.
(NONE, SPINAL ANESTHESIA, OR OTHER)
Any tissues or parts surgically removed may be disposed of by the hospital in accordance with accustomed practice.

I hereby certify that I have read and fully understand the above **Authorization for Medical and/or Surgical Treatment,** the reasons why the above-named surgery is considered necessary, its advantages and possible complications, if any, as well as

possible alternative modes of treatment, which were explained to me by Dr._____.
I also certify that no guarantee or assurance has been made as to the results that may be obtained.

Witness_____   Signed_____
(PATIENT OR NEAREST RELATIVE)

Witness_____   _____
(RELATIONSHIP)

Authorization must be signed by the patient, or by the nearest relative in the case of a minor; or when patient is physically or mentally incompetent.
FORM C-410   PHYSICIANS RECORD CO., BERWYN, ILLINOIS   PRINTED IN U.S.A.

Form courtesy of Physicians' Record Company

FIG. 6 – SPECIAL CONSENT FORM

Special Consents

A special consent or authorization form (Figure 6) is required for any nonroutine diagnostic or therapeutic procedures performed on the patient. This form provides written evidence that the patient agrees to the procedure(s) listed on the form. For the consent to be valid, the physician must discuss the procedures named, the risks, alternative procedures, and likely outcomes with the patient and/or guardian.

The *Conditions of Participation* require that the medical staff bylaws and rules and regulations state that a surgical operation may be performed only on consent of the patient or his legal representative, except in emergencies. Also they require (in the section on the Surgery department) that a properly executed consent form for operation be in the patient's medical record prior to surgery.

The JCAH requires that there be evidence of informed consent for procedures and treatments for which consent is required according to the policy developed by the medical staff, governing body, and law. When consent is not obtainable, the reason is to be documented in the record. See Chapter 17 for further discussion of consents/authorizations.

CLINICAL DATA

Clinical data are the second broad category of medical record information. Use of the word "clinical" refers to data reflecting the patient's illness(es) and treatment(s). Information which is the responsibility of or generated by physicians will be discussed first.

Admission and Discharge Form

The medical information which is part of the admission and discharge form (identification/summary sheet/face sheet—Figure 3) usually includes the provisional or admitting diagnosis, the final (principal) diagnosis, complications or other diagnoses, and procedures. The attending physician is responsible for supplying this information and attesting to the validity of the information by signing the form. There is no requirement that the provisional diagnosis must be on the admitting/discharge record. Its presence here is helpful for room assignment in those hospitals with specialized services. It also assists nursing service in beginning care for the patient. With the advent of the prospective payment system, patients with certain diagnoses are expected to be cared for on an outpatient basis. Only extenuating circumstances allow the federal government to reimburse the hospital for admitting and treating patients with these diagnoses. Therefore, it is important that the provisional diagnosis be provided at or before admission.

HISTORY

Family Name	First Name	Attending Physician	Room No.	Hosp. No.

CHIEF COMPLAINT
Concise statement of complaints with date of onset and duration of each. Record in order of importance.

PAST HISTORY

Measles	Influenza
Whooping cough	Pleurisy
Mumps	Tuberculosis
Chickenpox	Asthma
Tonsillitis	Arthritis
Scarlet fever	Amebiasis
Diphtheria	Lues
Rheumatic fever	Gonorrhea
Typhoid fever	Injuries
Malaria	Operations
Pneumonia	Other

FAMILY HISTORY
If living health of, and if deceased cause of death of father, mother, siblings, children. Any familial:

Cancer	Heart disease
Tuberculosis	Allergy
Diabetes	Arthritis
Hemophilia	Other
Kidney disease	

INVENTORY BY SYSTEMS

GENERAL

Nutrition	Tremor
Fever	Weight gain
Night sweats	Weight loss
Falling hair	Other

SKIN

Eruptions	Jaundice
Cyanosis	Other

HEAD

Headache	Syncope
Trauma	Other

EYES

Eyestrain	Lacrimation
Diplopia	Glasses (Date Last Checked)
Photophobia	Blurring
Inflammation	Other
	(over)

FORM D-219 (REV. 3/81)   PHYSICIANS' RECORD CO., BERWYN, ILL 60402 · PRINTED IN U.S.A   HISTORY (OVER)

Form courtesy of Physicians' Record Company

FIG. 7 – MEDICAL HISTORY (front)

The final (principal) diagnosis, other diagnoses, and procedures are to be written in full, without symbols or abbreviations, in acceptable terminology. The admission/discharge form may also provide such information as consultations, autopsy performance, presence of institutional (nosocomial) infections, allergies, or sensitivities.

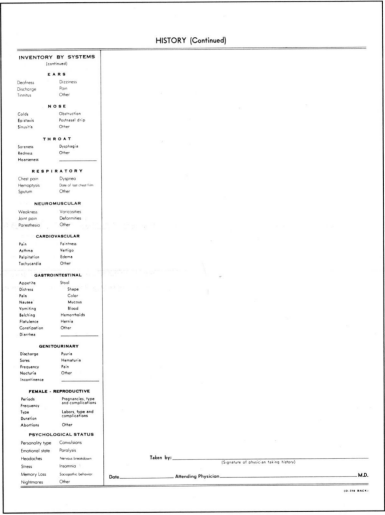

Form courtesy of Physicians' Record Company

FIG. 8 – MEDICAL HISTORY (back of Fig. 7)

The *Conditions of Participation* state that the provisional diagnosis is an impression reflecting the examining physician's evaluation of the patient's condition based mainly on physical findings and history. This is interpreted to be an admitting diagnosis recorded at the time of admission as a basis for beginning treatment.

Medical History

The medical history of the patient is baseline data which the physician uses to establish a provisional or tentative diagnosis on which to base the treatment of the patient (Figures 7 and 8). In the event that a reliable history cannot be elicited from the patient, the history must be obtained from the person best able to relate the facts. It is helpful to record the source of the history, i.e., the patient, parent, or friend. If the history and physical examination are performed by an intern, he should sign the reports which should also be countersigned by the resident and/or attending physician. If the attending physician does not agree with the data recorded, he adds his own findings and pertinent observations before signing. To promote uniformity and completeness in the medical record, each facility should adopt a standard outline for the history. The outline may be printed on the history form or it may be a blank sheet on which the physician records the data. Positive (the presence of a symptom) and negative data should be recorded. It is recommended that the terms "negative" or "normal" not be used except in summarizing stated facts. The data should reflect what the patient states. The physician's point of view may be expressed in the physical examination and subsequent notes. The following information is suggested content for the history.

1. Chief complaint: nature and duration of the symptoms that caused the patient to seek medical attention, as stated in the patient's own words.
2. Present illness: detailed chronological description of the development of the patient's illness from the appearance of the first symptom to the present time.
3. Past medical history: a summary of childhood and adult illnesses, such as infectious diseases, pregnancies, allergies and drug sensitivities, accidents, operations, hospitalizations, and current medications.
4. Psychosocial or personal history: marital status, dietary, sleeping, exercise patterns, use of coffee, alcohol, other

drugs and tobacco, occupation, environment, daily routine, religious beliefs, and outlook on life.

5. Family history: diseases among relatives in which heredity or contact may play a role, such as allergies, infectious diseases, mental, metabolic, endocrine, cardiovascular, renal diseases, or neoplasms. The health of immediate relatives, ages at death, and causes of death should be recorded.

6. Review of systems: a systemic inventory to reveal subjective symptoms which the patient either forgot to describe or which at the time seemed relatively unimportant. Generally an analysis of the subjective findings will indicate the nature and extent of the physical examination required. The following data are examples of items which the physician is to include. He uses his judgment in deciding when to limit or expand the information.

   a. General: usual weight, recent weight changes, fever, weakness, fatigue.

   b. Skin: rashes, eruptions, dryness, cyanosis, jaundice, changes in skin, hair or nails.

   c. Head: headache (duration, severity, character, location).

   d. Eyes: glasses or contact lenses, last eye examination, vision, glaucoma, cataracts, eyestrain, pain, diplopia, redness, lacrimation, inflammation, blurring.

   e. Ears: hearing, discharge, tinnitus, dizziness, pain.

   f. Nose: head colds, epistaxis, discharges, obstruction, postnasal drip, sinus pain.

   g. Mouth and throat: condition of teeth and gums, last dental examination, soreness, redness, hoarseness, difficulty in swallowing.

   h. Respiratory: chest pain, wheezing, cough, dyspnea, sputum (color and quantity), hemoptysis, asthma, bronchitis, emphysema, pneumonia, tuberculosis, pleurisy, last chest x-ray.

   i. Neurological: fainting, blackouts, seizures, paralysis, tingling, tremors, memory loss.

j. Musculoskeletal: joint pain or stiffness, arthritis, gout, backache, muscle pain, cramps, swelling, redness, limitation in motor activity.

k. Cardiovascular: chest pain, rheumatic fever, tachycardia, palpitation, high blood pressure, edema, vertigo, faintness, varicose veins, thrombophlebitis.

l. Gastrointestinal: appetite, thirst, nausea, vomiting, hematemesis, rectal bleeding, change in bowel habits, diarrhea, constipation, indigestion, food intolerance, flatus, hemorrhoids, jaundice.

m. Urinary: frequent or painful urination, nocturia, pyuria, hematuria, incontinence, urinary infections.

n. Genitoreproductive: Male–venereal disease, sores, discharge from penis, hernias, testicular pain or masses. Female–age at menarche; menstruation: frequency, type, duration, dysmenorrhea, menorrhagia; symptoms of menopause; contraception; pregnancies; deliveries; abortions; last Pap smear.

o. Endocrine: thyroid trouble, heat or cold intolerance, excessive sweating, thirst, hunger or urination.

p. Hematologic: anemia, easy bruising or bleeding, past transfusions.

q. Psychological: personality type, nervousness, mood, insomnia, headache, nightmares, depression.

The JCAH further states that in programs for children and adolescents, an evaluation of developmental age factors and consideration of educational needs should be included as appropriate. Qualified oral surgeons, who have been granted such privileges by the medical staff, may perform a complete history (and physical examination) on their patients. Dentists and podiatrists are responsible for documenting their patient's history pertaining to their respective areas. If a complete history has been recorded within a week prior to admission, such as in the office of a physician or a qualified oral surgeon or staff member, a legible copy of this report may be placed in the hospital medical record, provided there have been no changes since the original was recorded; or if there have been changes, these were documented at the time of admission. The history is to be completed within 24 hours of admission.

Physical Examination

The physical examination (Figure 9) is also baseline data about the patient which assist the physician in determining a

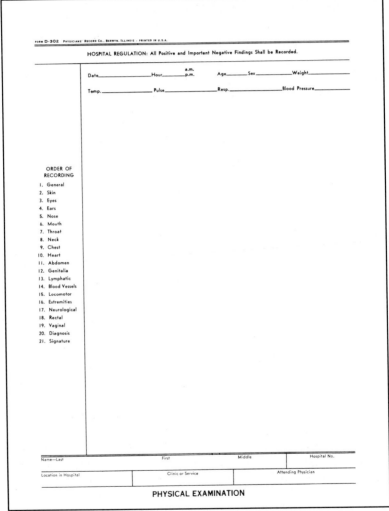

FORM D-302 PHYSICIANS' RECORD CO., BERWYN, ILLINOIS - PRINTED IN U.S.A.

HOSPITAL REGULATION: All Positive and Important Negative Findings Shall be Recorded.

Date_____Hour_____ a.m. p.m.   Age_____Sex_____Weight_____

Temp._____Pulse_____Resp._____Blood Pressure_____

ORDER OF
RECORDING
1. General
2. Skin
3. Eyes
4. Ears
5. Nose
6. Mouth
7. Throat
8. Neck
9. Chest
10. Heart
11. Abdomen
12. Genitalia
13. Lymphatic
14. Blood Vessels
15. Locomotor
16. Extremities
17. Neurological
18. Rectal
19. Vaginal
20. Diagnosis
21. Signature

Name—Last   First   Middle   Hospital No.

Location in Hospital   Clinic or Service   Attending Physician

PHYSICAL EXAMINATION

Form courtesy of Physicians' Record Company

FIG. 9 – PHYSICAL EXAMINATION

diagnosis. The examination should be comprehensive of all body systems. The degree of detail depends upon the age and sex of the patient, the patient's symptoms, other physical findings or laboratory data, and the specialty of the attending physician.

The diagnosis portion of the physical examination may be a statement of a provisional (tentative) diagnosis. The physician records his impression based on the subjective statements of the patient in the history and his objective findings in the physical examination. The physician may have several diagnoses which he considers as possibilities for the patient. The stating of several different diagnoses is referred to as the "differential" diagnosis.

Suggested content of the physical examination follows. Words in parentheses indicate sections which the physician may be likely to omit when the exam is entirely negative.

1. General Survey: apparent state of health, signs of distress, posture, weight, height, skin color, dress and personal hygiene, facial expression, manner, mood, state of awareness, speech.
2. Vital signs: pulse, respiration, blood pressure, (temperature).
3. Skin: color, its vascularity, any lesions, edema, moisture, temperature, texture, thickness, mobility and turgor, nails.
4. Head: hair, scalp, skull, (face).
5. Eyes: visual acuity and (fields), (position and alignment of the eyes), (eyebrows), (eyelids); (lacrimal apparatus); conjunctivas; scleras; (corneas), (irises); pupils: size, shape, equality, reaction to light and accommodation; extraocular movements; ophthalmoscopic exam.
6. Ears: (auricles), canals, tympanic membranes, hearing, discharge.
7. Nose and sinuses: airways, mucosa, septum, sinus tenderness, discharge, bleeding, smell.
8. Mouth: breath, (lips), teeth, gums, tongue, salivary ducts.
9. Throat: tonsils, pharynx, palate, uvula, postnasal drip.
10. Neck: stiffness, thyroid, trachea, vessels, lymph nodes, salivary glands.
11. Thorax, anterior and posterior: shape, symmetry, (respiration).
12. Breasts: masses, tenderness, discharge (nipples).
13. Lungs: (fremitus), breath sounds, adventitious sounds, friction, spoken voice, whispered voice.

14. Heart: location and quality of apical impulse, thrill, pulsation, rhythm, sounds, murmurs, friction rub, jugular venous pressure and pulse, carotid artery pulse.
15. Abdomen: contour, peristalsis, scars, rigidity, tenderness, spasm, masses, fluid, hernia, bowel sounds and bruits, palpable organs.
16. Genitourinary: scars, lesions, discharge, penis, scrotum, epididymis, varicocele, hydrocele.
17. Vaginal: external genitalia, Skene's and Bartholin's glands, vagina, cervix, uterus, adnexa.
18. Rectal: fissure, fistula, hemorrhoids, sphincter tone, masses, prostate, seminal vesicles, feces.
19. Musculoskeletal: spine and extremities, deformities, swelling, redness, tenderness, range of motion.
20. Lymphatics: palpable cervical, axillary, inguinal nodes; location; size; consistency; mobility and tenderness.
21. Blood vessels: pulses, color, temperature, vessel walls, veins.
22. Neurological: cranial nerves, coordination, reflexes, biceps, triceps, patellar, Achilles, abdominal, cremasteric, Babinski, Romberg, gait, sensory, vibratory.
23. Diagnosis.

The JCAH requires a report of a comprehensive current physical assessment. If one has been performed within a week prior to admission, such as in the office of a physician staff member, then a durable, legible copy of this report may be used in the patient's medical record if there have been no changes in the patient or if these changes have been documented at the time of admission. When the patient is readmitted within 30 days for the same or a related problem, an "interval" physical exam reflecting any changes may be used, provided the original physical exam is readily available. Prior to surgery the medical record must contain a current, thorough physical exam. The recorded physical exam is to be signed by a physician or, when given the privilege, a qualified oral surgeon. The physical exam is to be completed within 24 hours of admission.

In conjunction with the history and physical examination, the JCAH further requires that there be a statement of impressions or conclusions drawn from the aforementioned data and a statement of the course of action planned for the patient while in the hospital.

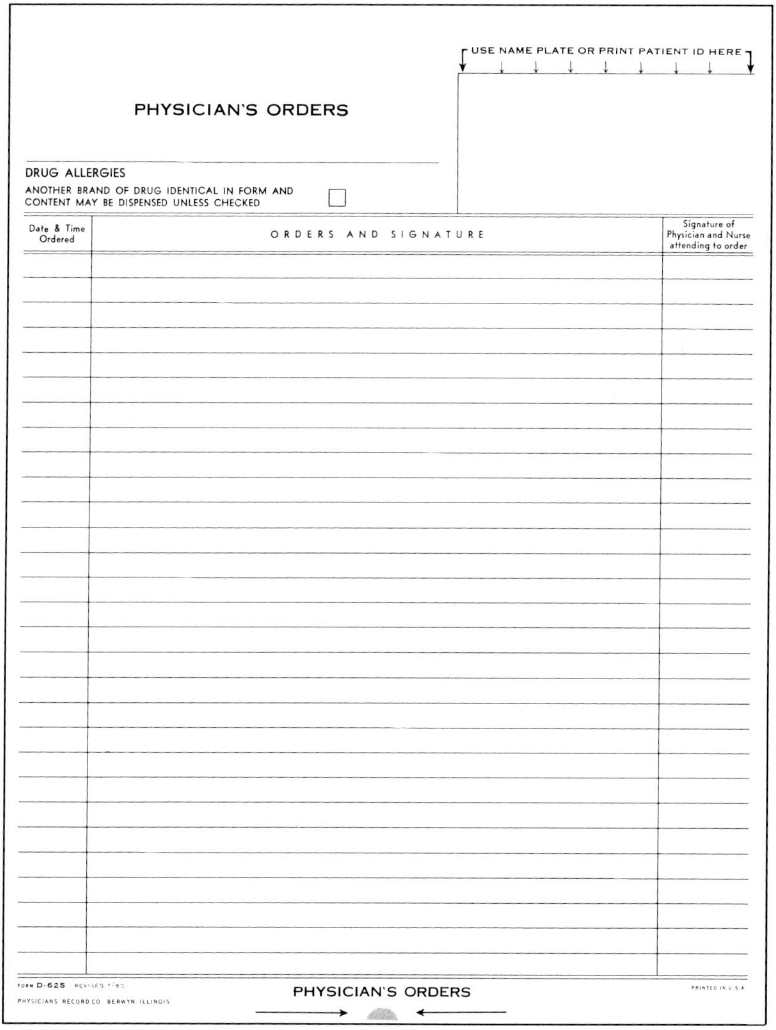
USE NAME PLATE OR PRINT PATIENT ID HERE

PHYSICIAN'S ORDERS

DRUG ALLERGIES

ANOTHER BRAND OF DRUG IDENTICAL IN FORM AND CONTENT MAY BE DISPENSED UNLESS CHECKED ☐

Date & Time Ordered	ORDERS AND SIGNATURE	Signature of Physician and Nurse attending to order

FORM D-625 REVISED

PHYSICIANS' RECORD CO. BERWYN, ILLINOIS

PHYSICIAN'S ORDERS

PRINTED IN U.S.A.

Form courtesy of Physicians' Record Company

FIG. 10 – PHYSICIAN'S ORDERS

Physician's Orders

The written or verbal orders constitute the attending physician's direction to nursing and ancillary services, and house staff, regarding all medications and treatments for the patient. The physician's orders (Figure 10) are to be dated and signed by the physician giving the order. Routine or "standing" orders

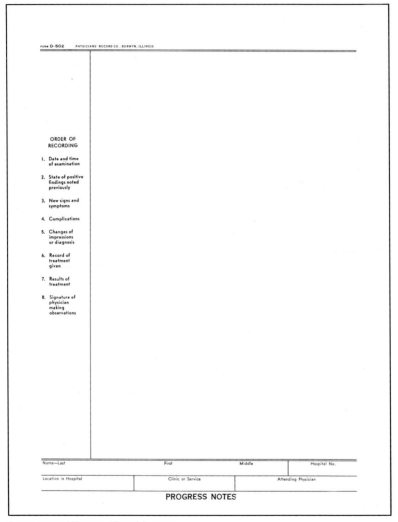

ORDER OF
RECORDING

1. Date and time
of examination

2. State of positive
findings noted
previously

3. New signs and
symptoms

4. Complications

5. Changes of
impressions
or diagnosis

6. Record of
treatment
given

7. Results of
treatment

8. Signature of
physician
making
observations

| Name—Last | First | Middle | Hospital No. |
| Location in Hospital | Clinic or Service | | Attending Physician |

PROGRESS NOTES

Form courtesy of Physicians' Record Company

FIG. 11 – PROGRESS NOTES

are a set of orders designed for routine care of patients with a certain diagnosis or procedure. When these are used as either a separate sheet or incorporated on the physician's order form, they are also to be signed by the physician. Most hospitals discourage the use of standing orders because the specified services may not be medically necessary for some patients. A discharge order should be written on every patient when the physician determines the patient may be released from the facility. Absence of a discharge order may indicate the patient left the hospital against medical advice (AMA), a fact which should be noted in the progress notes or discharge summary. Verbal orders of authorized practitioners may be allowed with certain limitations. Medical staff rules and regulations should state who may receive verbal orders and the time limits for affixing a signature to these orders. Medical staff rules and regulations may prohibit the use of such orders.

The JCAH specifies that the medical staff rules and regulations should define any category of verbal orders associated with any potential hazard to the patient, and require the responsible practitioner to sign such orders within 24 hours.

Progress Notes

Progress notes (Figure 11) are specific statements related to the course of the patient's illness, his response to treatment, and his status at discharge. The attending physician is responsible for recording his continuing observations of the patient's progress. Ancillary professionals, such as occupational, physical and respiratory therapists, also document the care they provide and the patient's response to treatment.

Generally an admission note, follow-up progress notes, and a final note are recorded. The admission note summarizes the general condition of the patient at the time of admission. Pertinent information about the patient not recorded in the history or physical examination should be recorded here. Subsequent progress notes are written as frequently as required by the patient's condition and medical staff rules and regulations. All treatments provided and the patient's response to each are to be included in the progress notes. Any complications which develop in the patient should also be documented in the progress notes. If the hospital has house officers, an end-of-service note is to be written as one house officer relinquishes the care of the patient to another. This note summarizes the patient's course of illness and treatment. The final note is a statement of the: patient's general condition on discharge, discharge instructions including patient activity, diet, medications, and time for follow-up visit to a physician. If the patient expires while in the hospital, the final note describes the circumstances regarding the patient's death, the findings, whether an autopsy was performed, and the cause of death.

Pathology Reports

Pathology reports (Figure 12) consist of a microscopic and/or macroscopic description of tissue expelled (as in an abortion), removed from a patient during surgery, or during a specialized procedure (biopsy) to provide tissue for pathological analysis, or after death when an autopsy (or necropsy) is performed. A request for tissue examination identifying the clinical diagnosis is sent with the tissue specimen to the pathologist. He examines the tissue and writes a report which includes as a minimum a descriptive diagnostic report of gross specimens received. The pathologist and the medical staff jointly decide which categories of specimens require only a gross description and diagnosis. When a microscopic evaluation is performed, any tissue diagnosis is to be based on the microscopic findings. The pathologist is responsible for signing the pathology report. Hospitals which contract with an outside agency for pathology services are to obtain the original pathology report for inclusion in the record.

In the autopsy report the pathologist documents a summary of the history of the patient's illness and treatment, a detailed report of gross (macroscopic) findings, microscopic findings, and anatomic diagnosis at autopsy. The provisional diagnosis should be recorded in the medical record within 3 days, and a complete autopsy protocol should be made part of the record within 90 days. The pathologist is responsible for signing the autopsy report.

Radiology Reports

The radiology and/or nuclear medicine reports are descriptions of diagnostic or therapeutic radiologic services. Diagnostic procedures can include: x-ray, radioactive scanning, thermography, xerography, and ultrasonography. With these methods, the results are projected into a form which can be visualized. A physician, usually a radiologist, writes or dictates a description of what he sees and the implications for the patient. This interpretation, which the radiologist signs, becomes the report. For therapeutic purposes, x-ray and radioactive materials may be administered. The amount of the dose, the date, and time

TISSUE REPORT

Clinical Diagnosis: Date:

Pathological Diagnosis:

Macroscopic Examination:

Microscopic Examination:

_____M.D.
SIGNATURE OF PATHOLOGIST

FORM D-1203   PHYSICIANS RECORD CO., BERWYN, ILLINOIS - PRINTED IN U.S.A.   TISSUE REPORT

Form courtesy of Physicians' Record Company

FIG. 12 – PATHOLOGY – TISSUE REPORT

are documented. At the end of the treatment, a summary of the treatment is provided and is signed by the radiologist and becomes part of the medical record.

The most common form of radiology report found in the record is the x-ray (Figure 13). Most hospitals combine the request and report for radiologic services on one form. Often the upper por-

X-RAY REPORT

Family Name	First Name		Home Phone	Room No.	Hosp. No.
Address		Occupation	Sex M F	Age—Years	X-Ray No.
Attending Physician			Date		O.P.D. No.

Submitted for (Please check) X-ray film ☐   Stereo ☐   Fluoroscopic exam. ☐   Complete exam. ☐   Discretion of Radiologist ☐   Treatment ☐

Dressings   may ☐   may not ☐   be removed   Previously rayed _____

Clinical Summary _____

Suspected pathology _____

Attending Physician _____ M.D.

Findings _____

_____ M.D.
Signature of Roentgenologist

FORM D-1904   PHYSICIANS' RECORD CO., BERWYN, ILLINOIS – PRINTED IN U.S.A.   X-RAY REPORT

Form courtesy of Physicians' Record Company

FIG. 13 – RADIOLOGY – X-RAY REPORT

tion contains the request. This portion contains the patient's name, hospital number and other identifying information, the part or region to be examined (which the attending physician documents), and the signature of the attending physician. The bottom portion usually provides space for the interpretation and the radiologist's signature.

The *Conditions of Participation* state that routine procedures such as x-ray are not considered consultations.

The JCAH requires, in general, that clinical observations including results of therapy and reports of procedures, tests and their results be contained in the medical record. All diagnostic and therapeutic procedures should be recorded and signed, including those from outside facilities, in which case the source facility is identified. Specifically the JCAH states that a radiologist will ordinarily provide a signed report; however, reports of specialized procedures performed by staff physicians who are not radiologists may be authenticated by them if they have been granted such privileges by the medical staff. The interpretations of radiographs taken outside of the hospital may be entered in the record if requested by the attending physician and if the quality of radiographs permits.

Consultation Report

Consultation reports (Figure 14) contain an opinion about a patient's condition by a physician other than the attending physician. This opinion, requested by the attending physician, is based on a review of the patient's medical record, an examination of the patient, and a conference with the attending physician. Many hospitals use a form which combines a request for consultation with the consultation report. In the request the attending physician indicates on which points he desires an opinion. The consultant records his findings, makes recommendations for the patient, and signs the report.

The *Conditions of Participation* require that the medical staff have established policies regarding the status of consultants. They further specify that a consultant must be well qualified by training, experience, and competence to give an opinion in the specialty in which his advice is sought. They also state that routine procedures, such as x-ray examinations, electrocardiogram determinations, tissue examinations, and proctoscopic and cystoscopic procedures are not normally considered to be consultations. The categories of patients for which consultations are required are (1) patients who are not good medical or surgical risks, (2) patients whose diagnoses are obscure, (3) patients whose physicians have doubts as to the best therapeutic measures to be taken, and (4) instances where there is a question

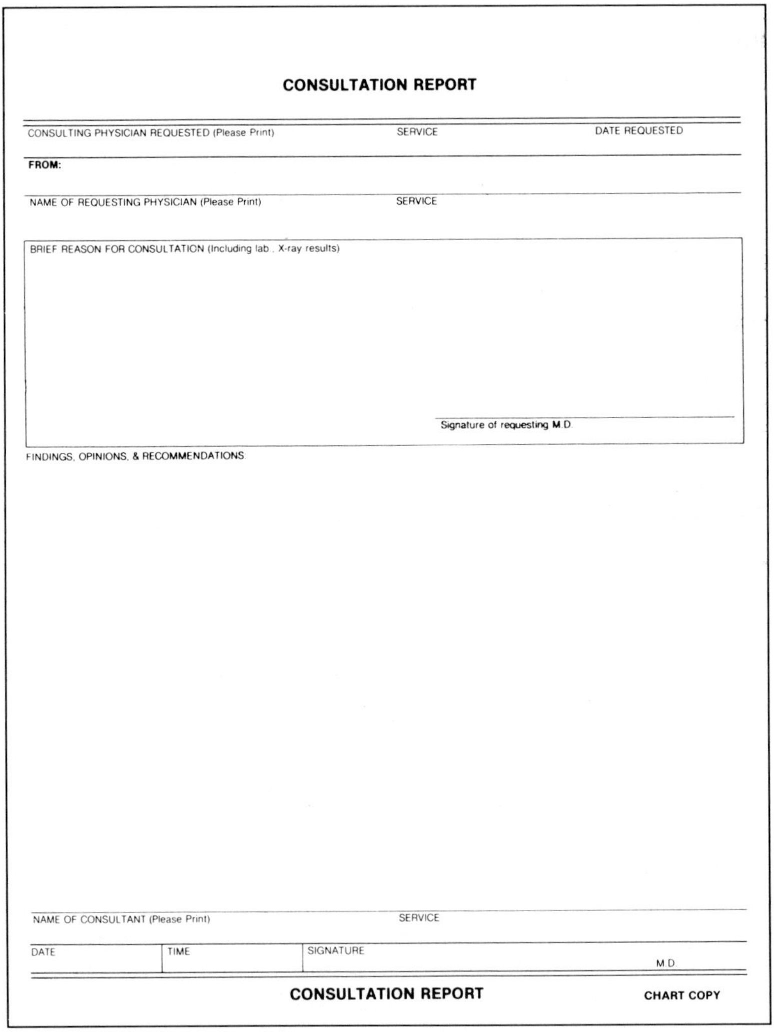

CONSULTATION REPORT

CONSULTING PHYSICIAN REQUESTED (Please Print) SERVICE DATE REQUESTED

FROM:

NAME OF REQUESTING PHYSICIAN (Please Print) SERVICE

BRIEF REASON FOR CONSULTATION (Including lab., X-ray results)

Signature of requesting M.D.

FINDINGS, OPINIONS, & RECOMMENDATIONS

NAME OF CONSULTANT (Please Print) SERVICE

DATE TIME SIGNATURE M.D.

CONSULTATION REPORT **CHART COPY**

Form courtesy of Physicians' Record Company

FIG. 14 – CONSULTATION REPORT

of criminal activity. The exception to this is when the admission is an emergency. The attending physician is responsible for requesting consultation.

Operative Data

Some hospitals group information generated from each surgical procedure. This collection of information is referred to as an

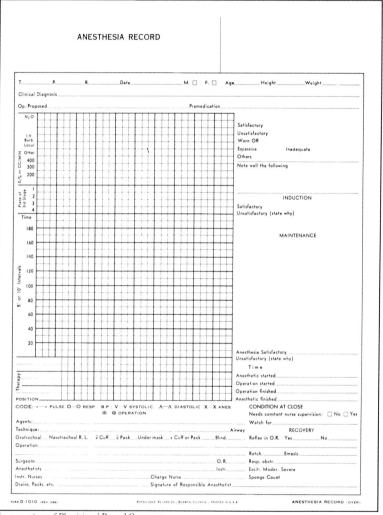

Form courtesy of Physicians' Record Company

FIG. 15 – ANESTHESIA REPORT (front)

operative set or section. The information usually contained in an operative section is: consent for surgery, preanesthesia and postanesthesia reports, the operative report, and if applicable, pathology report.

Anesthesia Report

When a patient undergoes a procedure which requires an anesthetic other than a local, an anesthesia report (Figures 15

ANESTHESIA STUDY

PREOPERATIVE	POSTOPERATIVE

Check negative conditions only. Record positive details below.

Resp._____ Urol._____

Circ._____ Neurol._____

G.I._____ Obst._____

Gyn._____ Metab._____

Positive:_____

COMPLICATIONS	R. O. N.	Op. Day	DAYS POSTOPERATIVE															Wks. P.O.	
		D	N	1	2	3	4	5	6	7	8	9	10	11	12	13	14	3	4
Nausea & Vomiting																			
Headache																			
Urinary retention																			
Backache																			
Laryngitis																			
Pulmonary																			
Shock																			

Remarks:_____

Anes. History

Urine_____ B.P._____

Hb._____ RBC_____ WBC_____

Other Lab. data_____

(O-1010 BACK)

FIG. 16 – ANESTHESIA REPORT (back of Fig. 15)

and 16) is required. This form documents the preoperative medication, the amount of concentration, time given, and effect. Additionally this form lists the anesthetic agent, the amount, the technique used to administer it, the effect and duration of the anesthetic, the temperature, pulse, respiration and blood pressure, blood loss, blood transfusions and intravenous fluids given, and notations of the patient's condition throughout the procedure.

Any treatments given which are not documented elsewhere and surgical manipulation which may affect the conduct of anesthesia and complications arising during administration of the anesthetic are documented on the form. The practitioner providing the anesthetic (nurse anesthetist or anesthesiologist) is responsible for recording the information and signing the anesthesia report.

In conjunction with the administration of anesthesia there must be recorded in the medical record a preanesthesia and a postanesthesia note. The preanesthesia note is often found in the progress notes and includes information on the choice of anesthesia, the medical procedure anticipated, the patient's previous drug history, past anesthetic problems and any potential anesthetic problems, a physical examination of the patient, summary of laboratory data, and preanesthesia medications.

The postanesthesia note may be in the progress notes, the recovery room report, or in the anesthesia report. The postanesthesia report documents the patient's condition after anesthesia, specifying the nature and extent of any anesthesia-related complications. It is documented and signed within 24 hours after surgery by the practitioner who administered the anesthetic.

Documentation of at least one postanesthetic visit which describes the presence or absence of anesthesia-related complications is required by the JCAH. A note made in the surgical or obstetrical suite or in the postanesthesia care unit does not ordinarily constitute a visit. The number of visits will be determined by the status of the patient. A visit should be made early in the postoperative period and again after complete recovery from anesthesia. Each note must specify the date and time. It is recommended that the postanesthesia note be made by a physician or qualified oral surgeon. All anesthesia personnel are encouraged to make postanesthesia notes for patients to whom they have administered anesthesia. It is acceptable for the physician or dentist who discharges the patient to make the documentation required if it is not feasible for anesthesia personnel to do so. It is recommended that the anesthesia records should be completed promptly and filed in the record within 24 hours of completion.

Recovery Room Record

Patients are taken to the recovery room for immediate post-operative or postanesthesia care. Pertinent data regarding the patient's condition on arrival and transfer from the recovery room, as well as information regarding the patient's condition and treatment while there, must be documented. This provides a complete record from the time the patient leaves the operating room until he arrives on the nursing unit. A form specifically designed for recording recovery room care is often used. This allows quick comparison of all required information, including vital signs, treatment, and progress. The postanesthesia note may be documented on this form. Depending on the content of a particular form, it may be signed by either the nurse or physician, or both.

The JCAH does not require a recovery room form. It states that when there is a postanesthesia care unit, the medical record data are to contain the patient's level of consciousness on entering and leaving the unit, the vital signs, status reports of infusions, surgical dressings, tubes, catheters, and drains. If there is no special care unit, similar information is to be documented in the medical record.

Operative Report

The medical records of all patients who had surgical procedures performed must include an operative report (Figure 17). A preoperative diagnosis should be recorded in the medical record prior to surgery. It is helpful, though not required, to have the preoperative diagnosis included on the operative report. This allows quick comparison of the preoperative diagnosis with the postoperative diagnosis, which is to be documented on this form. Also included in the operative report are a full description of the findings, both normal and abnormal, the organs explored, procedures, ligatures, sutures, number of packs, drains and sponges used, and names of surgeons and assistants. The date and duration of surgery and the condition of the patient at the completion of surgery should also be stated. The operative report should be written or dictated immediately after surgery, signed by the surgeon, and filed in the medical record as soon as possible after surgery. When there is a transcription and/or

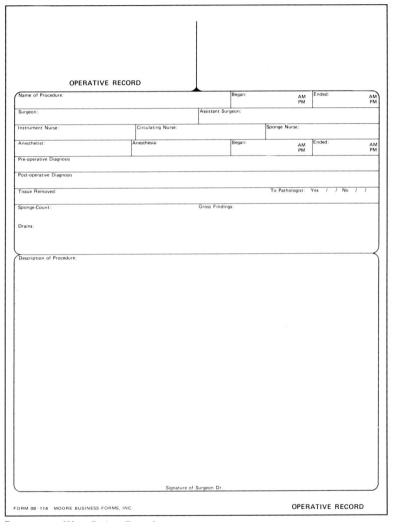

Form courtesy of Moore Business Forms, Inc.

FIG. 17 – OPERATIVE REPORT

filing delay, a comprehensive operative progress note should be entered in the medical record immediately after surgery to provide continuity of care.

Special Medical Reports

Electrocardiograph Report

The electrocardiogram (ECG, EKG) is a graphic tracing which represents the electrical changes in heart muscle as the heart beats. Surface electrodes on the patient transmit the impulses resulting from the depolarization and repolarization of the heart muscle. These changes are plotted against time on paper tape. The normal EKG shows five waves or deflections, which represent the electrical changes and are called P, Q, R, S, and T waves. The electrocardiograph report consists of the cardiologist's signed interpretation of an electrocardiogram. The actual graphic tracing may be filed in the medical record or in the EKG laboratory, available for reference if necessary.

Electromyographic Reports

The electromyograph report consists of the neurologist's or orthopedist's interpretation of an electromyogram (EMG). The EMG measures electrical activity in skeletal muscles at the motor unit level. The changes are transmitted via electrodes (surface or needle) to an oscilloscope for visual display. The EMG evaluates insertional activity (presence or absence of) and the activity with the muscle at rest and/or during stages of voluntary contraction. The muscles evaluated and the potentials and frequency evoked are stated in the report by the examiner. The interpretation of these measurements is the responsibility of the neurologist or orthopedist.

Discharge Summary

The discharge summary (or clinical resume–Figure 18) is a concise recapitulation of the patient's course in the hospital: the reason(s) for hospitalization; significant findings from examinations/tests; procedures; therapies provided and the response to these; condition at discharge; and instructions given regarding medications, physical activity, diet, and follow-up care. The description of the patient's condition upon discharge should be stated in a manner that allows comparison with the condition upon admission. Vague terms such as "improved" should be avoided. When preprinted instructions are given to the patient, this fact should be documented in the record; and a sample instruction sheet should be on file in the medical record department. All relevant diagnoses established by the time of dis-

DISCHARGE SUMMARY

Family Name   Room No.   Hosp. No.

Attending Physician   Date of Admission   Date of Discharge

Provisional Diagnosis:

Principal Diagnoses:

Additional Diagnoses:

Operative Procedures:

Brief History and Essential Physical
    Findings:

Significant Laboratory, X-ray and
    Consultation Findings:

Course in Hospital with Complications,
    if Any:

Condition, Treatment, Final Disposition
    on Discharge and Prognosis:

Special Instructions to Patient:
    (Diet, Medications, Follow-up
    Care, Physical Activity)

Date _____   Signed _____ M.D.

FORM D-103 (REV. 3/81)   PHYSICIANS RECORD CO. BERWYN, ILLINOIS - PRINTED IN U.S.A.   DISCHARGE SUMMARY

Form Courtesy of Physicians' Record Company

FIG. 18 – DISCHARGE SUMMARY

charge and all operative procedures should be recorded in acceptable terminology, which indicates topography and etiology as necessary. The discharge summary and the admission/discharge form may both contain listings of final diagnoses and procedures. Care must be exercised to insure that both listings are the same. A final progress note can substitute for a discharge summary in the following cases: patients who are hospitalized less than 48 hours with problems of a minor nature, normal newborns, and uncomplicated obstetrical deliveries. The discharge summary should be written or dictated immediately after the discharge of the patient.

Nursing Data

The second type of clinical data found in the medical record is nursing data generated by the registered nurse, licensed practical nurse, and the nurse's aide. Some forms, such as the recovery room record discussed earlier, contain data documented by both nurses and physicians. There are, however, a number of forms in the medical record which are the sole responsibility of nursing personnel. A nursing assessment or nursing care plan for each patient is required. This document includes statements of the nursing measures to be taken which will facilitate the medical care provided. Although traditionally nursing care plans were not filed in the medical record, today most hospitals include nursing assessments with the permanent medical record.

Nurses' Notes

The nurses' notes (Figure 19) are narrative entries made by nursing personnel regarding their observations of the patient, care and treatment given the patient, and the patient's response to the therapy. The nurses' notes should describe the patient's needs, problems, and activities in terms of the patient's actual behavior. As much as possible, nurses' entries should contain objective data, such as stating the milliliters of fluids taken rather than subjective terms such as intake "poor" or "good."

Any subjective data should be in the form of statements made by the patient, such as complaints of pain or how he feels emotionally. The nurses' notes usually consist of an admission note, subsequent notes as required by the patient's condition and hospital regulations, and a discharge note.

The admission note includes the time of admission, how the patient arrived (wheelchair, stretcher, or walking), symptoms, signs, treatment instituted, time and type of specimen sent to the laboratory, and the time the attending physician was notified of patient's admission. The discharge note should con-

NURSES' NOTES				
Family Name	First Name	Attending Physician	Room No.	Hosp. No.
Intern		Day Nurse		Night Nurse
Date	Treatment and Medicines		Food	Remarks

FORM D-804   PHYSICIANS RECORD CO., BERWYN, ILLINOIS - PRINTED IN U.S.A.   NURSES' NOTES

Form courtesy of Physicians' Record Company

FIG. 19 – NURSES' NOTES

tain time of discharge, how the patient left and with whom, discharge instructions, and if transferred to another facility, the name of the facility. If the patient leaves without a discharge order and against the advice of the physician, this should be noted and the reason. If the patient dies, the note should describe when life functions apparently ceased, the time the physician was notified, and the time a physician pronounced the patient dead.

Historically nurses' notes have been written in different colors of ink (black, green, and red) to indicate the nursing shift on which the entry was made. This is no longer considered advisable because of the increased frequency of photocopying and microfilming records. Red and green ink do not photocopy or microfilm well. It is recommended that black or dark blue ink be used to make entries. The nurse providing the care is responsible for making and signing the entries. Often the nurse will sign with first initial, last name, and professional status (RN or LPN).

The JCAH states that clinical observations in the nurses' notes should contain pertinent, concise, meaningful observations, and information which reflects the patient's status. Nursing documentation should address the patient's needs, problems, capabilities, and limitations. Nursing intervention and patient response must be noted. The JCAH encourages standardization of routine care and repeated monitoring documentation, such as personal hygiene given, medications administered, temperature, pulse, and respiration.

Graphic Sheet

The graphic sheet (vital sign or TPR sheet—Figure 20) is used to record several different parameters regarding the patient. Most commonly, the temperature, pulse, respiration, and blood pressure measurements are charted on this form. Other information which may be included is intake and output of fluids (and solids). One form usually provides space for charting and parameters, six times a day for several days. The patient's condition may require more frequent measuring of the vital signs. An additional form may be needed to allow for frequent documentation. Signatures of the individuals making these observations are usually not required.

Medication Sheet

The medication sheet (Figure 21) provides documentation of the medicines given orally, topically, by injection, inhalation,

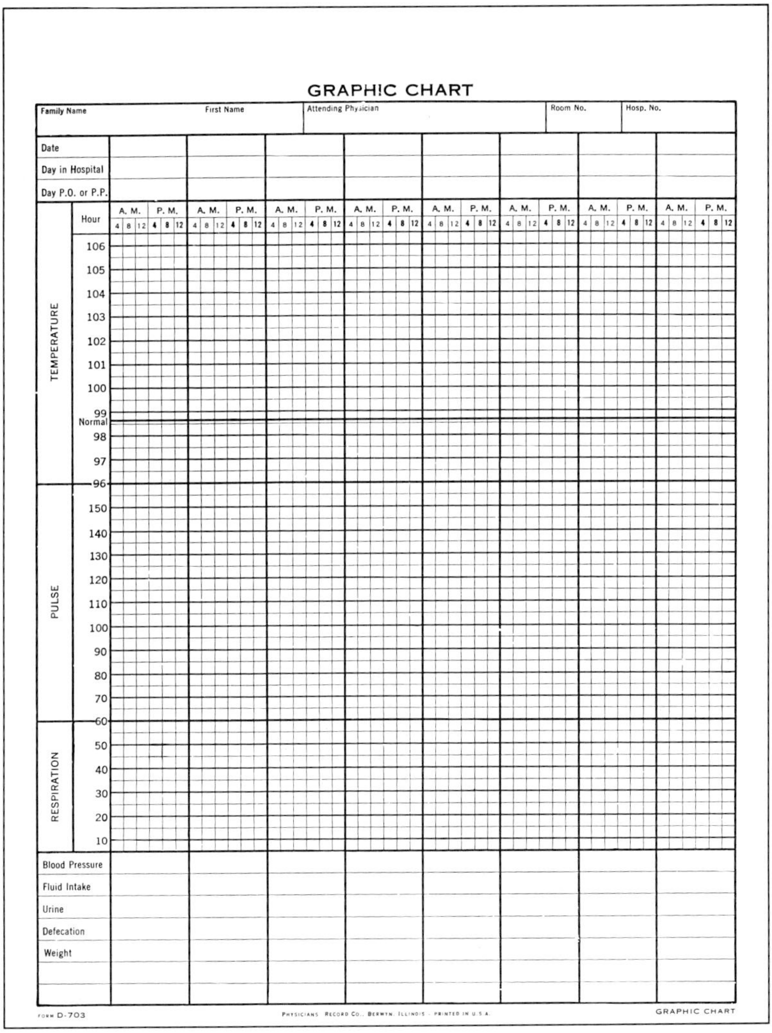
GRAPHIC CHART

Family Name | First Name | Attending Physician | Room No. | Hosp. No.

Date
Day in Hospital
Day P.O. or P.P.
Hour — A. M. 4 8 12 P. M. 4 8 12

TEMPERATURE: 106, 105, 104, 103, 102, 101, 100, 99 Normal, 98, 97, 96
PULSE: 150, 140, 130, 120, 110, 100, 90, 80, 70, 60
RESPIRATION: 50, 40, 30, 20, 10

Blood Pressure
Fluid Intake
Urine
Defecation
Weight

FORM D-703 PHYSICIANS RECORD CO., BERWYN, ILLINOIS - PRINTED IN U.S.A. GRAPHIC CHART

Form courtesy of Physicians' Record Company

FIG. 20 – GRAPHIC CHART

and infusion. The date, time, name of drug, dose, and route by which it was given are documented after the drug has been administered. Intentional omission of medication is also documented in the medical record; and the reason for such is noted in the nurses' notes, such as in preparation for surgery. The professional giving the drug initials the entry.

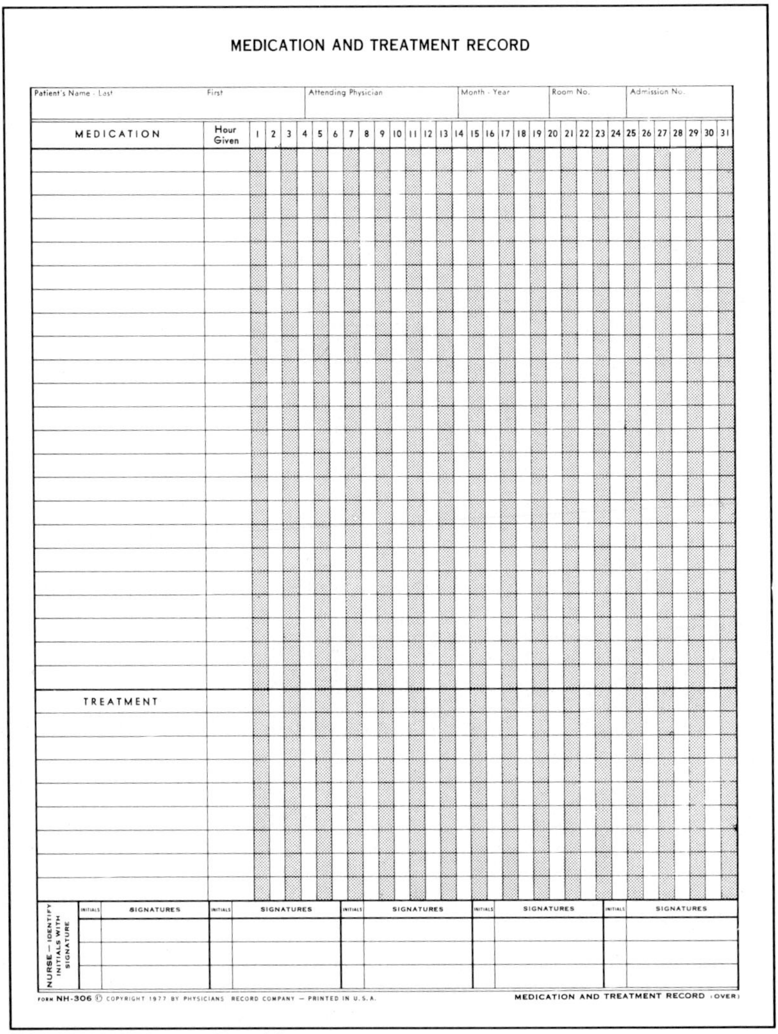
MEDICATION AND TREATMENT RECORD

Patient's Name - Last | First | Attending Physician | Month - Year | Room No. | Admission No.

MEDICATION	Hour Given	1	2	3	4	5	6	7	8	9	10	11	12	13	14	15	16	17	18	19	20	21	22	23	24	25	26	27	28	29	30	31
TREATMENT																																

NURSE — IDENTIFY INITIALS WITH SIGNATURE	INITIALS	SIGNATURES	INITIALS	SIGNATURES	INITIALS	SIGNATURES	INITIALS	SIGNATURES	INITIALS	SIGNATURES

FORM NH-306 © COPYRIGHT 1977 BY PHYSICIANS RECORD COMPANY — PRINTED IN U.S.A. MEDICATION AND TREATMENT RECORD (OVER)

Form Courtesy of Physicians' Record Company

FIG. 21 – MEDICATION SHEET

Miscellaneous Reports

Nursing service personnel in specialized care units of the hospital, such as the intensive care unit (ICU), coronary care unit

(CCU), or postanesthesia room (PAR–recovery room) may be responsible for documenting observations about the patient on specialized forms. These forms allow for more frequent recording of observations and may be used in addition to or in place of routine forms.

Ancillary Data

The ancillary data contained in the medical record refer to that information generated by health professionals other than physicians and nurses. The most common ancillary forms are medical laboratory, physical therapy, respiratory therapy, and social service reports.

Medical Laboratory Reports

The medical laboratory reports (Figure 22) consist of various types of analyses or examinations of body substances such as blood, urine, and stool. The medical laboratory usually provides: blood bank, blood chemistry, hematology, microbiology, serology, and urinalysis tests and reports. The attending physician orders the test(s) on the physician's order sheet. Nursing service fills out a requisition for the test. The appropriate specimen is obtained from the patient and sent, along with the requisition, to the medical laboratory. The test is performed by a medical technologist or bacteriologist. After completion of the test, the results are documented on the appropriate report form, the form dated and signed by the professional performing the test, and the report is sent back to the nursing unit. Laboratory reports are commonly recorded on small slips of paper which are then placed on a collection sheet in the medical record, as shown in Figure 22. An increasing use of automation, however, can provide computer printouts of multiple test results; and when this system is used, these computer printouts become part of the medical record.

Reports should be designed to facilitate comparison of each determination with pertinent reference values and sequential and related analyses. Another way to provide the reference values is to include a current list of such in the medical record. When tests are performed in an outside laboratory, the name of the laboratory should be on the report filed in the medical record. The JCAH states that reports of clinical laboratory examinations should be completed promptly and filed in the medical record within 24 hours of completion if possible.

The medical record should contain complete and accurate information about blood transfusions. The American Association of Blood Banks (AABB) in its *Technical Manual,* specifies that

LABORATORY REPORTS

| MISCELLANEOUS LABORATORY | | | | A123456 |

(Form image: Miscellaneous Laboratory order slip)

MISCELLANEOUS LABORATORY order form with fields:

ROUTINE / Preop.; Date Needed / Not Emergency But Needed By / Time / Date / Emergency Only Ordered By Physician Report to Go Directly to M.D.

DATE REQUIRED · SPECIMEN DRAWN BY · REQUESTING PHYSICIAN · DATE · NURSE · TIME

ORDER ONLY ONE TEST ON THIS SLIP   ☐ OUTPATIENT

Specimen_____
Examination Desired_____
REPORT:

REPORTED BY   DATE REPORTED

MISCELLANEOUS LABORATORY

☐ OUTPATIENT

CROSSMATCH RECORD		UNIT NUMBER					BLOOD BANK PRODUCTS SPECIFY UNIT		
PATIENT		DONOR		SALINE COMPATIBLE	ALBUMIN COMPATIBLE	COOMBS COMPATIBLE	ANTIBODY SCREEN	FRESH FROZEN PLASMA · PLATELET CONCENTRATE · FIBRINOGEN	
GROUP	TYPE	GROUP	TYPE					SALT-POOR ALBUMIN · CRYOPRECIPITATE	

PLASMA PROTEIN FRACTION (5%) 250 cc.
RhoGAM
LOT OR UNIT NO.

| Dᵘ | | STARTED BY | | STOPPED BY | |
| DATE GIVEN | TIME STARTED | TIME FINISHED | cc. ADMINISTERED |

REPORTED BY
DATE REPORTED

REACTION TO TRANSFUSION ☐ YES ☐ NO   IF YES, USE SEPARATE REPORT FORM

BLOOD TRANS. – BLOOD BANK PROD.

FORM D-408 PHYSICIANS RECORD CO BERWYN ILLINOIS   LABORATORY REPORTS

Form courtesy of Physicians' Record Company

FIG. 22 – MEDICAL LABORATORY REPORTS

the transfusion form, which becomes part of the patient's record, should have the name and identification number of the intended recipient and the donor identification number. Notation of ABO and Rh groups of the patient and donor should be the same on the label of the blood bag as on the transfusion form. The transfusionist who administers the blood, checks identification information at the patient's bedside and documents on the transfusion form that this information has been checked. In addition, the transfusionist notes on the transfusion form whether the compatibility tag identifies the person performing the test and the interpretation of results. After the transfusionist checks the identifying information, he must sign the transfusion form to indicate that the identification was correct and to identify himself as the person who started the transfusion. Notation of the date and time of transfusion, the nature of the transfusion product, its identification number, and the patient's condition at the start of transfusion should be recorded in the patient's medical record. After transfusion of each unit of blood, the patient care personnel (nurse) records the time, the volume and type of component given, the patient's condition, and the identity of the person who stops the transfusion and observes the patient.

Physical Therapy

Physical therapy reports (Figures 23 and 24) describe assessments and treatments including the use of exercise, heat, cold, water, electricity, ultrasound, and other physical means to restore the patient to useful activity. The assessment or treatment is ordered by the physician on the physician's order sheet or on a requisition which is sent to the physical therapy department by nursing service. The therapist providing the service documents the treatment given and the patient's response, and dates and signs the report.

The initial report contains objective data regarding: behavior; joint evaluation; muscle/motor evaluation; respiratory evaluation; functional evaluation; and other evaluations, such as posture, skin, reflexes, prosthetics, orthotics, sensation, and edema, as necessary. Goals and recommended procedures to achieve these goals should be included.

The progress notes or reports also are stated objectively to allow comparison to the initial findings and demonstrate progress toward the goals. Continual reassessment and adjustment of the treatment program should be done in consultation with the physician and documented. Education of the patient and/or patient's family also should be documented. A discharge note

PHYSICAL THERAPY EVALUATION

Date______
Initial______
Interim______
Final______

PATIENT NAME	Patient Number	Age:

DIAGNOSIS:

TO:

Physical Therapy Plan of Treatment has been reviewed with

______patient
______family
______other agency personnel involved with patient's care

GOALS

Short Term:	Long Term:
1.	1.
2.	2.
3.	3.

PHYSICAL THERAPY PLAN OF TREATMENT:
1.
2.
3.
4.
5.

The PT Plan of Treatment is recommended pending physician's approval

______, R.P.T.

The PT Plan of Treatment is amended and or approved by:

______ Date ______
Physician

KEY: I: Independent A: Needs Assist S: Needs Supervision for Safety U: Unable NA: Not Applicable

FUNCTIONAL ASSESSMENT		**Comments:** If applicable remark on frequency, speed, assistive devices.
BED ACTIVITIES:		
1. Rolls, turns in bed		
2. Moves sideways in bed		
3. Comes to sitting position		
4. Sitting balance		
TRANSFERS:		
1. Wheelchair to and from bed		
2. Toilet		
3. Tub		
4. Car		
AMBULATION:		
1. Wheelchair mobility		
2. Comes to standing position		
3. Standing balance		
4. Initiates steps		
5. Textures (carpets, outside)		
6. Dynamic balance (movement)		
7. Stairs		
8. Uses elevators		
ACTIVITIES OF DAILY LIVING:		
1. Feeds self		
2. Uses toilet		
3. Dresses self		
4. Bathes self		
BEHAVIOR (Items below rated + or −)		
1. Alert		
2. Oriented to time, place, direction		
3. Disoriented		
4. Cooperative		
5. Confused		
6. Safety awareness		

(OVER)

Form courtesy of Physicians' Record Company

FIG. 23 – PHYSICAL THERAPY REPORTS (front)

or summary when service is discontinued is documented to explain therapies provided and the patient's response to these.

The JCAH requirements for Rehabilitative Services contain

generic medical record content requirements which apply to the services usually combined to provide rehabilitation. These include physical therapy, occupational therapy, speech pathology,

EXERCISE TOLERANCE

a) Pulse Rate:	b) Respiration	c) Blood Pressure
Before Exercise_____	Rate_____	Before Exercise_____
After Exercise_____	Quality_____	After Exercise_____

Endurance   General Posture

SPEECH IMPAIRMENT	AUDITORY IMPAIRMENT	VISUAL IMPAIRMENT
☐ Yes ☐ No	☐ Yes ☐ No	☐ Yes ☐ No

SKIN CONDITION   SENSATION

GAIT ANALYSIS

MOBILITY   ASSISTIVE DEVICE

STRENGTH	RANGE OF MOTION
A. TRUNK	A. TRUNK
B. EXTREMITIES	B. EXTREMITIES

COMMENTS/RECOMMENDATIONS:

Frequency_____ Duration_____

Therapist_____

Form courtesy of Physicians' Record Company

FIG. 24 – PHYSICAL THERAPY REPORTS (back of Fig. 23)

audiology, prosthetic and/or orthotic device fabrication and fitting, and others.

The JCAH requirements for medical record content include a written plan of care for each patient by the appropriate therapist in which the treatment objectives and short-term and

PLEASE USE BALL POINT PEN AND BEAR DOWN

DATE	PHYSICIAN'S ORDERS

1. OXYGEN CONCENTRATION (CIRCLE ONE)
   ROOM AIR , AIR DILUTION , 100%

2. LENGTH OF RX. (CIRCLE ONE)
   5 MIN. , 10 MIN. , 15 MIN.
   OTHER__________

3. CM H20 PRESSURE (CIRCLE ONE)
   10 CM , 15 CM , 20 CM,
   OTHER__________

4. MEDICATION (CHECK ONE)
   _____ 3cc N/S
   _____ 2.5cc N/S, .5cc BRONKOSOL
   _____ 1.5cc N/S, .5cc BRONKOSOL
   1cc MUCOMYST
   _____ 2.5cc N/S, .3cc ALUPENT
   _____ 1.5cc N/S, .3cc ALUPENT
   1cc MUCOMYST
   _____ 4cc ETHYL ALCOHOL
   _____ OTHER (SPECIFY)

(I PPB-HAND HELD · INCENTIVE SPIROMETRY)

5. FREQUENCY (CIRCLE ONE)
   OD., BID., TID., QID., ______ QHR.

6. COUGH, DEEP BREATHE Pt. X 3

7. D/C Rx. IF PULSE >120, UNLESS SPECIFIED.__________

8. CHARTS WILL BE FLAGGED AFTER 3 DAYS. IF NOT REORDERED, Rx. D/C'D.

BE SURE TO IMPRINT PATIENT'S NAME BELOW

THERAPEUTIC OBJECTIVES OF RESPIRATORY THERAPY

DATE: ______

PATIENT:__________ ROOM:______

DIAGNOSIS:__________

( ) IMPROVE DISTRIBUTION OF VENTILATION
( ) DELIVERY OF AEROSOL MEDICATION
( ) PREVENT OR TREAT ATELECTASIS
( ) IMPROVE ARTERIAL OXYGENATION
( ) IMPROVE OR PROMOTE COUGH
( ) MOBILIZE SECRETIONS
( ) OTHER:__________

PHYSICIAN__________ DATE______

OTHER RESPIRATORY ORDERS:__________

FORM N01 SPEEDIPLY• PAT D MCP• PAT D MBF 28

Form courtesy of Moore Business Forms, Inc.

FIG. 25 – RESPIRATORY THERAPY REPORT

long-term rehabilitation potential are stated. The record should contain documentation on assessment of rehabilitative progress and an estimate of further rehabilitation.

Respiratory Therapy Report

The respiratory therapy report (Figure 25) documents the assessments and treatments of the patient and the patient's response to these. The treatments provided by respiratory therapy include administration of oxygen, therapeutic gases, aerosols and humidity, mechanical ventilation, and emergency resuscitation. Evaluations and examinations provided by respiratory therapy include various pulmonary function tests such as spirometry, lung volume measurements, and arterial blood analysis. The JCAH states that respiratory therapy services shall be ordered by a physician and should state the type, frequency and duration of treatment, and as appropriate, the type and dose of medication, the type of diluent, and oxygen concentration. This and any related respiratory consultation should be placed in the medical record. All respiratory therapy services should be documented in the record including the type of therapy, date and time of administration, effects of therapy, and any adverse reactions. Upon discharge, the physician should document a timely, pertinent summary of the overall results of respiratory therapy and the need for long term oxygen therapy.

Social Service Record

Social service reports are developed by the social worker caring for the patient. The social worker has access to and knowledge of a wealth of information about the patient, some of which is sensitive, personal data which are not recorded in the social service report for the medical record. The Society of Social Work Directors of the American Hospital Association recommends in its book *Documentation by Social Workers in Medical Records* that the social service record should contain background, social information, and problems identified by the patient, his family, and the social worker. A plan of action, progress reports, and a discharge note should be documented in the medical record.

Special Records

Special care units established in the hospital give specialized care to certain groups of patients such as those in the coronary care unit, in intensive care, in kidney dialysis, in a psychiatric unit, or in a rehabilitation unit. Wherever possible, regular medical record forms are used; but in some instances special forms must be developed to document the needed data.

The previous sections have covered the content of medical rec-

SHORT-STAY RECORD

HISTORY	REPORT OF OPERATION
Past History	Preoperative Diagnosis
Present Complaint	Postoperative Diagnosis
	Operation
PHYSICAL EXAMINATION	
General Appearance — nutrition — pallor	Surgeon
	Assistant
Head — Eye, Ear, Nose and Throat	Anesthetist
	Anesthetic
	Condition during Anesthesia
Heart — is murmur present?	Operation: Date _____ Began _____ Ended _____
is there enlargement?	Immediate Postoperative Condition
Lungs — are respirations normal?	
rales _____ dullness	Hemorrhage, Shock, etc.
Abdomen — distension?	
is spleen enlarged?	
is liver enlarged?	Findings
Adenopathy — neck	
axilla	
groin	
Genitalia	
	Procedure
Extremities — Bones and joints	

FINAL DIAGNOSIS: _____

RESULTS: Discharged Alive: ☐   Died: ☐ Under 48 hours   ☐ Over 48 hours

Signed _____ M.D., Attending Physician

FORM D-1880   PHYSICIANS' RECORD CO., BERWYN, ILLINOIS - PRINTED IN U.S.A.   SHORT-STAY RECORD (OVER)

Form courtesy of Physicians' Record Company

FIG. 26 – SHORT-STAY RECORD (front)

ords as they are used for inpatients in hospitals. The following section will touch on some special categories of patients: the short-stay, obstetric, and newborn patients.

Short-Stay Records

The short-stay or short-form record (Figures 26 and 27) may be used for patients who are hospitalized for conditions of a

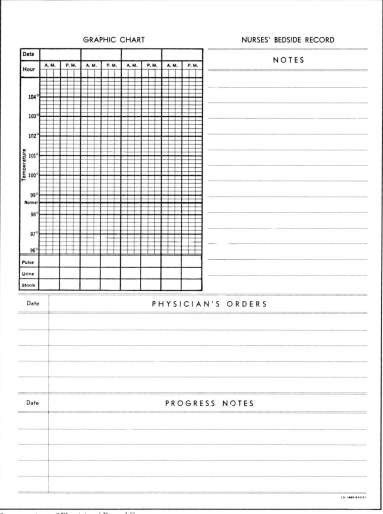

GRAPHIC CHART   NURSES' BEDSIDE RECORD

Date

Hour

Temperature
104°
103°
102°
101°
100°
99° Normal
98°
97°
96°

Pulse
Urine
Stools

Date   PHYSICIAN'S ORDERS

Date   PROGRESS NOTES

NOTES

Form courtesy of Physicians' Record Company

FIG. 27 – SHORT-STAY RECORD (back of Fig. 26)

minor nature which require less than 48 hours of hospitalization. The short-stay record should contain identification data, a description of the patient's condition, pertinent physical findings, an account of the treatment given and the patient's response to each, and any other data, such as laboratory tests or consultations necessary to justify the diagnosis and treatment.

Health History Summary Date:	HOLLISTER maternal/newborn RECORD SYSTEM	PATIENT IDENTIFICATION Patient's name _____

Age____ Race____ Religion____ | Marital status ____ | Years married ____ Education ____ Occupation ____
Home address ____ | Home tel. ____ | Work tel. ____
Nearest relative ____ | Relative's employer ____ | Work tel. ____
Referring physician ____ | Attending physician ____

Medical History	Patient	Family	Check and detail positive findings including date and place of treatment. Precede findings by reference number.	Sensitivities (detail positive findings)
1. Congenital anomalies				30. ☐ None known
2. Genetic diseases				31. ☐ Antibiotics
3. Multiple births				32. ☐ Analgesics
4. Diabetes mellitus				33. ☐ Sedatives
5. Malignancies				34. ☐ Anesthesia
6. Hypertension				35. ☐ Other
7. Heart disease				**Preexisting Risk Guide**
8. Rheumatic fever				Indicates pregnancy/outcome at risk
9. Pulmonary disease				36. ☐ Age < 15 or > 35
10. GI problems				37. ☐ < 8th grade education
11. Renal disease				38. ☐ Cardiac disease (class I or II)
12. Other urinary tract problems				39. ☐ Tuberculosis, active
13. Genitourinary anomalies				40. ☐ Chronic pulmonary disease
14. Abnormal uterine bleeding				41. ☐ Thrombophlebitis
15. Infertility				42. ☐ Endocrinopathy
16. Venereal disease				43. ☐ Epilepsy (on medication)
17. Phlebitis, varicosities				44. ☐ Infertility (treated)
18. Nervous/mental disorders				45. ☐ 2 abortions (spontaneous/induced)
19. Convulsive disorders				46. ☐ ≥ 7 deliveries
20. Metabol./endocrine disorders				47. ☐ Previous preterm or SGA infants
21. Anemia/hemoglobinopathy				48. ☐ Infants ≥ 4,000 gms
22. Blood dyscrasias				49. ☐ Isoimmunization (ABO, etc.)
23. Drug addiction				50. ☐ Hemorrhage during previous preg.
24. Smoking/alcohol				51. ☐ Previous preeclampsia
25. Infectious diseases				52. ☐ Surgically scarred uterus
26. Operations/accidents				53. ☐ ____
27. Blood transfusions				Indicates pregnancy/outcome at high risk
28. Other hospitalizations				54. ☐ Age ≥ 40
29. No known disease				55. ☐ Diabetes mellitus

Menstrual History	Onset age	Cycle q days	Length days	Amount	L M P	mo/day/yr quality

56. ☐ Hypertension
57. ☐ Cardiac disease (class III or IV)
58. ☐ Chronic renal disease

Pregnancy History	Grav	Term	Pret	Abort	Live	E D C	mo/day/yr

59. ☐ Congenital/chromosomal anomalies

No	Month/year	Sex	Weight at birth	Wks. gest	Hrs. in labor	Type of delivery	Details of delivery. Include anesthesia and maternal or newborn complications. Use Risk Guide numbers where applicable
1							
2							
3							
4							
5							
6							
7							
8							

60. ☐ Hemoglobinopathies
61. ☐ Isoimmunization (Rh)
62. ☐ Drug addiction/alcoholism
63. ☐ Habitual abortions
64. ☐ Incompetent cervix
65. ☐ Prior fetal or neonatal death
66. ☐ Prior neurologically damaged infant
67. ☐

Initial Risk Assessment
68. ☐ No risk factors noted
69. ☐ At risk
70. ☐ At high risk

Signature

FIG. 28 – ANTEPARTUM RECORD

It is not necessary to have a discharge summary when using the short-stay record.

Regular forms (i.e., other than the short-stay) are to be used for records of: obstetric patients, patients who develop complications during hospitalization, or who die during hospitalization. In the latter two situations, if the short-stay form was originally used, it is discontinued and regular forms are used.

Obstetric Data

A complete hospital obstetric record includes several special forms: antepartum (prenatal) record, labor and delivery record, and postpartum record. The American College of Obstetrics and Gynecology identifies recommended content for these forms in its *Standards for Obstetric–Gynecologic Services.*

Antepartum Record

The antepartum or prenatal data (Figures 28-30) are started in the obstetrician's office or obstetric clinic, preferably very early in the pregnancy. The antepartum record should contain the following data:

Health history – including menstrual history, past pregnancies, number of full-term pregnancies, premature pregnancies, spontaneous and induced abortions, number of living children, spacing of previous pregnancies, length of gestation, route of delivery, sex and weight of newborn and any complications, drug sensitivities, blood transfusions, blood group and Rh type, diabetes and other metabolic disorders, vascular disease, sexually transmitted diseases, convulsive disorders, gynecologic abnormalities, and serious injuries. The previous administration of Rh immune globulin should be specifically noted.

Family history – presence or absence of metabolic disorders, cardiovascular diseases, malignancy, congenital abnormalities, mental retardation, and multiple births in immediate relatives.

Social history – patient's occupation and work environment, ethnic origin, educational and religious background.

Physical examination – neck, breasts, heart, lungs, abdomen, pelvis, size of uterus, configuration and capacity of bony pelvis, rectum, and extremities.

Laboratory tests performed as early in the pregnancy as possible – hemoglobin or hematocrit, urinalysis, blood group and Rh type, irregular antibody screen, rubella antibody titer, cervical cytology, and syphilis screen.

Risk assessment – including a problem list and recommendations for management, with special attention to such high risk factors as cesarean section, operation on the uterus or cervix,

Initial Pregnancy Profile Date:	HOLLISTER® maternal/newborn RECORD SYSTEM	PATIENT IDENTIFICATION Patient's name_____

History Since LMP Patient	Check and detail all positive findings below. Precede findings with symptom number.	**15. Nutritional Assessment**
1. Headaches		☐ Adequate ☐ Inadequate
2. Nausea/vomiting		
3. Abdominal pain		Remarks: _____
4. Urinary complaints		
5. Vaginal discharge		
6. Vaginal bleeding		
7. Edema (specify area)		
8. Febrile episode		**16. Medications Since LMP**
9. Rubella exposure		
10. Other viral exposure		(Rx, non-Rx, vitamins) ☐ **None**
11. Drug exposure		
12. Radiation exposure		Describe: _____
13. Other		
14. Last ☐ **None** contraceptive		
Type _____		
Last used _____		

Initial Physical Examination	Height	Weight	Pregravid weight	B.P.	Pulse	OPTIONAL

SYSTEM	Normal	ABN	Check and detail all positive findings below. Use reference numbers.
17. Skin			
18. EENT			
19. Mouth			
20. Neck			
21. Chest			
22. Breast			
23. Heart			
24. Lungs			
25. Abdomen			
26. Musculoskeletal			
27. Extremities			
28. Neurologic			
Pelvic Examination			
29. Ext. genitalia			
30. Vagina			
31. Cervix			
32. Uterus (describe)			
33. Adnexa			
34. Rectum			
35. Other			

Bony Pelvis	36 Diag. conj.	37 Shape sacrum	38 S.S. notch	39 Ischial spines
	40 Pubic arch	41 Trans. outlet	42 Post sag. diam.	43 Coccyx

44. Classification: ☐ Gynecoid   ☐ Android   ☐ Anthropoid   ☐ Platypelloid
45. Estimation: ☐ Adequate   ☐ Borderline   ☐ Contracted

Exam by

FIG. 29 – ANTEPARTUM RECORD

diabetes, hypertension, medical indication for termination of pregnancy, premature onset of labor, history of prolonged labor suggesting dystocia, multiple gestation, two or more abortions, use of drugs, alcohol and tobacco, and congenital abnormalities.

It is recommended that a copy or satisfactory abstract of the current prenatal information be available in the labor and de-

Prenatal Flow Record	HOLLISTER® maternal/newborn RECORD SYSTEM	PATIENT IDENTIFICATION Patient's name_____

Risk Guide for Pregnancy and Outcome

Preliminary Risk Assessment (detail risk factors from the HHS below)	Initial Prenatal Screen			Additional Lab Findings		
	Mo day	Test	Result	Mo/day	Test	Result
☐ (0) No risk factors noted	/	Hct/Hgb		/	Hct/Hgb	
☐ (1) At risk	/	Patient's Blood type and Rh		/	Hct/Hgb	
☐ (2) **High risk**	/	Father's Blood type and Rh		/		

Continuing Risk Guide (enter dates first noted and revise RISK STATUS)

Mo/day	Potential risk factors	Mo/day	High risk factors				
/	3. Preg. without familial support	/	18. Diabetes mellitus	/	Antibody		Blood sugar
/	4. Second pregnancy in 12 months	/	19. Hypertension			/	
/	5. Smoking (≥ 1 pack per day)	/	20. Thrombophlebitis	/	Serology	/	Bacteriuria
/	6. Rh negative (nonsensitized)	/	21. Herpes (type 2)	/	Rubella titer	/	
/	7. Uterine/cervical malformation	/	22. Rh sensitization	/	Urinalysis micro	/	
/	8. Inadequate pelvis	/	23. Uterine bleeding	/	Pap test	/	
/	9. Venereal disease	/	24. Hydramnios	/	G.C.	/	
/	10. Anemia (Hct < 30%; Hgb < 10%)	/	25. Severe preeclampsia				
/	11. Acute pyelonephritis	/	26. Fetal growth retardation				
/	12. Failure to gain weight	/	27. Premature rupt. membranes				
/	13. Multiple pregnancy (term)	/	28. Multiple pregnancy (preterm)				
/	14. Abnormal presentation	/	29. Low/falling estriols				
/	15. Postterm pregnancy	/	30. Significant social problems				
/	16.	/	31. Alcohol and drug abuse				
/	17.	/	32.				

| G | T | P | A | L | L M P | mo/day/yr | E D C | mo/day/yr |

☐ Initial prenatal instruction — Quickening date _____ mo/day/yr
☐ Attends prenatal classes
☐ Cesarean section — Anesthesia _____
☐ For sterilization
☐ Breast ☐ Bottle Feeding — Baby's physician _____
☐ Circumcision

Physician's signature _____

This record is copyrighted by Miller Communications, Inc. and may not be reproduced without permission of Hollister Incorporated, the exclusive licensee under said copyright.

FIG. 30 – ANTEPARTUM RECORD

livery area by the estimated 36th week of pregnancy and arrangements made to obtain it as soon as possible if admission is necessary prior to this time.

Labor and Delivery Record

Specialized forms are used to document the patient's progress from the time of admission through labor and delivery to the

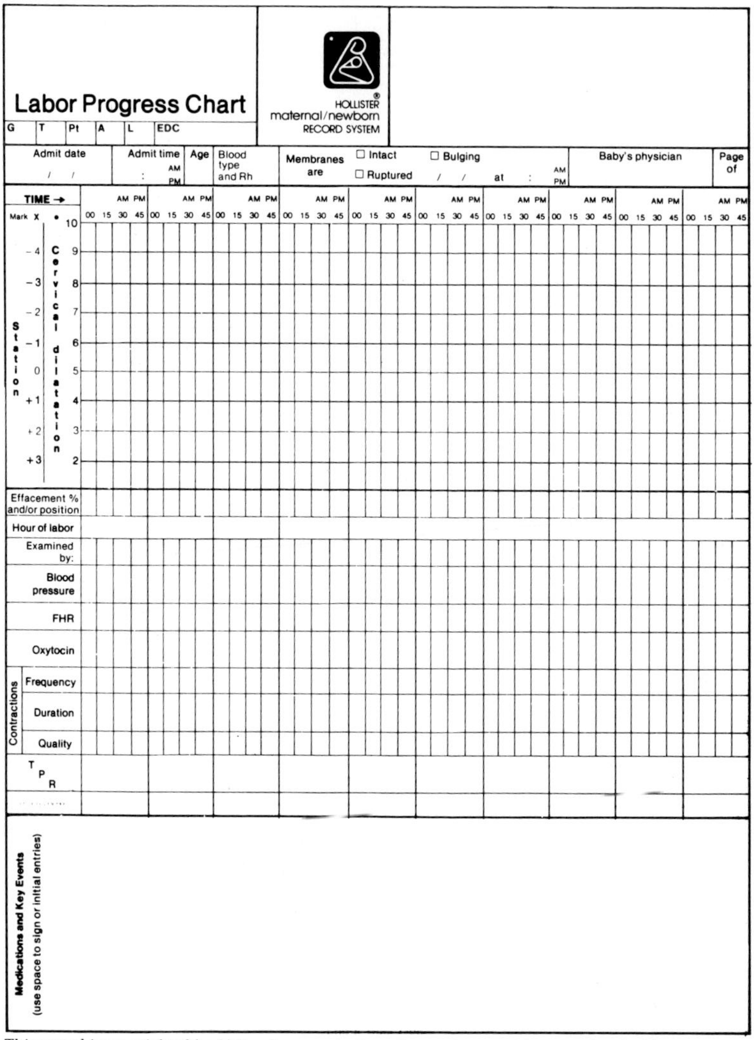

This record is copyrighted by Miller Communications, Inc. and may not be reproduced without permission of Hollister Incorporated, the exclusive licensee under said copyright.

FIG. 31 – LABOR AND DELIVERY RECORD

postpartum period. These may be called Labor and Delivery Record, Labor and Delivery Summary and may consist of several forms depending on the arrangement of data (Figures 31 and 32). The antepartum record should be reviewed as soon as possible after admission and notations made regarding: parity, estimated date of delivery, blood group, Rh type, serologic tests

---

Labor and Delivery Summary

HOLLISTER® maternal/newborn RECORD SYSTEM

Labor Summary

G	T	Pt	A	L	Type and Rh

Presentation
- ☐ Vertex
- ☐ Face or brow
- ☐ Breech _____
- ☐ Transverse lie   ☐ Compound
- ☐ Unknown

Position

Complications   ☐ **None**
- ☐ No prenatal care
- ☐ Preterm labor (≤ 37 wks.)
- ☐ Postterm (≥ 42 wks.)
- ☐ Febrile (≥ 100.4°) when admitted
- ☐ PROM (≥ 12 hrs. preadmit)
- ☐ Meconium
- ☐ Foul smelling fluid
- ☐ Hydramnios
- ☐ Abruption
- ☐ Placenta previa
- ☐ Bleeding-site undetermined
- ☐ Toxemia (mild) (severe)
- ☐ Seizure activity
- ☐ Precipitous labor (< 3 hrs.)
- ☐ Prolonged labor (≥ 20 hrs.)
- ☐ Prolonged latent phase
- ☐ Prolonged active phase
- ☐ Prolonged 2nd stage (> 2.5 hrs.)
- ☐ Secondary arrest of dilatation
- ☐ Cephalopelvic disproportion
- ☐ Cord prolapse
- ☐ Decreased FHT variability
- ☐ Extended fetal bradycardia
- ☐ Extended fetal tachycardia
- ☐ Multiple late decelerations
- ☐ Multiple variable decelerations
- ☐ Acidosis (pH < 7.2)
- ☐ Anesthetic complications
- ☐ _____

Induction   ☐ **None**
- ☐ ARM   ☐ Oxytoc. ☐ _____

Augmentation   ☐ **None**
- ☐ ARM   ☐ Oxytoc. ☐ _____

Monitor   ☐ **None**

	FHT	UC
External	☐	☐
Internal	☐	☐

Medications   Total dosage

Time of last narcotic   :

Delivery Data

Method of Delivery
Cephalic
- ☐ Spontaneous   Type
- ☐ Low forceps
- ☐ Mid forceps
- ☐ Rotation _____ to _____
- ☐ Vacuum extraction
Breech
- ☐ Spontaneous
- ☐ Partial extraction (assisted)
- ☐ Total extraction
- ☐ Forceps to A.C. head
Cesarean (details in operative notes)
- ☐ Low cervical: transverse
- ☐ Low cervical: vertical
- ☐ Classical
- ☐ Cesarean hysterectomy

Placenta
- ☐ Spontaneous
- ☐ Expressed
- ☐ Manual
- ☐ Adherent
- ☐ Ut. exploration

Blood loss
- ☐ < 500 ml.
- ☐ > 500 ml. Specify amount detail in Remarks
(_____ ml.)

Configuration
- ☐ Normal
- ☐ Abn. _____
Weighed (no) (yes) _____ gms.

Cord
- ☐ Nuchal cord x _____
- ☐ True knot
- ☐ ② ③ Umbilical vessels
Cord blood to (lab) (refrig.) (discard)

Episiotomy
- ☐ **None**   Suture
- ☐ Median _____
- ☐ Mediolateral
- ☐ Other _____

Laceration
- ☐ **None**
- ① ② ③ ④ Degree perineal
- ☐ Vaginal
- ☐ Cervical
- ☐ Uterine rupture
- ☐ Other _____

Surgical Procedures   ☐ **None**
- ☐ Tubal ligation   ☐ Curettage
- ☐ Other _____

Delivery Data (cont.)

Delivery Anesthesia   ☐ **None**
1 = Local   2 = Pudendal   3 = Paracervical
4 = Epidural   5 = Spinal   6 = General

Delivery Room Meds.   ☐ **None**

Chronology   Date

EDC	/ /		
ADMIT TO HOSPITAL	/ /		
MEMBRANES RUPTURED	/ /		
ONSET OF LABOR	/		
COMPLETE CERVICAL DIL.	/		
DELIVERY OF INFANT	/		
DELIVERY OF PLACENTA	/		

Infant Data

Apgar Scores   Heart rate / Respiration / Muscle tone / Reflex irritation / Skin color / Totals

1 min						
5 min						

Resuscitation ☐ **None** spontaneous respiration
- ☐ Oxygen
- ☐ Bag and mask
- ☐ Intubation
- ☐ Ext. cardiac massage
- ☐ Other _____
_____ mins. to sustained respiration

Infant Data (cont.)

Medications
- ☐ **None**
- ☐ Volume expander
- ☐ Sodium bicarbonate
- ☐ Drug antagonists
- ☐ Umbilical catheter
- ☐ Other _____

Initial Newborn Exam
- ☐ **No observed abnormalities**
- ☐ Gross congenital anomalies
- ☐ Mec. staining   ☐ Trauma
- ☐ Petechiae   ☐ Other
Describe _____

Basic Data
ID bracelet no. _____
Hospital record no. _____
- ☐ Male   ☐ Female
Birth order: _____ of ① ② ③ ④
Record procedures whether done in the delivery room or nursery
Weight _____ Length _____
- ☐ Vitamin K
- ☐ AgNo₃ 1% or _____
by: _____

Output
- ☐ Urine
- ☐ Meconium
- ☐ Gastric _____ (ml.)
- ☐ Living at transfer to:

Deceased   Date
- ☐ Antepartum   mo / day / yr
- ☐ Intrapartum   Time
- ☐ Neonatal (in deliv. room)

Remarks: _____

Nurse

Assisting   Attending   Date completed   / /

This record is copyrighted by Miller Communications, Inc. and may not be reproduced without permission of Hollister Incorporated, the exclusive licensee under said copyright.

FIG. 32 – LABOR AND DELIVERY SUMMARY

for syphilis, rubella titer, and other important laboratory data. There should be an evaluation performed and documented by the admitting physician. If the patient has not had prenatal care, the evaluation should include a complete history, or an updated history if she has had prenatal care.

The updated history should include: time of onset of contractions, status of membranes, presence of any significant bleeding, time and content of last ingestions, drug intake, known allergies, use of contact lenses or eyeglasses, and presence of dentures. Notation should be made of attendance in childbirth classes, use and choice of analgesia or anesthesia, and plans for breast or bottle feeding. The extent of the admitting physical examination will depend on the condition of the patient. It should include the patient's blood pressure, pulse, temperature, frequency, quality and duration of uterine contractions, notation of leaking of amniotic fluid or unusual bleeding, pelvic examination, degree of cervical dilatation, effacement, fetal position, presentation, station of the presenting part, and heart rate. When there are no complications, trained nursing personnel may perform the initial pelvic examination.

During normal labor, the assessment of the quality of uterine contractions, fetal heart tones, and examination of the pelvis are done frequently to detect evidence of abnormality and to assess progress of labor. The patient's blood pressure, temperature, pulse, intake and output, and the fetal heart rate are also assessed frequently. Any significant sign or symptom, such as bleeding or meconium staining, should be evaluated by the physician.

Delivery data are recorded, such as: type of delivery, type forceps used, blood loss, description of placenta and cord, episiotomy, laceration, anesthesia and other medications, and chronology of the labor and delivery. Data about the infant are also documented: apgar scores (which rate the infant at one minute and five minutes after birth), sex, weight, length, onset of respiration, abnormalities, and treatment to eyes.

Electronic fetal heart rate monitoring may be done prior to and during delivery. The tracings are part of the medical record and should include patient name, hospital number, and date and time of admission and delivery. Relevant data such as examinations, changes in position of the patient, medications, and the corresponding times should be recorded on the tracings.

Postpartum Record

The postpartum record (postpartum progress notes) contains information about the condition of the mother after delivery. It usually starts immediately after the patient is moved from the delivery room. Hospitals may use a regular progress note form, nurses' notes, or a special postpartum record to record this data. The information recorded is specific to postdelivery cases, such as: lochia, condition of breasts, fundus, perineum, medications, treatment, intake and output, and other pertinent information regarding progress. The observations and documentation are completed by nursing personnel as frequently as the patient's condition requires. Each entry is dated and timed.

Newborn Data

A healthy newborn record contains a few routine forms such as the admission and discharge form, and specialized forms such as birth history, newborn identification form, and newborn physical examination and nursing record. The newborn's condition such as prematurity or anomalies may require more detailed observations and specialized forms.

Birth History

The birth history (history of newborn delivery) may be a form (or forms) which is also used in the mother's medical record, as shown in Figures 31 and 32, or may be a separate form. The maternal information to be recorded is: previous obstetric history; medical history; diseases during this pregnancy; mother's blood group and Rh type; tests for syphilis, gonorrhea, herpes, and dates performed; drugs taken during pregnancy, labor and delivery; duration of ruptured membranes and labor, including length of the second stage; method of delivery and indications for such; placental abnormalities; and estimated amount and description of amniotic fluid. The newborn data recorded include: results of measurements of fetal maturity and well-being, apgar scores at one and five minutes, description of resuscitation, description of abnormalities, and problems occurring from birth until transfer to the admission/observation area of the nursery.

This information may be compiled by the nurse and physician, with each signing his own entries.

Newborn Identification

While the newborn is still in the delivery room, two identical bands indicating the mother's admission number, the newborn's sex, and the date and time of birth are placed on the wrist or ankle. An identification form with information about the mother and infant and an identification band number are prepared. The birth records and identification bands should be checked by both the nurse and responsible physician before the newborn leaves the resuscitation area of the delivery room. Footprinting and fingerprinting may also be used for newborn identification. Techniques such as sophisticated blood typing are now available and appear to be more reliable. Specific forms are required for each of these methods. Usually the nurse in charge of the delivery room is responsible for preparing and securing the identification bands and may prepare the identification sheet. Usually both the physician and nurse sign the identification form.

Newborn Physical Examination

The newborn's condition is assessed as soon as possible after birth. The initial physical examination (Figure 33) should include: date and time of birth; date, time and age at examination; sex; racial origin; birth weight, length, and head and chest circumferences; temperature; general appearance (e.g., activity, tone, cry); skin (e.g., pallor, cyanosis); head (size and shape of skull, molding, caput, hematoma, sutures, fontanels, size and position of jaw); facies; eyes; nose; mouth and pharynx; neck; thorax; lungs (respiratory rate and pattern, quality and distribution of breath sounds); heart murmur; circulation and peripheral pulses; abdomen; genitalia; anus; extremities; spine; neurological (posture, movements, state of consciousness, reflexes, symmetry, active and passive tone); and estimate of maturity.

The attending physician should examine the apparently normal infant no later than 12 hours after birth. The normal newborn is also examined at least every three days during hospitalization and within 24 hours prior to the infant's discharge from the hospital. The results of these examinations are recorded in the infant's chart and signed by the physician.

Newborn Progress Notes

The newborn progress notes refer to information compiled by the nurses in the newborn nursery. This information may be

---

Initial Newborn Profile

HOLLISTER®
maternal/newborn
RECORD SYSTEM

1. Basic Data (entered by nursing personnel)

Mother's name ____   G   T   P   A   L

LMP ___ mo / day / yr

EDC ___ mo / day / yr   Delivery date ___ mo / day / yr   Time of birth ___ AM PM

Apgar at   1 min   5 min   Sex: □ Male □ Female □ Ambiguous

2. Physical Examination

Date of exam ____   Time of exam ___ AM PM   Baby's age at exam ___ hrs

Temperature ____   Respiration rate ____

Femoral pulse   □ Normal   □ Absent/weak   □ Delayed

(Code ☑ = No abnormalities   ◎ = Abnormalities present)

1 □ Reflexes   6 □ Thorax   11 □ Genitals
2 □ Skin color, lesions 7 □ Lungs   12 □ Anus
3 □ Head/Neck   8 □ Heart   13 □ Trunk/Spine
4 □ Eyes   9 □ Abdomen   14 □ Extremities/Joints
5 □ ENT   10 □ Umbilicus   15 □ Tone/Appearance

Description of abnormal findings — Please describe your findings objectively. Reserve your impressions or diagnoses for part 3 below. Please begin your findings with the reference number preceding each category.

_____
_____
_____
_____
_____
_____
_____
_____

3. Impressions and Diagnosis

Initial Risk Estimate □ No risk factors noted □ Low risk □ Medium risk □ High risk

_____
_____
_____
_____
_____
_____
_____

Newborn Risk Indicators — Please review these along with the prior risk information available to you, in order to arrive at your Initial Risk Estimate in part 3.

Observable at birth	Within 24 hrs. postpartum
□ **No risk factors noted**	□ **No risk factors noted**
□ Abnormal presentation	□ Abdominal distension
□ Multiple birth	□ Vomiting
□ Low birth weight	□ Failure to pass meconium (if skin not stained)
□ Resuscitation at birth	
□ 1 min. Apgar ≤5	□ Melena
□ 5 min. Apgar ≤7	□ Apneic episodes
□ Placental abnormalities	□ Tachypnea (transient)
□ Two cord vessels	□ See-saw breathing
□ Difficult catheterization	□ Cyanosis
□ ≥20ml. of gastric aspirate	□ Petechiae/Ecchymoses
□ Small mandible with cleft palate	□ Jaundice
□ Grunting	□ Pallor
□ Deep retractions	□ Plethora
□ Imperforate anus	□ Fever
□ Pallor	□ Hypothermia
□ Jaundice	□ Arrhythmias
□ Plethora	□ Murmur
□ Convulsions	□ Lethargy
□ Decreased tone	□ Tremors (jitters)
□ Congenital malformations	□ Convulsions

4. Maturity Evaluation

Gest. age by dates ___ wks   Weight ___ lbs ___ gms ozs   Chest circ ___ cm
Gest. age by exam ___ wks   Length ___ cm   Head circ ___ cm

This infant is   □ Pre-term (<37 weeks)   □ SGA
classified as   □ Term (37-42 weeks)   □ AGA
                 □ Post-term (>42 weeks)   □ LGA

5. Plans: diagnostic and therapeutic

_____
_____
_____
_____
_____
_____
_____
_____
_____
_____
_____

Signature: _____

FIG. 33 – NEWBORN PHYSICAL EXAMINATION

written in narrative progress notes or may be entered on a flow chart, such as the newborn flow record (Figure 34), which is designed to allow for easier comparison of data. The American

Academy of Pediatrics recommends that until the newborn's vital signs are stable (usually the first 6-12 hours after birth) there must be frequent recording of: temperature, heart, and

This record is copyrighted by Miller Communications, Inc. and may not be reproduced without permission of Hollister Incorporated, the exclusive licensee under said copyright.

FIG. 34 – NEWBORN PROGRESS NOTES

respiratory rates; notations of color (cyanosis, jaundice); adequacy of peripheral circulation; type of respiration; state of consciousness; and presence of irritability, or twitching. Time of voiding and meconium stool should be noted. Weight should be measured and documented daily.

Other data usually recorded include: amount and type of intake and output, condition of the umbilical stump, any treatments or medications given, and any other pertinent observations.

Observations for the healthy newborn are made and recorded every eight hours until discharge. The specific time of observation is documented, and the entries are signed by the nurse making the observations.

The JCAH requirements contain one statement regarding newborn records. When oxygen is prescribed for newborn infants, its use should be recorded at least as an oxygen concentration percentage and at regular defined intervals, in accordance with the written policy of the newborn nursery.

SUMMARY

A medical record must be maintained on every person who receives hospital services. The admission office begins the medical record, and all departments which provide care to the patient add forms to the record to document the services given. The medical record department processes the medical record and determines when it is complete. The completed medical record is retained in the medical record department for future reference and safekeeping.

The medical record may be organized in one of several ways: source-oriented, problem-oriented, or integrated. Certain data must be documented in the medical record and in the manner required by licensing, certifying, and accrediting agencies. Some of the requirements for medical record content are very specific regarding the data to be included on particular forms; other requirements state that the data are to be documented in the medical record. Except where specifically stated in the requirements of the approving agencies, the content of medical record forms is an individual determination made by each hospital.

The medical record administrator with a knowledge of medical record content requirements can provide significant assistance to the hospital in providing quality care and meeting the requirements of licensing, certification, and accreditation agencies.

STUDY QUESTIONS

1. Describe the flow of information into the medical record.
2. Describe briefly the processing of the medical record within the medical record department.
3. Define: source-oriented, problem-oriented, and integrated medical record formats.
4. State the JCAH requirement involving the use of abbreviations and symbols in the medical record.
5. Describe the proper method for correcting errors in the medical record.
6. State the three situations in which a final progress note can substitute for a discharge summary, according to the JCAH requirements.
7. Name three medical record forms which are usually the sole responsibility of nursing service.
8. State the four categories of patients for whom a consultation should be provided.
9. Name four types of special records maintained by hospitals.

REFERENCES

Accreditation Manual for Hospitals. Joint Commission on Accreditation of Hospitals. Chicago, Illinois, 1984.

American Association of Blood Banks. *Technical Manual.* Philadelphia, Pennsylvania: J. B. Lippincott Co., 1981.

ANDERSON, LEROY. "Standardization of the Physical Therapy Record." *Medical Record News.* Vol. 47 (April, 1977), pp. 92-94.

BATES, BARBARA. *A Guide to Physical Examination.* Philadelphia, Pennsylvania: J. B. Lippincott Co., 1983.

Conditions of Participation—Hospitals. U.S. Department of Health and Human Services, Social Security Administration, Washington, D.C., 1974.

DRIPPS, ROBERT D., ECKENHOFF, JAMES E., and VANDAM, LEROY D. *Introduction to Anesthesia.* Philadelphia, Pennsylvania: W. B. Saunders Co., 1982.

EGAN, DONALD F. *Fundamentals of Respiratory Therapy.* Saint Louis, Missouri: C. W. Mosby Co., 1977.

Guidelines for Perinatal Care. American Academy of Pediatrics and American College of Obstetrics and Gynecologists. Evanston, Illinois, 1983.

HEBERT, LAUREN A. "Basics of Medicare Documentation for Physical Therapy." *Clinical Management in Physical Therapy,* Vol. 1, No. 3, (1981), pp. 13-14.

Hospital Care of Newborn Infants. American Academy of Pediatrics. Evanston, Illinois, 1977.

LEWIS, LUVERNE WOLFE. *Fundamental Skills in Patient Care.* Philadelphia, Pennsylvania: J. B. Lippincott Co., 1984.

MAHONEY, ELIZABETH ANNE et al. *How to Collect and Record a Health History.* Philadelphia, Pennsylvania: J. B. Lippincott Co., 1976.

RAMBO, BEVERLY, and WOOD, LUCILE A. *Nursing Skills for Clinical Practice.* Philadelphia, Pennsylvania: W. B. Saunders Co., 1982.

SHERMAN, JACQUES L., and FIELDS, SYLVIA K. *Guide to Patient Evaluation.* Garden City, New Jersey: Medical Examination Publishing Co., Inc., 1978.

SKURKA, MARGARET F., and CONVERSE, MARY E. *Organization of Medical Record Department in Hospitals.* American Hospital Association, 1984.

STOELTING, ROBERT K., and MILLER, RONALD D. *Basics of Anesthesia.* Livingston, New York: Churchill, 1984.

WEED, LAWRENCE L. *Medical Records, Medical Education, and Patient Care.* Cleveland, Ohio: The Press of Case Western Reserve University, 1970.

chapter 4

MEDICAL RECORDS IN AMBULATORY CARE, HOME CARE, AND HOSPICE PROGRAMS

Health care provision in the United States is changing. Care is no longer exclusively provided in an inpatient setting or in a physician's office. Instead, care may be provided in a variety of ambulatory care settings or in a patient's home or place of residence. Patients, the health care consumers, now have choices as to hospitals and physicians. Increasingly, ambulatory care and home care are chosen as alternatives to hospitalization or institutionalization just as ambulatory care through a health maintenance organization, urgent care center, etc., is chosen as an alternative to an office visit to a private physician.

There are several factors that influence the increased utilization of these alternative forms of health care. A primary factor is the effort by the government, third-party payers, and the business community to contain or reduce health care costs. Hospitals recently began to be reimbursed by Medicare through a prospective payment system (presently Diagnostic Related Groups). This system provides hospitals with a financial incentive to discharge patients earlier, and with these early inpatient discharges come an increased need for home care and/or more intensive outpatient follow-up. Pressures to reduce costs have also resulted in increased reimbursement coverage for out-of-hospital services, and in some cases, insurance policies actually demand certain treatment be provided on an outpatient basis.

Integral to cost-containment is the concern over the effect of the tremendous growth in the elderly population. The U.S. Census Bureau has projected a doubling in the age group 65 and over between 1980 and 2020 with an even more rapid increase in the 85 years and older age groups. In order to meet the health care needs of this elderly population without massive increases in health care expenditures, cost-containment measures must be implemented and, therefore, utilization of alternatives to expensive inpatient care will continue to increase. In the future, however, the cost of these alternatives will be more closely scrutinized. In fact, prospective payment systems for ambulatory care and home care are presently being investigated; and there is discussion regarding the future development of some form of capitation system. A capitation system would reimburse an individual or a provider one fixed amount regardless of the number of, or nature of, services provided. Such a system would hope to eliminate an aggregate increase in Medicare health care expenditures.

Two other factors that will continue to influence increased utilization of alternatives are consumerism and scientific and technological advances. There is a trend toward alternative health care by the consumer. Patients are demanding more in terms of information and convenience; and for many, alternative care (i.e., home care, hospice care, and ambulatory care) is preferred to inpatient care. Scientific and technological advances have allowed care previously performed in the hospital (e.g., dialysis, cancer chemotherapy, hyperalimentation, etc.) to be provided in the home or in an ambulatory setting. These advances, therefore, have made alternatives to inpatient care feasible.

This chapter will discuss health record requirements and data needs for ambulatory care, home care, and hospice care. Ambulatory care theoretically encompasses home care and hospice home care, since ambulatory care is defined by the American Hospital Association as the "provision of health care services to outpatients and to other patients who do not require admission to the hospital as inpatients." In this chapter, however, care provided in an outpatient setting (as opposed to a home setting) is referred to as ambulatory care; since this care is very different from home care and hospice home care both in its provision and in its record documentation and management.

Medical record professionals must become active in helping to improve record documentation and systems in ambulatory care, home care, and hospice care. Medical record professionals can provide valuable assistance in the development of integrated inpatient, outpatient, home care, and hospice record systems. Integrated systems improve the continuity of patient care and eliminate the need for unnecessary duplication of tests or examinations. When patient care data are readily available, care can be less costly and of higher quality.

Medical record professionals must provide input and/or develop policies for providers regarding appropriate record content and format; exchange of patient data between providers; confidentiality of data; and the collection of comprehensive, uniform data and statistics. When employed in an inpatient facility, the medical record practitioner should be familiar with the provision of ambulatory, home care, and hospice care in the community served by the facility in order to act as a knowledgeable resource person on the entire spectrum of health data needs.

AMBULATORY CARE

Ambulatory care can be provided in a hospital in a freestanding setting or on site in an ambulatory care facility in a business, prison, or university. In 1975 the National Center for Health Statistics documented that the majority of physicians' visits (68 percent) was provided in a free-standing setting, the doctor's office. The majority of ambulatory care visits probably still occurs in doctors' offices; but this, as will be described, is changing.

HOSPITAL-BASED AMBULATORY CARE

The provision of ambulatory care in hospitals has increased. *Hospital Ambulatory Care: Making It Work* cites the following growth statistics:

- In 1980, 46 percent of hospitals were operating an organized ambulatory care program compared to 37 percent in 1970;
- Hospital outpatient visits exceeded 221 million in 1981, a 183 percent increase since 1963; and
- Medicare expenditures for hospital outpatient services (excluding payments to physicians) were $1.9 billion in 1980 compared to $93 million in 1970, a 1,950 percent increase.

The American Hospital Association defines an outpatient as a "person who receives medical, dental, or other health-related services in a hospital or other health care institution but who is not lodged there." Hospital outpatients are generally categorized as clinic outpatients, emergency outpatients, and referred outpatients.

The *Glossary of Hospital Terms* defines these three types of outpatients as follows:

Clinic Outpatient – An outpatient who is admitted to the clinical service of the hospital for diagnosis or treatment on an ambulatory basis in a formally organized unit of a medical or surgical specialty or subspecialty. In this group, the clinic assumes overall medical responsibility for the patient.

Emergency Outpatient – A patient who is admitted to the emergency, accident, or equivalent service of the hospital for diagnosis and treatment of a condition that requires immediate medical, dental, or allied services.

Referred Outpatient – An outpatient who is admitted exclusively to a special diagnostic or therapeutic service of the hospital for diagnosis or treatment on an ambulatory basis. In this group, the responsibility for medical care remains with the referring physician.

A clinic outpatient often receives care as follow-up to a period of hospitalization or confinement. Periodic visits may be scheduled with one or several specialty clinics or outpatient departments related to the type of illness or injury from which the person is convalescing.

Emergency outpatients are different from clinic outpatients in that they require immediate care to sustain life or prevent critical consequences. These patients are most often seen first in the hospital's emergency service or department. If a patient arrives at the emergency department who does not require immediate medical care, he is often referred to an outpatient or specialty clinic. This frees emergency service personnel to deal with true emergency situations. Even patients who receive critical measures in the emergency department may be referred to outpatient clinics for return visits or to their family physician.

A referred outpatient utilizes the hospital for the sole purpose of receiving diagnostic tests or other services which may not be available in the physician's office. These patients leave when the test or service is completed. No further treatments or visits are scheduled, since follow-up care is the responsibility of the patient's physician.

OUTPATIENT RECORDS

Hospital Clinic Outpatient Records

Clinic outpatients often receive hospital-based ambulatory care services over an extended period of time. Entries which document the care provided should be made each time an outpatient returns to a clinic for care or treatment. For this reason it is very important that the patient's record be available at all times. The JCAH states a unit record system should be used. That is, all inpatient and ambulatory care records (including emergency records) relating to one patient should be integrated or filed together. If this system is not feasible, a system must be established either to consolidate a patient's records at the time of admission or scheduled outpatient visit, or to incorporate pertinent medical information (e.g., discharge summaries, operative reports, and pathology reports) in the ambulatory care record. A complete health picture of the patient must be available to everyone contributing to the patient's continuing care.

Outpatient record entries should be arranged so that preceding remarks can be quickly scanned for the necessary medical data. Progress notes are usually arranged in chronological order. Referencing may be made to individual problems or conditions by use of the problem-oriented method of recording discussed in other chapters. Thus, data particular to one injury, such as a hip fracture, can be readily scanned by problem number and name. The JCAH requires documentation of a summary list of significant past surgical procedures, past and current diagnoses and problems, and currently and recently used medications. This list must be in the same location in each patient record.

Both the federal government and the Joint Commission on Accreditation of Hospitals list a number of specific data items essential to a good clinic outpatient record. The Medicare *Conditions of Participation: Hospitals* state that at least enough information must be included to ensure continuity of care; including the patient's medical history, physical findings, laboratory and diagnostic test results, diagnosis, and treatment record.

The JCAH specifies the following information should be documented in the record at the time of each ambulatory care visit:

- Patient identification.
- Relevant history of the illness or injury, and physical findings.
- Diagnostic and therapeutic orders.
- Clinical observations, including results of treatment.
- Reports of procedures, tests, and results.
- Diagnostic impression.
- Patient disposition and any pertinent instructions given for follow-up care.
- Immunization record.
- Allergy history.
- Growth charts for pediatric patients.
- Referral information to and from agencies.

In addition, the Joint Commission requires that complete findings of techniques used in every operation are accurately written or dictated immediately after the procedure. This report must be authenticated by the individual who performed the procedure.

In addition to the standards of the JCAH and Medicare, individual states may also have regulations related to ambulatory care records. The medical record practitioner should be thoroughly familiar with all applicable regulations in his state. Other specific items of medical data included on the clinic forms will be dictated by the type of outpatient services rendered. An outpatient department record form which can be used to document required visit information is shown in Figures 1 and 2.

Emergency Records

Because of the nature of emergency medical treatment, the information entered on the emergency outpatient record differs somewhat from the clinical outpatient record. Adequate information for dealing with life and death situations must be readily available. Record systems must be developed to integrate the information obtained and the care given prior to the patient's arrival at the emergency department. Records of patients who were formerly treated as inpatients or outpatients should also be made available for emergency care.

The *Medicare Conditions of Participation: Hospitals* specify items considered essential for treating emergency service patients. Included are patient identification; history of disease or

---

OUTPATIENT DEPARTMENT GENERAL RECORD

Name_____ Sex_____ Age_____ Race____ Case number_____

Address_____ Date: OPD registration_____
      CITY OR VILLAGE   COUNTY

Family index name_____ Hospital numbers_____

Clinic enrollment

Date	DIAGNOSIS	Physician's Signature
	I	
	II	
	III	
	IV	

HISTORY   PHYSICAL EXAMINATION   RECOMMENDATIONS

Date_____

Signature_____ M.D.

FORM R-502   PHYSICIANS' RECORD CO., BERWYN, ILLINOIS · PRINTED IN U.S.A.   OPD GENERAL RECORD (OVER)

Form courtesy of Physicians' Record Company

FIG. 1 – AMBULATORY CARE RECORD (front)

injury; physical findings; laboratory and x-ray reports, if any; and diagnosis, treatment and disposition of the case. The physician in charge of the case must sign the emergency outpatient record to validate its contents.

The Joint Commission requires that a medical record be kept each time a patient receives treatment from the emergency service. The physician responsible for the emergency service pro-

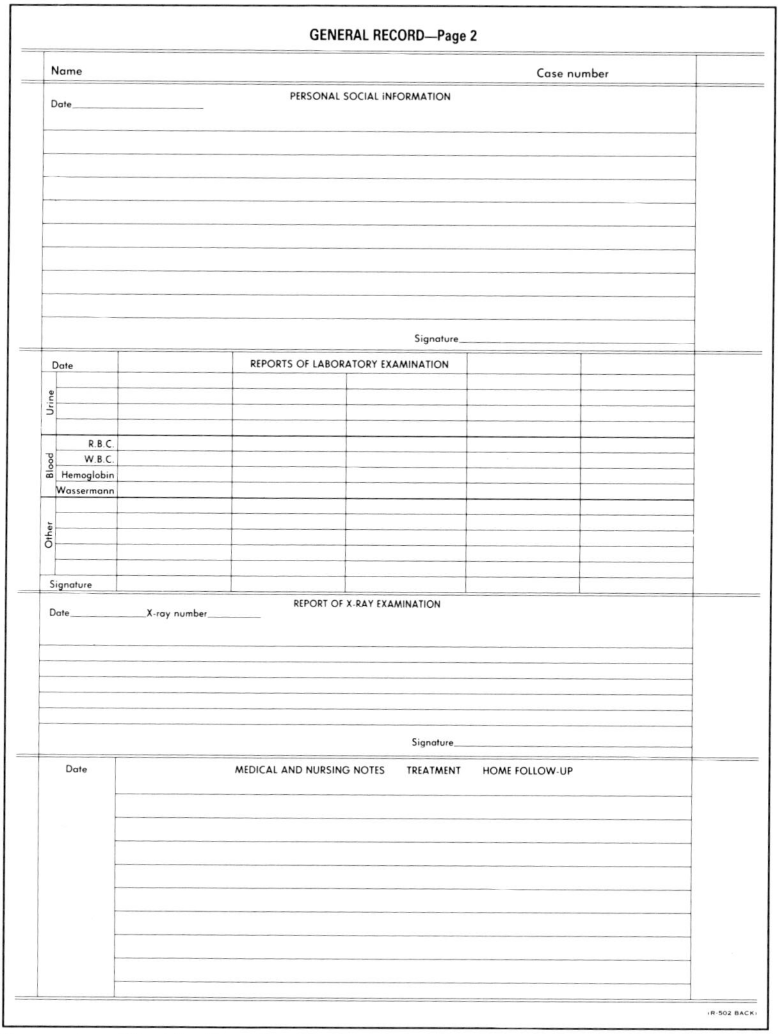

GENERAL RECORD—Page 2

Name		Case number

Date_____   PERSONAL SOCIAL INFORMATION

Signature_____

Date		REPORTS OF LABORATORY EXAMINATION		

Urine

Blood — R.B.C. / W.B.C. / Hemoglobin / Wassermann

Other

Signature

Date_____   X-ray number_____   REPORT OF X-RAY EXAMINATION

Signature_____

Date	MEDICAL AND NURSING NOTES TREATMENT HOME FOLLOW-UP

(R-502 BACK)

Form courtesy of Physicians' Record Company

FIG. 2 – AMBULATORY CARE RECORD (back of Fig. 1)

vided should authenticate the medical record. Items that should be documented include:

- Patient identification. When this is not available, a reason should be stated in the medical record.

- Time and means of arrival.

- Pertinent history of the present illness or injury, physical findings, and vital signs.

- Emergency care given to the patient prior to arrival.

- Diagnostic and therapeutic orders.

- Clinical observations including results of treatment.

- Reports of procedures, tests, and results.

- Diagnostic impression.

- Conclusion at the termination of treatment, which includes final disposition, patient's condition on discharge or transfer, and any instructions given to the patient or family for follow-up care.

- A patient leaving against medical advice.

A copy of the emergency service treatment form is usually sent to the patient's physician for his use in providing follow-up care. A complete record of all the care given to the patient ensures the hospital of adequate legal protection. An emergency record similar to the one shown in Figure 3 can assure this complete documentation.

The content of emergency service records is often mentioned in state regulations. These requirements should be reviewed by medical record professionals when developing emergency service medical records and record-retrieval procedures.

Referred Outpatient Records

Records for referred outpatients may only include the results of the tests or services received. Complete medical and health information is not necessary as the patient returns to his own physician for further care. If the referred outpatient has been either an inpatient or ambulatory care patient on a previous occasion, his records should be filed with existing hospital medical records.

OTHER HOSPITAL-BASED AMBULATORY CARE PROGRAMS

Ambulatory Surgery Facilities

An ambulatory surgery facility is defined by the American Hospital Association as a "free-standing or hospital-based facility, with an organized professional staff, that provides surgical services to patients who do not require an inpatient bed." Ambulatory surgery facilities are commonly referred to as surgicenters. Hospital surgicenters may be located at the hospital or may be satellite facilities located physically separate from the hospital. Surgicenters may also be free-standing facilities which are often operated for profit and owned by physicians or investor-owned companies.

Surgicenters have only recently been approved for Medicare reimbursement. Medicare regulations as well as third-party payers encourage the performance of certain surgical procedures on an ambulatory basis rather than on an inpatient basis. Medical record requirements for hospital-based surgicenters can be found in the JCAH *Accreditation Manual for Hospitals* and in the August 5, 1982, Federal Register, Vol. 47, No. 151.

Satellite Ambulatory Care Units

These units are physically separated from the hospital and may provide comprehensive care or services for special populations or for special needs (e.g., family planning, sports medicine, maternal and child care, preventive care, etc.). These units may also be primary care centers and provide walk-in minor emergency care and basic health services. The basic health services provided by primary care centers may consist of family medicine, general internal medicine, and/or pediatrics. Medical record requirements are the same for these satellite units as for other hospital outpatient units. Of special concern in satellite units, however, is the flow of information between the satellite and the hospital. A system must be implemented to assure the indexing of a patient's ambulatory and inpatient care encounters, and records of these encounters must be readily accessible.

FREE-STANDING AMBULATORY CARE FACILITIES

There are many types of free-standing ambulatory care facilities. The doctor's office provides a large percentage of free-

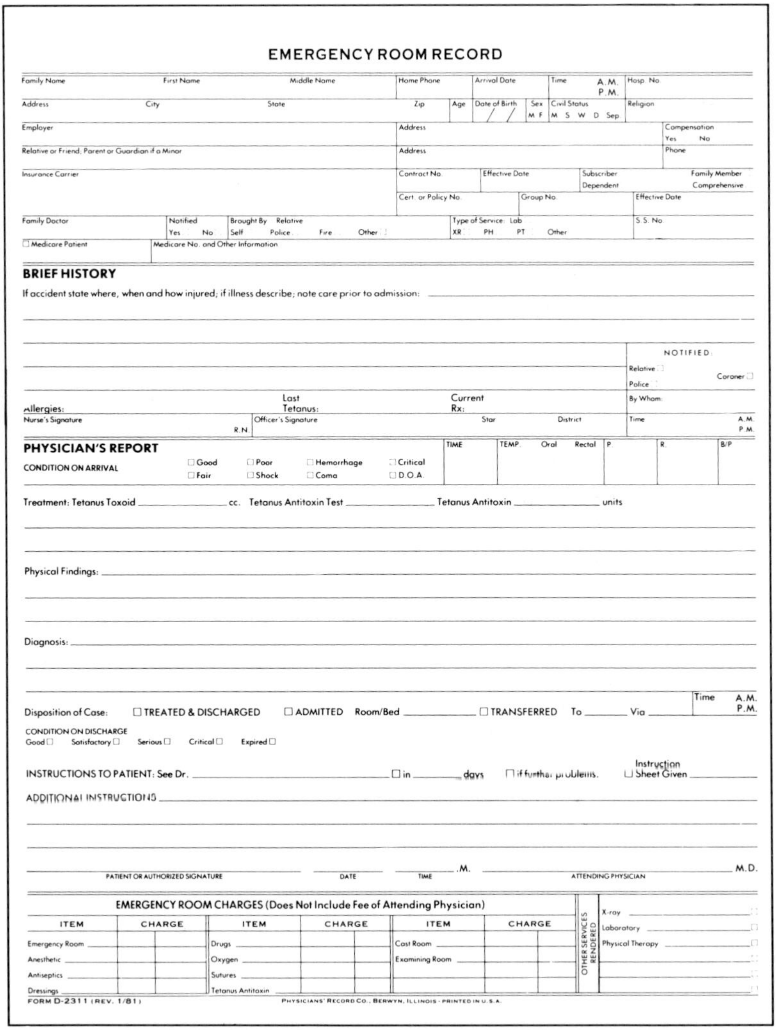

EMERGENCY ROOM RECORD

Family Name | First Name | Middle Name | Home Phone | Arrival Date | Time A.M. P.M. | Hosp. No.

Address | City | State | Zip | Age | Date of Birth / / | Sex M F | Civil Status M S W D Sep. | Religion

Employer | Address | Compensation Yes No

Relative or Friend; Parent or Guardian if a Minor | Address | Phone

Insurance Carrier | Contract No. | Effective Date | Subscriber Dependent | Family Member Comprehensive

Cert. or Policy No. | Group No. | Effective Date

Family Doctor | Notified Yes No | Brought By Relative Self Police Fire Other | Type of Service: Lab XR PH PT Other | S.S. No.

☐ Medicare Patient | Medicare No. and Other Information

BRIEF HISTORY

If accident state where, when and how injured; if illness describe; note care prior to admission: ______

NOTIFIED: Relative ☐ Police ☐ Coroner ☐ By Whom:

Allergies: | Last Tetanus: | Current Rx:

Nurse's Signature R.N. | Officer's Signature | Star | District | Time A.M. P.M.

PHYSICIAN'S REPORT

CONDITION ON ARRIVAL ☐ Good ☐ Fair ☐ Poor ☐ Shock ☐ Hemorrhage ☐ Coma ☐ Critical ☐ D.O.A. | TIME | TEMP. Oral Rectal | P. | R. | B/P

Treatment: Tetanus Toxoid ______ cc. Tetanus Antitoxin Test ______ Tetanus Antitoxin ______ units

Physical Findings: ______

Diagnosis: ______

Disposition of Case: ☐ TREATED & DISCHARGED ☐ ADMITTED Room/Bed ______ ☐ TRANSFERRED To ______ Via ______ | Time A.M. P.M.

CONDITION ON DISCHARGE
Good ☐ Satisfactory ☐ Serious ☐ Critical ☐ Expired ☐

INSTRUCTIONS TO PATIENT: See Dr. ______ ☐ in ______ days ☐ if further problems. ☐ Instruction Sheet Given ______

ADDITIONAL INSTRUCTIONS ______

______ PATIENT OR AUTHORIZED SIGNATURE ______ DATE ______ TIME .M. ______ ATTENDING PHYSICIAN M.D.

EMERGENCY ROOM CHARGES (Does Not Include Fee of Attending Physician)

ITEM	CHARGE	ITEM	CHARGE	ITEM	CHARGE	OTHER SERVICES RENDERED
Emergency Room		Drugs		Cast Room		X-ray ☐
Anesthetic		Oxygen		Examining Room		Laboratory ☐
Antiseptics		Sutures				Physical Therapy ☐
Dressings		Tetanus Antitoxin				☐

FORM D-2311 (REV. 1/81) PHYSICIANS' RECORD CO., BERWYN, ILLINOIS - PRINTED IN U.S.A.

Form courtesy of Physicians' Record Company

FIG. 3 – EMERGENCY RECORD

standing ambulatory care. This office may be a solo practice, a private group practice, a health maintenance organization, or a preferred provider organization. Public health departments often provide ambulatory care through neighborhood health centers, and increasingly, free-standing facilities are emerging that are for profit and operated by investor-owned companies.

Neighborhood Health Centers

Neighborhood health centers (also known as community health centers) are specifically designed to bring health care to the economically disadvantaged. Residents in poverty areas will often not seek necessary medical services, due to either lack of money or the unavailability of primary care physicians. If the condition persists, the patient will eventually arrive at the hospital's emergency service for treatment. Neighborhood health centers attempt to provide medical care in these poverty-stricken areas.

Treatment in the neighborhood health center is generally family centered. Indirectly, illnesses may result from crowded living conditions, unsanitary facilities, and other social and economic factors. Family care teams are used by the center to provide continuity of care to families combatting these types of problems. In such a system, the health care team usually includes an internist, pediatrician, nurse, and social worker. Continued emphasis is placed on preventive medicine procedures and education. Patients must be brought to understand the relationship between illness and living conditions.

Group Practice

The AHA defines a group practice as a "combined practice of three or more physicians and/or dentists who share office space, equipment, records, office personnel, expenses, and income." A group practice may be a single specialty (i.e., all dentists, all gynecologists, etc.), or it may be a multispecialty and provide comprehensive care. Most group practices do not have any medical record professional support. Increasingly, however, the need for this support is being recognized; and medical record professionals are now providing consultation services to group practices.

Health Maintenance Organizations

Health maintenance organizations (HMOs) emerged as an attempt to control health care costs. Federal legislation in 1973 provided financial support to HMOs that met federal regulations and this furthered the growth of HMOs. The AHA defines a HMO as an "organization that has management responsibility for providing comprehensive health care services on a prepayment basis to voluntarily enrolled persons within a designated population." A fixed premium is paid by members in return for the availability of all services included under the plan. Most plan options are comprehensive in nature. HMO plans include coverage of inpatient services, emergency services, and ambulatory care services. In addition, there are provisions for regular medical and dental checkups, immunizations, and other preventive measures aimed at retaining good health. Eyeglasses, hearing aids, and prosthetic devices may also be covered.

Preferred Provider Organizations

Preferred provider organizations (PPOs) are also a response to escalating health care costs. PPOs are established by a panel consisting of health care providers or insurers. PPOs are similar to HMOs because a benefit package is offered to subscribers. The benefit package offered may include physician and hospital services as well as other services. The PPO panel contracts with providers to offer care to PPO subscribers at a negotiated cost that is usually discounted. Subscribers are free to use providers not affiliated with the PPO, but there is a financial incentive to use the contracted provider.

Unlike HMOs, PPOs utilize a fee-for-service system; so, there is a potential for cost increases even with a lower cost per individual service. For this reason, utilization review of both inpatient and ambulatory care is essential if costs are to be reduced or contained. A PPO is also different from a HMO, because it is not itself an entity. There is no central location to store a patient's record or to coordinate care. Each provider has a separate record of patient care provided. The PPO obtains information regarding each provider's services and charges through claims submitted and, in some cases, through abstracts completed by the provider.

Urgent Care Centers

These centers are often open 12 to 16 hours a day, seven days a week and offer convenient care for routine or minor emergency problems such as sprains, sore throats, etc. Some urgent care centers also handle industry-related urgent care. Urgent care centers that handle only industry-related urgent care are called occupational medical clinics. Urgent care centers are staffed by physicians and provide some laboratory and radiology services. These centers attract patients that would otherwise go to an emergency room or to a physician's office. Medical record professionals should refer to their state's regulations regarding these centers.

ON-SITE AMBULATORY CARE

On-site ambulatory care is care provided in a nonhospital setting such as a business, a university, or a prison. Industrial health clinics emphasize maintenance of employee health and safety; and student university health centers treat students and, sometimes, faculty within the college or university. Treatment may range from first aid to general medical care; and in the case of industrial health clinics, it may include preemployment physicals and other programs such as stress management. Joint Commission ambulatory health standards as well as standards from the Accreditation Association for Ambulatory Health Care, Inc., are applicable to most on-site ambulatory care settings. In addition, *Standards for Health Services in Jails* and *Standards for Health Services in Prisons* are available from the American Medical Association. The National Commission on Correctional Health Care has recently published *Standards for Health Services in Juvenile Confinement Facilities*. Medical record professionals should also refer to any applicable state or federal regulations.

MEDICAL RECORDS IN FREE-STANDING FACILITIES

Medical record standards for free-standing facilities are found in JCAH's *Ambulatory Health Care Standards Manual* and in the Accreditation Association for Ambulatory Health Care's *Accreditation Handbook for Ambulatory Health Care*. Both groups accredit free-standing ambulatory care facilities such as private

group practices, neighborhood health centers, health maintenance organizations, urgent care centers, ambulatory surgery
centers, etc.

To assure the ongoing provision of effective medical care,
JCAH requires free-standing ambulatory care medical records
to contain a summary list of significant past-surgical procedures
and past and current diagnoses or problems. The list should be
conspicuously documented in each patient's record. The list
should not repeat recurring problems or diagnoses and must include any significant surgical conditions, significant medical
conditions, any allergies and untoward reactions to drugs, and
currently or recently used medications.

In addition, all entries in the patient's record (for each visit)
should be identified with the patient's name and number (when
applicable) and should include:

  — Date, department, and provider name and profession.
  — Chief complaint or purpose of visit.
  — Diagnosis or medical impression.
  — Studies ordered.
  — Therapies administered.
  — Disposition, recommendations, and instructions to patient.
  — Signature or initials of practitioner.

Many states have regulations applicable to some free-standing
ambulatory settings, and medical record professionals should be
familiar with these as well as with any applicable federal regulations.

Format of Ambulatory Care Records

The arrangement of information in the patient's ambulatory
care record should be convenient for those who must refer to
it on a daily basis. The ambulatory care record should provide
a ready means of communication among all providers. As discussed in an earlier chapter, either the source-oriented, integrated, or problem-oriented method of recording may be used.
In the source-oriented method, forms are filed in chronological
order and placed in separate sections of the record by the type
of form or service rendered. In an integrated record, progress
notes are entered in strict chronological order by all providers
of care, regardless of service. Problem-oriented progress notes

are useful when a patient is seen for multiple problems at one time, and reference must be made to the treatment course of each.

Each ambulatory care facility should decide on a suitable format based on individual needs and preferences. The medical record professional can assist the facility in choosing a suitable format and recommending necessary changes in the arrangement of health records.

Computerized Ambulatory Care Records

The use of computerized ambulatory care medical records has been examined now for many years. The COSTAR (Computer Stored Ambulatory Record) system was developed by the Laboratory of Computer Science at Massachusetts General Hospital in collaboration with the Harvard Community Health Plan in the 1960s. It has been operational since 1969, and in November, 1982 there were over 50 COSTAR sites. The COSTAR system is a comprehensive medical information system for ambulatory care which allows for the capture and storage of narrative medical information. Use of the system can result in a paperless record although printed record copies can be generated. The system is directory-based and thus allows for coded/standardized data. Data can be collected by clinical staff on encounter forms and later entered into the computer by clerical staff, or data can be entered directly by clinical staff. The quality of the data base in this system has been questioned; and, to assure higher data accuracy, direct entry is preferable. Methods have now been developed that allow for more data precision in a user-friendly manner. Implementation of the COSTAR system requires a major personnel and financial commitment.

Other ambulatory care medical record systems in use include TMR (The Medical Record) and STOR (Summary Time Oriented Record). TMR is a flexible computerized ambulatory care medical record system developed at the Duke University Medical Center. Like the COSTAR system, data can be collected on various forms by clinical staff and then entered into the computer by other staff. The system has the capacity to substitute for the paper record; and the Division of Nephrology of Durham, North Carolina's Veterans Administration Hospital was the first site to use the system as such.

STOR is a computerized ambulatory care medical record system used at the University of California at San Francisco (UCSF). The system has on-line features and can produce hard copy. In November, 1984 the system had been implemented in all the arthritis and renal clinics at UCSF, and the system contained over 1,800 patient records. This system has replaced the paper medical record for about 85 percent of the visits to these clinics. There have been problems with the accuracy of this system's data base due to information being transcribed in a free-text form, and a system has been added to the program in an attempt to improve the data quality.

In addition to the above, several computer systems are now available for use in physicians' offices. One such system allows the physician to store, track, and analyze medical records. It is a dictionary-driven system which incorporates the problem-oriented medical record system.

The medical record professional should be familiar with the various ambulatory care computer record systems available and, if employed in an ambulatory care setting, should be actively involved in planning and implementing any such system. Key considerations when implementing a computerized record system are: (1) Who is the system for – the provider, the administrator, or the researcher? (2) How should the data be structured for ease of access? and (3) What type of patients will be included in the system – cardiac patients, pediatric patients, etc.?

It must be emphasized that the systems described above are presently implemented in a small number of ambulatory care facilities. The medical record professional is more likely to be involved in implementing a more limited ambulatory care computer system such as those described in the "Collection of Ambulatory Care Data" section below.

Analysis of Ambulatory Care Records

The accuracy and completeness of ambulatory care records are just as important to the patient, physician, and other health care providers as are inpatient records. Medical record personnel may be delegated the task of quantitative review of the records after each patient visit or episode of care. A careful review of entries should be made to ensure that all required data are present and signed by the appropriate persons. If a hospital's ambulatory care record is not filed in the medical record department, responsibility for quantitative analysis may be delegated to employees supervising records in the ambulatory care area itself.

A review of the quality of data entered in ambulatory care records should be performed by the medical staff on an ongoing basis. The medical record department may be asked to assist in performance of this function, or it may be delegated to a medical staff committee. Specific requirements for quality control reviews of a hospital's ambulatory care records may be found in the appropriate sections of the JCAH's *Accreditation Manual for Hospitals.* For example, the "Emergency Services" section requires daily review by the medical director or designee of at least a sample of emergency medical records of patients seen during the previous 24 hours as well as a review of the records of patients receiving blood transfusions and antibiotics. Record review requirements for free-standing or on-site ambulatory care records can be found in the applicable accreditation standards cited earlier in this chapter and in applicable government regulations.

QUALITY ASSURANCE

Requirements for ambulatory care quality assurance programs are found in the applicable JCAH standards and in the *Accreditation Handbook for Ambulatory Health Care.* The Health Maintenance Organization Act of 1973, P.L. 93-222, requires federally funded HMOs to have a quality assurance program; and requirements for these programs have been published by the federal office of HMOs (OHMO).

For many reasons, quality assurance methods for ambulatory care may differ from those used for inpatient care as ambulatory care is different in scope, provision, and documentation. Ambulatory care medical records of some providers may not be good data sources for quality assurance studies since they may be brief; poorly organized; and illegible or incomplete, often containing no mention of relevant care by other providers. In addition, retrieval of records by diagnoses, problems, or by reasons for visits may not be possible since coding and indexing may not be performed. Quality assurance activities are also limited by staffing and funding. Staff that is available to conduct quality assurance studies may have little formal training in medical terminology, anatomy and physiology, medical records, etc.

Quality assurance methods established must utilize available data and must be easily understood by the persons involved. Medical record professionals should be active in helping to establish ambulatory care quality assurance programs as well as procedures for coding, indexing, and data collection.

Collection of Ambulatory Care Data

Routine collection of patient information assists the ambulatory care facility in analyzing its patterns of care and the demographics of its patient population. Through the implementation of an appropriate coding and indexing system, the information contained in the patient's health record can be compiled for administrative, research, and educational uses.

Computers can assist the ambulatory care facility to collect and retrieve timely, comprehensive data. Ambulatory care computer modules now address functions such as registration, appointment scheduling, medical data entry (used to document information on a patient encounter), and accounts receivable/billing. With the growth of ambulatory care and the resultant increased demand for ambulatory care information systems, it is expected that the systems available will be improved; and the applications will be broader (as described earlier).

Minimum Uniform Data Set

Adequate patient information in ambulatory care records is vital to the continuing treatment of patients. Many times visits are months apart, and the patient may not see the same professional staff member twice. The most reliable vehicle to relay a total picture of the patient's medical history and needs is the medical record. Guidelines for content of ambulatory care records have been established by the Department of Health and Human Services. These essential data items, contained in the *Uniform Ambulatory Medical Care Minimum Data Set*, are required for participation in many federal health and funding programs; but they also provide a basis for collecting patient health information in other ambulatory care facilities as well. Additional items of information will be collected by most facilities in accordance with their own specialty and treatment needs, since this basic data set only specifies minimal data collection requirements.

Three categories of data items are included in the minimum basic data set – patient information, provider information, and encounter information. The patient's name, residence, date of birth, sex, race and ethnic background would be included in the patient information section of ambulatory care records.

The health care provider is characterized by name and professional address, identification number, type of practice (e.g., solo, group, neighborhood health center, etc.), and the profession serving the patient (e.g., doctor, nurse, dentist, etc.). More detailed information is required to clearly identify the patient-provider encounter. These items are listed below:

- Date, place and reason for encounter.

- Diagnostic services.

- Problem, diagnosis, or assessment.

- Therapeutic services.

- Preventive services.

- Disposition.

- Expected principal source of payment.

- Total charges.

Classification Systems for Ambulatory Care

Classification systems for ambulatory care are described in Chapter 12. Regardless of the classification system used, it should meet the reporting needs of the facility. Requests for data are continually received from various accrediting and licensing agencies. Research and educational needs of the facility's professional staff can be met if proper methods of data collection have been implemented. Administration uses patient information from the health record for the completion of report and survey forms, studying patient populations and utilization of facility and services, and determining staffing and equipment needs.

Statistical Definitions

Once health record information has been coded and indexed, it is available for data retrieval purposes. A comparison of data items is only meaningful if comparable units of measure are used. The accurate definition of terms for use in outpatient statistics has long been debated. Recording patient information meaningful to the field of ambulatory care requires the use of a number of distinct units of measure. The medical record professional should refer to the *Glossary of Hospital Terms* and to the AHS's *Hospital Administration Terminology* for standard ambulatory care definitions and statistical formulas.

The AHA gives the following definitions for ambulatory care events:

Outpatient Visit – all services provided an outpatient in the course of a single appearance in an outpatient or inpatient unit.

Occasion of Service – specific identifiable act of service provided a patient, such as performance of a test, medical examination, treatment, or procedure.

Encounter – instance of direct contact between a patient and a professional hospital staff member responsible for assessing and treating the condition of the patient or providing social work services.

Episode of Hospital Care – measure of the services provided in a continuous course of care by a hospital to a patient for a particular medical problem or condition, such as a sequence of emergency, inpatient, and outpatient services.

The differences noted in the above definitions point out some of the difficulties in collecting ambulatory care statistics. An outpatient visit may involve one or more outpatient occasions of service to the individual, depending on how many tests are done or outpatient units visited. Encounters may be with professional personnel responsible for the patient's care or with ancillary personnel, such as social workers, who assist in the care of the patient. Patients may have several encounters during one visit, and an ambulatory care facility needs to maintain data on the number and types of these encounters. An episode of care statistic may be used to record a series of visits to the facility for one continuing condition. Because of the differences expressed in each of these units of measure, many ambulatory care facilities find it useful to record data on outpatient visits, encounters, occasions of service, and episodes of care in order that accurate patterns of care are documented and readily available.

HOME CARE

"Home care" and "home health care" for all practical purposes are interchangeable terms that describe services (medical and nonmedical) provided to patients and their families in their home or place of residence. Many persons and organizations prefer to use the term home care as it suggests a broader provision of services, and we will use this term throughout this chapter. Many home health care definitions, however, are not literal so they also reflect this broad array of services. An example is the American Medical Association's definition which states home health care is:

> Any arrangement for providing, under medical supervision, needed health care and supportive services to a sick or disabled person in his home surroundings. The provision of nursing care, social work, therapies (such as diet, occupational, physical, psychological, and speech), vocational and social services, and homemaker/home health aide services may be included as basic components of home health care. . . .

Home care is fast becoming an integral component of the health care delivery system in the United States. Because of the reasons mentioned in the beginning of this chapter (i.e., cost containment measures, the increasing elderly population, consumerism, and improved health care technology), the number of home care providers is rapidly increasing. In response to the Medicare prospective payment system, many hospitals are now vertically integrating by offering home care services to their patients. Hospital patients are being discharged earlier than previously, and home care is becoming more "high tech" in response to this and in response to the availability of technological innovations.

There are currently over 4,000 Medicare certified home health agencies, but it has been estimated by the National Association for Home Care that there are over 17,000 home care providers who may offer one or more home care services. These other providers may be noncertified home health agencies, home care staffing companies, or home care equipment companies. Equipment companies often furnish durable medical equipment directly to patients and are, therefore, often responsible for patient education regarding the equipment's use. A home care staffing company may furnish selected services such as the services of home health aides, companions, or homemakers. These companies may provide some services at a patient's request or may provide services in conjunction with a home health agency and/or in response to doctors' orders. Home health agencies provide a broader range of services; and to be Medicare certified, a home health agency must provide skilled nursing care and at least one of the following therapeutic services – physical, speech, or occupational therapy; medical social services; or home health aide services. The Health Care Financing Administration (HCFA) defines five major Medicare provider home health agency categories: (1) hospital or provider-based, (2) proprietary, (3) private nonprofit, (4) government (state or local health and welfare departments), and (5) voluntary nonprofit (visiting nurse associations).

MEDICAL RECORDS IN HOME CARE

The smooth flow of patient information is particularly important to home care. Because the providers of care perform their services in the patient's home, they are physically removed from the other professionals of the sponsoring hospital or agency. Information must be available for these providers to make their visit, and information regarding their visits must be efficiently incorporated in the patient's medical record. Procedures and documentation must assure that the medical record at any time reflects an accurate, current picture of the patient's status and the services being provided. On referral to and from home care, there must be efficient, complete information exchange between providers. In hospital-based programs, patient indexes should contain data on the patients who are receiving home care. There should be a unit record, which means that home care records of discharged patients should be filed together with other hospital records. The medical record in home care is a vital communication tool and, as such, helps to assure continuity of patient care.

Medical record documentation in Medicare certified home health agencies is now virtually dictated by the *Medicare Con-*

ditions of Participation for Home Health Agencies. The conditions require that all care provided be based on a written plan of treatment. The plan must be established by the attending physician in conjunction with agency staff, and it must be reviewed by agency personnel and the attending physician at least once every 60 days and as often as the severity of the patient's condition requires. The physician's signature is required on all initial and on all subsequent plans of treatment. The plan of treatment must document all pertinent diagnoses, including mental status, types of services and equipment required, frequency and duration of visits, prognosis, rehabilitation potential, functional limitations, activities permitted, nutritional requirements, medications and treatments, any safety measures to protect against injury, instructions for timely discharge or referral, and any other appropriate items. A home care plan of treatment form is shown in Figure 4. All drugs and treatments administered must be ordered in writing by a physician. A home health agency must provide skilled nursing service by or under the supervision of a registered nurse, and progress notes must reflect the provision of this skilled nursing care. Documentation by the therapist must also reflect the provision of skilled care, and documentation must show that any social services provided helped the patient's medical condition. When aides provide patient care, the medical record must document supervisory visits at appropriate intervals by the registered nurse or therapist. Patients receiving home care must be homebound (unable to leave residence without major assistance), and medical record documentation must reflect this homebound status. The conditions also require home care records to include appropriate identifying information, copies of summaries sent to physicians, and a discharge summary.

The National League for Nursing also has an accreditation program for home health agencies, and primarily voluntary nonprofit and government agencies participate in this program. The League's standards require that service records be maintained for each patient, and they outline what each record should contain. The League has an *Administrator's Handbook for Community Health and Home Care Services* which contains some home care record forms and some record management guidance.

The National Homecaring Council represents and accredits

agencies providing homemaker/home health aide services. Its standards contain some record keeping guidance for these home care providers.

| Provider No.
Month of Service _____
Pharmacy No. _____ | HOME CARE DEPARTMENT
MEDICAL INFORMATION REPORT
PLAN OF TREATMENT | Home Care No. _____
HICN _____
Start of Care Date _____
Date of Birth _____ |

Name _____ Address _____ Phone _____
M.D. _____ Address _____ Phone _____

Diagnosis: 1. _____ Date of Onset of Illness _____

2. _____ Prognosis for Rehab. _____

3. _____ Mental Status _____

Hospital Adm. Date _____ D.C. Date _____ Allergies _____

Reason for Homebound: _____

Functional Limitations: _____ Equip/Ass't Devices _____

Services Required:	Frequency of visits	Anticipated Length of service	No. of visits made during month	Diet _____
Skilled Nursing	___	___	___	Lab. Work _____
Speech Therapy				
Physical Therapy	___	___	___	Activity Level _____
Occupational Therapy				
Med. Soc. Serv.	___	___	___	Supplies Needed _____

OTHER PHYSICIAN ORDERS: _____

PROBLEMS	GOALS	PLAN OF TREATMENT

MEDICATIONS/CHANGES

SUMMARY/PROGRESS REPORT   V.S. Range: B/P _____ Resp. _____
                                          Pulse _____ Temp. _____

R.   DATE _____

This will certify that this patient is homebound and in need of Home Health Services as outlined above. The information on this form is contained in the Physician's Plan of Treatment on file in our agency.

_____ DATE _____   _____ M.D. DATE _____
Supervisor   Physician Signature

Form courtesy of Physicians' Record Company

FIG. 4 – HOME CARE – PLAN OF TREATMENT

The medical record professional should also refer to Public Health Service guidelines and to any applicable state regulations. It must be emphasized that state regulations may be the only mandatory requirements that home care providers must meet if they are not accredited or Medicare certified.

ANALYSIS OF HOME CARE RECORDS

Home care records should be reviewed throughout a patient's care episode, not just at discharge from home care. Some items that should be monitored are (1) the presence of initial assessments and care plans, (2) the prompt return of care plans and orders sent to the attending physicians for signature and review, (3) the documentation of care plan reviews at, as a minimum, 60-day intervals, and (4) the documentation of all visits. If visits are not documented or not documented properly (i.e., do not reflect skilled nursing care), agencies can lose Medicare reimbursement money. Many agencies, therefore, monitor visit documentation very closely.

To assure that established policies are followed in providing services, the *Medicare Conditions of Participation for Home Health Agencies* require that there be quarterly record reviews and, to assure a simplified record format with minimal data duplication, the National League for Nursing requires that a mechanism be established for the regular review and updating of record format.

The JCAH accredits hospital-based home care programs and has requirements for record documentation. The JCAH requires documentation of a care plan that conforms to the physician's orders. The plan must be reviewed at least every 60 days. The care plan should contain reference to at least the following:
- All pertinent diagnoses;
- Prognosis, including short-term and long-term objectives of treatment;
- Types (such as nursing, other therapeutic, and/or support services) and frequency of services to be provided, including any medication, diet, treatment, procedures, equipment, and transportation required;
- Functional limitations of the patient;
- Activities permitted;
- Safety measures required to protect the patient from injury; and
- Sociopsychological needs of the patient.

The JCAH also requires that the patient's primary physician be sent a written summary report at least every 60 days and that a copy of this report be filed in the medical record. According to JCAH a patient's completed home care record must become part of his hospital unit medical record. The following information must be included in the home care record:

— Designation of the physician having primary responsibility for the patient's care.
— The composition of the patient's household and the name of a person who will assume responsibility for his care if such is required.
— The suitability or adaptability of the patient's residence for the provision of the required health care services.
— Signed and dated progress notes for each home visit, including a description of signs and symptoms; treatment, service, or medication rendered; patient reaction; any change in the patient's condition; and any patient/family instruction given.
— Copies of all transfer and summary reports.
— Upon discharge from the home care program, a discharge report, including summary statement, disposition, and, if applicable, referral.

QUALITY ASSURANCE

Quality assurance in home care presently focuses largely on program evaluation rather than on the quality assessment of patient care. Both types of evaluations are important and should be reflected in a home care program's quality assurance plan. The JCAH requires the monitoring and evaluation of the quality and appropriateness of patient care services as well as the resolution of any identified problems. Objective criteria, developed by a home care program's staff, must be used to perform the required monitoring and evaluation. Medicare requires an annual review of a home health agency's total program but does not require an evaluation of patient care. The National League for Nursing has standards for evaluation which address program evaluation, the quality of care delivered by each discipline, and utilization review.

Collection of Home Care Data

To assure availability of standard data for program evaluation, quality of care assessment, research, and for numerous administrative functions, each individual home care program must document standard, uniform data for each of its patients. Home care computer systems are available for assistance with data collection and processing. There are programs available that produce reports summarizing an agency's activity, its patient profile, its employees' activities, its referral sources, etc. Many home care agencies use computers for management of accounts receivable and for billing, and many computer systems have word processing capabilities enabling patient reports such as the care plan to be generated.

Minimum Uniform Data Set

Uniform data must also be recorded if meaningful comparisons are to be made between home care providers and if data are to be available for health care planning. In 1980 a *Long Term Health Care Minimum Data Set* was recommended for use to the Department of Health Education and Welfare (now Department of Health and Human Services) by the National Committee on Vital and Health Statistics. This data set was intended for use by home health agencies as well as other providers specializing in long term care. This data set was never formally adopted and is now being reviewed for revision by a National Subcommittee on Uniform Minimum Health Data Sets. Medicare-certified providers document the standard data required by Medicare, and, to date, this Medicare data has been the only data available for analysis of home care provided in the United States.

Classification Systems for Home Care

The classification system used by a home care provider should meet the needs of the provider as well as the requirements of its reimbursement source(s). Coding should be complete and should be performed according to a particular system's coding instructions. Coding must not only reflect the requirements of the reimbursement source(s). There must be indexing of assigned codes so data and medical records are easily retrievable for quality assurance studies, research, etc.

Statistical Definitions

There are no standard agreed-upon home care statistical definitions. A standard definition for a home care visit or a home care length of stay does not exist. For Medicare reimbursement purposes, a visit is each time a health worker furnishes home health services to the beneficiary. Therefore, if two different care givers see a patient on the same day it would be two visits; but if a nurse provides several services during the same visit, only one visit could be charged.

HOSPICE PROGRAMS

Hospice programs offer dying persons and their families or significant others an alternative. Unlike traditional care for terminal illness, a hospice provides palliative medical care to the terminal patient and psychosocial and spiritual support to the patient and his family. Hospice care and support are provided by an interdisciplinary team (which includes volunteers) in the patient's home or residence and in an inpatient setting. The care setting is dependent on the patient's condition and on the support available in the home. Most hospice patients have a primary care person assigned, and this is the person mainly responsible for looking after the patient in the home. This person may be the next of kin but need not be. Generally, patients receive inpatient care when acute symptom management is required or when the primary care person needs a respite. Most hospice patients spend the majority of their hospice stay at home, and many receive both home care and inpatient care during a hospice care episode. Sometimes care is not provided directly by a hospice but arranged or contracted for with a home health agency or an inpatient facility. Regardless, the patient still remains a hospice patient; and the hospice coordinates his care.

A patient's family is provided support before and after his death. Most hospice programs follow survivors for at least a year after a patient's death. The level of support provided to survivors is largely dependent on the assessed needs as well as on the survivors' desire for support. Support may be provided by professional staff but is often provided by volunteers.

The number of hospice programs has increased from 59 operating programs in 1978 to presently, according to a 1984 JCAH provider profile, 1,429 programs either providing care or in the developmental stage. Of the 1,429 programs profiled by JCAH, 38 percent were owned by hospitals, 21 percent by community home health agencies, 2 percent by long term care facilities, 1 percent by psychiatric facilities, and 38 percent were based in the community and independently owned.

MEDICAL RECORDS IN HOSPICE PROGRAMS

Hospice medical records document information on the patient and his family or significant other(s). Records must contain the patient's and the primary care person's identifying information. To assure well-coordinated, continuous hospice care, it is vital that records be well documented. The hospice record is the communication tool between the various interdisciplinary team members and between the hospice and the contracted inpatient facility or home health agency.

In 1984 the Foundation of Record Education of AMRA completed a W. K. Kellogg Foundation-funded hospice project. The primary objective of this project was to develop a model hospice medical record. This model record is available in *A Medical Record Handbook for Hospice Programs*. The model record forms are not copyrighted and medical record professionals are encouraged to copy and use the forms or to adapt the forms to a particular hospice's needs. The hospice handbook contains many other guidelines, several of which will be referred to later in this section. The guidelines and the model record were developed by a Hospice Project Advisory Committee which consisted of professionals employed by hospice programs, as well as representatives from various organizations (JCAH, AHA, AMA, and the National Hospice Organization). The documentation guidelines in the handbook were intended to provide guidelines to all hospices, not just those opting for JCAH hospice accreditation or hospice Medicare certification. Therefore, medical record professionals should ensure hospices are documenting in accordance with these guidelines even if they are not required to meet JCAH or Medicare documentation requirements. The handbook also addresses several hospice record management concerns. For instance, it recommends that the hospice record become part of the patient's unit record when the hospice is based in a hospital or a home health agency; and that the patient index file contain information on the patients receiving hospice care as well as the survivors being followed through bereavement programs.

The JCAH recently began an accreditation program for hospice programs, and its *Hospice Standards Manual* contains medical record documentation requirements. The JCAH states that the hospice record should contain patient and family identifying data, all pertinent diagnoses, the patient's prognosis, the designation of the attending physician, and the designation of the family member or other primary care person to be contacted in the event of emergency or death. There should be a medical history and, when the patient is an inpatient, a physical examination. Assessment information should include a physical assessment, which notes chronic or acute pain and other physical symptoms and their management, and a functional assessment which describes any functional limitations and any activity restrictions. A psychosocial assessment of the patient/family, to include an assessment of spiritual needs, is also required. There should be ongoing assessment of the patient's/family's needs. Figures 5 and 6 display the model Activities of Daily Living forms which contain functional and activity assessments, as well as other required assessment information. An interdisciplinary care plan must document a patient's/family's problems and needs and realistic, achievable goals and objectives to address these problems and needs. The plan must also document the discipline responsible for implementing the plan, the frequency of the team services planned, the medications prescribed, and the equipment required. It must be reviewed at least every 30 days, and care plan reviews must be documented in the record. A summary is required when a patient expires, is discharged from the hospice program, or is transferred between inpatient and home care. Survivors must be assessed for pathologic grief reactions, and this assessment along with any other bereavement documentation must be included in the patient/family record.

Medicare regulations generally require the same documentation as JCAH standards. Differences primarily reflect signature and time requirements. The Medicare regulations prescribe a specific hospice organizational structure and state that a hospice must maintain control of a patient's care when he receives care by a contracted inpatient facility. The contracted inpatient facility must follow the care plan established by the hospice, and the hospice record must at least include a summary of all inpatient services provided.

A. FUNCTIONAL ASSESSMENT (Record Code For Each Function.)

ASSESSMENT CODES: 1 = Can Do Alone   2 = Can Do With Assistance   3 = Unable To Do   4 = Not Determined

FUNCTION	CODE	COMMENTS
1. BATHING OR SHOWERING		
2. SHAMPOOING		
3. NAIL CARE		
4. HAIR CARE		
5. DRESSING		
6. BOWEL AND BLADDER		
7. TRANSFERRING IN AND OUT OF BED OR CHAIR		
8. WALKING		
9. STAIRS		
10. MOBILITY OUT OF HOME		

11. DOES PATIENT HAVE A HISTORY OF FALLS? _____

B. PATIENT CARE REQUIREMENTS

	YES	NO	COMMENTS
1. CATHETER			
2. COLOSTOMY/ILEOSTOMY			
3. OXYGEN/RESPIRATORY EQUIPMENT			
4. WALKER			
5. WHEELCHAIR			
6. COMMODE			
7. HOSPITAL BED			
8.			
9.			

C. SUITABILITY OF PATIENT/FAMILY RESIDENCE

1. STAIRS ___ ___ COMMENTS: _____
    YES NO

2. SAFETY HAZARDS ___ ___ DESCRIBE: _____
    YES NO

3. SAFETY MEASURES NEEDED: _____

4. ADEQUACY OF ENVIRONMENT: _____

ACTIVITIES OF DAILY LIVING
(Page 1 of 2)

Imprint Patient Identification or Write-In Information Below

Patient's Name

Medical Record No.

Hospice Project/FORE of AMRA 5/84 Form #4

FIG. 5 – HOSPICE CARE (page 1 of 2)

Medicare reimburses hospices at four different rates for the following care levels: routine home care, continuous home care, inpatient respite care, and general inpatient care. Continuous home care (8 hours or more of continuous, predominantly nursing care) and general inpatient care (care for acute symptom management that cannot be performed in the home) are the

---

D. ACTIVITIES

1. CURRENT ACTIVITIES (Describe): _____

_____

_____

2. LIMITATIONS IMPOSED BY ILLNESS (Describe): _____

_____

E. REFERRAL(S) FOR HOME ASSISTANCE (e.g. home health aide, homemaker, etc.)

_____

F. DIETARY

1. ROUTE OF FOOD INTAKE: ☐ By Mouth ☐ Feeding Tube ☐ IV ☐ Other_____

2. ALTERATIONS IN TASTE/SMELL: _____

3. APPETITE: _____

4. ALCOHOL INTAKE: _____ 5. FOOD RESTRICTIONS: _____

6. FOOD/FLUID LIKES/DISLIKES: _____

7. MEAL PATTERNS: _____

8. COMMENTS: _____

_____

G. REST/SLEEP (Check yes or no for each.)

SYMPTOM	YES	NO	COMMENTS/DESCRIPTION
1. SLEEP DISORDERS			
2. CHANGES IN SLEEP HABITS			
3. SLEEP AIDS			
4. NAPS			
5.			

H. WHAT DOES PATIENT ESPECIALLY WANT FROM HOSPICE? _____

_____

I. SOURCE(S) OF INFORMATION: _____

Date: _____ Information Recorded By _____

Signature and Title

ACTIVITIES OF DAILY LIVING
(Page 2 of 2)

Imprint Patient Identification or Write-In Information Below

Patient's Name

Medical Record No.

Hospice Project/FORE of AMRA 5/84 Form #4

FIG. 6 – HOSPICE CARE (page 2 of 2)

---

more intensive care levels, and when this care is provided, the medical record must justify that this care was needed.

The National Hospice Organization has hospice program standards but has no formal accreditation program. The program standards state that accurate and current records should be kept on all patients. State hospice regulations should also be referred to for record documentation requirements. It must again be stressed that all hospices should, at a minimum, document in accordance with the documentation requirements in *A Medical Record Handbook for Hospice Programs.* The model hospice record, as printed, should meet JCAH hospice standards and hospice Medicare regulations if documented per instructions and if standards and regulations are adhered to regarding frequency, signatures, and time requirements for documentation.

ANALYSIS OF HOSPICE RECORDS

The JCAH and Medicare have no requirements for medical record review. *A Medical Record Handbook for Hospice Programs* states that each hospice should have a system to review medical records on a frequent, ongoing basis. It is recommended that records be reviewed shortly after admission (within five days of an inpatient admission and within ten days of a home care admission), on discharge, and on an ongoing basis (every 30-60 days). Specific items to be reviewed are outlined in the handbook. The handbook also recommends that volunteer documentation be filed in the medical record and that it be reviewed and initialed by the volunteer coordinator and the team nurse coordinator prior to filing.

QUALITY ASSURANCE IN HOSPICES

The JCAH requires hospices to monitor and evaluate the quality and appropriateness of hospice program services. There should be routine collection of information pertaining to the delivery of interdisciplinary team services. This information should be assessed (using objective criteria), and important problems regarding care delivery or opportunities to improve patient/family services should be identified. Once problems or opportunities are identified, action must be taken and the effectiveness of this action evaluated. At least annually there should be documented evidence that quality assurance program findings resulted in action taken relating to patient/family services, administration or supervision, or in-service and/or continuing education. The quality assurance program's findings and conclusions should be coordinated, to the degree possible, with any inpatient facility or agency providing services (through contract or arrangements) to a hospice program's patients/families.

The JCAH also requires a hospice to monitor allocation of its resources and to resolve any identified problems. To do this a hospice must use objective criteria to review a randomly selected sample of medical records. This review should monitor concerns such as:

1. the appropriateness of the level of services and the team services provided,
2. the appropriateness of admission,
3. stays exceeding six months, and
4. delays in providing team service.

Utilization review should result in documented action being taken. The utilization review plan should be reviewed at least annually and revised as appropriate.

Medicare regulations require hospices to conduct ongoing assessments of the quality and appropriateness of the services provided. Services provided through arrangements or contracts must be assessed. There must be documentation of the mechanisms used to monitor care, the problems identified and resolved, and the suggestions made for improving care.

Collection of Hospice Data

Hospices must collect data in a uniform manner if services are to be evaluated and comparisons made within and among hospice programs. Data on the care provided by hospice programs are needed for both internal and external planning. There are presently few computer systems that are specifically developed for hospice data collection. A hospice management information system was recently developed by the Hospice Foundation of Miami, Florida, through a project funded by the Arthur Vining Davis Foundation. The system is capable of collecting and processing patient demographic, diagnostic, and care information. A plan of care can be printed, and the system can be used to provide up-to-date patient care information to the on-call nurse.

Minimum Uniform Data Set

In conjunction with the FORE of AMRA hospice project, a uniform hospice minimum data set was developed and recommended for use. Hospices should record the demographic and assessment data set items in their medical records and the service data set items in the record or elsewhere. The hospice handbook contains a form that can be used to collect service data. The data categories are listed below.

Demographic/Assessment Items
1. Personal identification
2. Social Security number
3. Sex
4. Birth date
5. Race and ethnicity
6. Marital status
7. Usual living arrangements and primary care person information
8. Principal and other significant diagnoses (coded)
9. Basic patient functional assessment
10. Patient care requirements
11. Patient orientation; time, place, and person
12. Memory; recent, and remote

Service Items
1. Provider identification
2. Referral source
3. Episodes of care–length of stays
4. Direct services–number of visits per service
5. Principal source of payment for services
6. Charges

Classification Systems for Hospices

The FORE of AMRA hospice project reviewed several existing classification systems and recommended that hospice programs use the *International Classification of Diseases, Ninth Revision, Clinical Modification (ICD-9-CM)* to code a patient's and a survivor's diagnoses and problems (see Chapter 12). Hospices should also maintain diagnosis and problem indexes. In hospital-based programs, coding and indexing should be coordinated with the hospital's medical record department. *A Medical Record Handbook for Hospice Programs* contains detailed guidance for hospice coding and indexing.

Statistical Definitions

There are two recognized hospice care episodes. The first episode begins with the patient's/family's admission to the hospice program and ends at the time a patient dies or is discharged from the hospice program. This episode includes all home care and inpatient care provided to the patient either directly or through contract with an inpatient facility or home health agency. The second care episode begins with the survivor's admission to bereavement follow-up (the day following a patient's death) and ends when the survivor is discharged from bereavement follow-up.

As previously mentioned, the recommended service data set items should be recorded by all hospices. From this data, the minimum statistics listed below should be calculated.

- Average Daily Census, preferably by type of service provided (home care, bereavement, inpatient).
- Average Length of Patient's Hospice Stay (the first hospice episode).
- Average Number of Total Days of Inpatient Care and Home Care Received by Patients/Families.
- Average Length of Bereavement Follow-up (the second hospice episode).

The hospice handbook contains formulas for the above statistics. Hospices that are Medicare certified should calculate a separate statistic that reflects the aggregate number of home care days and inpatient days received by Medicare patients. This is necessary because Medicare will not reimburse hospices at the inpatient care rate when, in a given year, the aggregate inpatient care days exceed 20 percent of the total care days.

SUMMARY

Ambulatory care, home care, and hospice care are integral components of the health care delivery system in the United States, and in recent years utilization of these alternative forms of health care has increased markedly. Medical records maintained for ambulatory care, home care, and hospice care assume a vital role in ensuring the continuity of patient care. The more diversified the health care delivery system becomes, the more important a role the medical record plays in providing the necessary link in continuous patient care. Medical record professionals must take an active role in the development of quality records and record management procedures in a variety of health care settings.

STUDY QUESTIONS

1. According to the JCAH, what data elements should be recorded in hospital-based ambulatory care records? In free-standing ambulatory care records?
2. What record system should be used for the maintenance of hospital-based ambulatory care records and home care records and hospice records? Why?
3. What are the Medicare documentation requirements for home care records? The JCAH requirements for home care records?
4. What are the JCAH documentation requirements for hospice care records?

AMBULATORY CARE REFERENCES

Accreditation Handbook for Ambulatory Health Care. Accreditation Association for Ambulatory Health Care, Inc. Skokie, Illinois, 1982.

Accreditation Manual for Ambulatory Health Care/85. Joint Commission on Accreditation of Hospitals, 1984.

Accreditation Manual for Hospitals/85. Joint Commission on Accreditation of Hospitals, 1984.

AVERY, MAURINE and IMDIEKE, BONNIE. *Medical Records in Ambulatory Care.* Maryland: Aspen Systems Corporation, 1984.

BARNETT, G. O. et al. "COSTAR – A Comprehensive Medical Information System for Ambulatory Care," in Blum, B Ed. *Proceedings of the Sixth Annual Symposium on Computer Applications in Medical Care.* New York: Computer Society Press, 1982, pp. 8-18.

Bibliography on Ambulatory Care. FORE Library, American Medical Record Association, 1983.

BURNS, LINDA A. "A Perspective on Hospital Ambulatory Care," in Meshenberg, K. and Burns, L., Eds. *Hospital Ambulatory Care: Making It Work.* Chicago, Illinois: American Hospital Association, 1983.

CAMPBELL, BERNICE C., RRA. "Confidentiality of Health Records in Emergency Medical Services Systems." *Medical Record News.* June, 1975.

CARMICHAEL, P. L. et al. "Design of an Office Medical Record Module," in Cohen, G. S., Ed. *Proceedings of the Eighth Annual Symposium on Computer Applications in Medical Care.* New York: Computer Society Press, 1984, pp. 433-436.

Conditions of Participation: Health Maintenance Organizations. Federal Insurance for the Aged. U.S. Department of Health, Education and Welfare, Social Security Administration, Washington, D.C.

Conditions of Participation: Home Health Agencies. Federal Insurance for the Aged. U.S. Department of Health, Education and Welfare, Social Security Administration, Washington, D.C.

Conditions of Participation: Hospitals. Federal Insurance for the Aged. U.S. Department of Health, Education and Welfare, Social Security Administration, Washington, D.C.

Consolidated Standards Manual/85 for Child, Adolescent, and Adult Psychiatric, Alcoholism, and Drug Abuse Facilities and Facilities Serving the Mentally Retarded/Developmentally Disabled. Joint Commission on Accreditation of Hospitals, 1984.

DAVY, JANE D. "Preferred Provider Organizations." *The American Journal of Occupational Therapy* 38, May, 1984, pp. 327-329.

EBERHANDY, JEANETTE. "Information Requirements for Health Maintenance Organizations, Clinical Data Needs and Automated Medical Records," in Cohen, G. S., Ed. *Proceedings of the Eighth Annual Symposium on Computer Applications in Medical Care.* New York: Computer Society Press, 1984, p. 417.

Glossary of Hospital Terms. American Medical Record Association, 1985.

HAMMOND, W. E. et al. "Differing Philosophies on Data Capture among Specialty Groups," in Cohen, G. S., Ed. *Proceedings of the Eighth Annual Symposium on Computer Applications in Medical Care.* New York: Computer Society Press, 1984, p. 477.

Hospital Administration Terminology. American Hospital Association. Chicago, Illinois, 1982.

HUMPHREY, ANN G. "Long-Term Care Policies Beginning to Take Shape." *Nursing Homes* 33 No. 5, November/December, 1984, pp. 34-36.

LINN, NORMAN and PUGLIESE, D. "Trends in Ambulatory Care Information System." *Computers in Health Care* 4 No. 1, January, 1983, pp. 26-32.

McLATCHEY, J. G. et al. "The Capturing of More Detailed Medical Information in COSTAR, in Cohen, G. S., Ed. *Proceedings of the Eighth Annual Symposium on Computer Applications in Medical Care.* New York: Computer Society Press, 1984, pp. 329-336.

McNERNEY, WALTER J. "Financing Ambulatory Health Care Services." *The Journal of Ambulatory Care Management* 7 No. 4, November, 1984, pp. 1-3.

MOXLEY, J. and ROEDER, P. "New Opportunities for Out-of-Hospital Health Services." *The New England Journal of Medicine* 310 No. 3, January 19, 1984, pp. 193-197.

PALMER, R. HEATHER. *Ambulatory Health Care Evaluation: Principles and Practice.* American Hospital Association. Chicago, Illinois, 1983.

Principles for Accreditation of Community Mental Health Programs. Joint Commission on Accreditation of Hospitals, 1976.

REED, JEANNE M., RRA. "Medical Record Practitioners in Neighborhood Health Centers." *Medical Record News.* February, 1972.

ROEMER, MILTON I. *Ambulatory Health Services in America: Past, Present and Future.* Maryland: Aspen Systems Corporation, 1981.

Standards for Health Services in Jails. American Medical Association, 1979.

Standards for Health Services in Juvenile Confinement Facilities. National Commission on Correctional Health Care. Chicago, Illinois, 1984.

Standards for Health Services in Prisons. American Medical Association, 1979.

U.S. Bureau of the Census. *America in Transition: An Aging Society.* Washington, D.C.: Government Printing Office, 1983.

VANMETRE, J. E. et al. "A Method for Improving the Quality of Data in STOR," in Cohen, G. S., Ed. *Proceedings of the Eighth Annual Symposium on Computer Applications in Medical Care.* New York: Computer Society Press, 1984, pp. 425-428.

HOME CARE REFERENCES

Accreditation Manual for Hospitals. Chicago, Illinois: Joint Commission on Accreditation of Hospitals, 1985, pp. 35-41.

Bibliography on Recordkeeping Systems: Home Health. FORE Library. American Medical Record Association, 1983.

"Conditions of Participation: Home Health Agencies." *Code of Federal Regulations.* Title 42 Section 405. pp. 1201-1230, (Subpart L).

KLEFFEL, D. "Home Health Record Systems: A Challenge to the Medical Record Profession." *Topics in Health Record Management: Ambulatory Care 1* (1981), pp. 33-44.

LAMMY, S. "Home Health Care: A Sound Alternative." *Michigan Hospitals* 19 No. 6, June, 1983, p. 25.

MORRIS, M. and FORSECA, J. "Home Care Today–An Interview." *American Journal of Nursing* 84 No. 3, March, 1984, p. 341.

"NAHC Responds to Senate Questions." *Caring* 3 No. 4, April, 1984, p. 6.

National League for Nursing. *Administrator's Handbook for Community Health and Home Care Services.* New York: NLN, 1984.

National League for Nursing. *Criteria and Standards Manual for NLN/ APHA Accreditation of Home Health Agencies and Community Nursing Services.* 7th Ed. New York: NLN, 1980.

National League for Nursing. *Policies and Procedures for NLN/APHA Accreditation of Home Health Agencies and Community Nursing Services.* New York: NLN, 1980.

RYDER, C. F. "Basic Data Requirements for Home Health Care." *Medical Care,* May, 1976, pp. 46-52.

SPIEGEL, A. D. *Home Healthcare: Home Birthing to Hospice Care.* Maine: National Health Publishing, 1983.

Statement on Home Health Care. American Medical Association. Chicago, Illinois, 1973.

U.S. Department of Health and Human Services. *Long-Term Health Care: Minimum Data Set.* Maryland, 1980.

HOSPICE REFERENCES

Bibliography on Recordkeeping Systems: Hospice Care. FORE Library. American Medical Record Association, 1984.

Federal Register 48 No. 243, December 16, 1983.

Hospice Standards Manual. Chicago, Illinois: Joint Commission on Accreditation of Hospitals, 1983.

"JCAH Hospice Provider Profile," 1984. Unpublished.

MILLER, S. C. *A Medical Record Handbook for Hospice Programs.* Chicago, Illinois: Foundation of Record Education of the American Medical Record Association, 1984.

————. "Hospice Medical Record Documentation and Management: Opportunity for Improvement." *Topics in Health Record Management* 5 No. 3, March, 1985.

Standards of Hospice Program of Care. Virginia: National Hospice Organization, 1979.

ZIMMERMAN, J. M. *Hospice: Complete Care for the Terminally Ill.* Maryland: Urban & Schwarzberg, 1981, p. 9.

chapter 5

HEALTH RECORDS IN
LONG TERM CARE FACILITIES

Providing patient health records is as important a goal in the operation and management of long term care facilities as it is for hospitals. In addition to their major function as a communication tool for those who give patient care, records also reflect the quality of care rendered; they provide information about patients to meet requirements of licensing, certifying and accreditation agencies; and they are used in cases where legal action is taken.

The content of health records and the procedures for their maintenance in long term care facilities are similar to those in hospitals. But even though the records are similar, the individual needs of each institution should be considered when organizing a health record system for long term care. The system should not duplicate the hospital medical record system because of the differences in recording data between acute, short term hospital care and the recording needs for patients who may be in the long term care facility for months or even years.

This chapter will describe long term care records, whether maintained in a free-standing facility or in one which is connected to or affiliated with a hospital. If a long term care facility or unit is part of or connected to a hospital, the record systems should be compatible with each other, even though the compilation of records, requirements, maintenance and statistics will be judged and monitored by different standards, different regulations, different modes of preparation, and different treatment modalities. If a unit record is maintained, the acute hospital portion is usually separated from the long term care portion by a divider, and separate statistics are compiled.

Some considerations in planning a record system for long term care facilities are: What is the basic content of the health record? How does it differ from an acute care record? What are the minimum standards for health records in long term care facilities? What system is most appropriate for maintaining these records?

The medical record practitioner should be aware that long term care facilities are an integral part of the health care delivery system. The major focus of long term care changed in 1965 with the passage of the Medicare Act (PL 89-97). Before that time, most long term care facilities were places for patients to stay who had little hope of recovery or rehabilitative potential. The federal *Conditions of Participation*, developed under the Medicare program, changed this focus and put more stringent requirements on patient care and the rehabilitative aspects of care. These *Conditions of Participation* and related state regulations should be carefully reviewed when developing procedures for the maintenance of health records.

THE LONG TERM CARE SETTING

The setting of long term care includes a wide range of services. A life care center or residential facility offers an alternative to completely independent living, with the residents being provided with living quarters and basic services such as meals, activities, and coordination of health care services. Such residents are not, in the technical sense, patients. In a facility which has more than one component, it will be important to differentiate residents (those who live independently in private quarters) from patients (those who are admitted to a designated component to receive medical and supportive care).

The term "nursing home" is a generic one, commonly used by the lay public to denote a health care facility for the convalescent and/or aged patient. The more proper designation indicates level of care, usually specified in the pertinent licensure regulations for a specific facility. All health care facilities of this type must be licensed by the state which will indicate the designation: skilled nursing facility, intermediate care facility, convalescent center, or similar term. A particular facility may be licensed to provide more than one level of care, with a certain percentage of beds/rooms and with specific physical facilities designated for each level of care. The skilled level of care is the most comprehensive level, with patients at that level needing continuous nursing service and a variety of support services on a routine basis. The gradation of care generally follows this pattern in a mixed facility: residential care, convalescent short stay care at either intermediate or skilled levels, long stay intermediate care, and long stay skilled level care. It is possible for a patient to move within these levels of care according to specific episodes. Generally, state regulatory agencies and their related reimbursement agencies have a point system for assessing the appropriate level of care. Administrative, social service, and nursing personnel have access to such systems; the medical record personnel will find it useful to acquaint themselves with such protocols. This ranking of level of care will affect utilization review requirements and will be useful in setting up the required content of the health record and the related statistical indicators.

Some current trends in the care of the aged are having an impact on the long term care facility. Newer outreach programs include home care components, based in the facility and respite care programs of very short stay, primarily developed to give the family or primary care taker a short term alternative to continuous care of the patient in the home. As hospitals experience the impact of pressures to shorten the length of stay, convalescent care at long term care facilities reemerges as a practice.

THE PATIENT POPULATION

Given such a variety of setting options, the patient population will vary from one institution to another. Some general characteristics may be noted. First of all, the primary patient population remains that of the frail and/or ill elderly person who is no longer able to live independently. These individuals usually are advanced in years, have generalized chronic physical deterioration associated with the aging process, and need a variety of supportive services to maintain the normal activities of daily living. Such patients will also have a variety of chronic, long term diagnostic conditions which require regular physician and nursing and other professional health care services. This class of patients comes to the facility either for a convalescent stay, such as a posthospitalization stay for several weeks or months, or for a prolonged stay, often for the "balance of life" when there is no other living arrangement available whereby the patient can receive the diffuse level of services needed due to age and/or illness. The medical record documentation process will, therefore, be characterized by ongoing, repeated documentation of chronic care, interspersed with particular major medical episodes; the documentation process will reflect months, and often years of continuous care.

The other mix of patients, those who come to the facility for comparatively shorter stays, often will have more specific and time-limited diagnostic situations which totally or partially resolve during the convalescent stay. The rehabilitative program is geared to returning these individuals to independent living. The age pattern may vary with this group who are not necessarily drawn primarily from the frail elderly population.

THE LEGAL, REGULATORY, AND ACCREDITING STANDARDS

Fundamental to the operation of a long term care facility is its proper license by the state agency empowered to regulate such facilities. As noted in earlier discussion, this license to operate denotes the specific range of care to be offered, e.g., skilled or intermediate care. The state licensure agency issues regulations which include specific areas of medical record content and practice. During the annual review for licensure renewal, all the significant aspects of the health record content and system are reviewed. Should an area be noted as not in compliance, the facility must file its plan of correction, specifying the manner and time frame in which it will bring the practices into compliance. A properly developed medical record system should reduce, even eliminate, any such noncompliance. Ongoing chart review and related monitoring processes will help reduce any noncompliance with respect to documentation by the direct patient care givers.

The second major set of regulations stems from those issued by the federal government in connection with the Medicare-Medicaid amendments to the Social Security Act. The *Conditions of Participation for Skilled Nursing Facilities (Subpart K)* specify these details. These regulations apply to all facilities that participate in Medicare-Medicaid programs. As with state regulations, there is periodic review for compliance; and a facility found not in compliance must take the necessary measures to correct any deficiency.

The third set of standards flows from voluntary participation in the Joint Commission on Accreditation of Hospitals program of accreditation. This accreditation body has developed standards for long term care facilities. Facilities which wish to have accreditation status, apply to the JCAH, participate in the site visit survey, and, if found in compliance, are issued the accreditation certificate appropriate to the facility's level of care. Unlike the state and federal regulations, compliance with the JCAH is voluntary; a facility may withdraw from this program, although this rarely happens.

Although a particular facility may not seek JCAH status, medical record personnel will find it useful to obtain such standards as a reference because they represent common professional practice. A particular facility's policies may be more stringent than the state and federal regulations. JCAH guidelines provide a basis for such policy development.

An alternative to JCAH accreditation is provided by the American Health Care Association which has its own standards. Some facilities, particularly proprietary groups, participate in this association's activities. Their guidelines should be obtained for use in such facilities.

THE PROFESSIONAL AND ADMINISTRATIVE STAFF

Ownership of a facility may include not-for-profit community, religious, philanthropic, or fraternal sponsorship. It may also include governmental sponsorship, as in a county or city facility. Ownership may be private, for profit, either by an individual, a corporate group, or a corporate conglomerate. The licensure regulations require that ownership/sponsorship be specified.

In any case, there will be a designated chief executive officer responsible for the day-to-day running of the facility. In large facilities there may be assistant administrators to work with the CEO. Under Medicare regulations and related state regulations, the administrator of a long term care facility must be licensed by the state.

A medical director will coordinate the work of the medical staff and provide oversight for the medical and professional care rendered. Each individual patient is assigned an attending physician responsible for his care.

The director of nursing service plays a key role in long term care. Because of the diffuse nature of care in many facilities, physician presence is more limited than in the acute care situation. The role of the director of nursing service as a primary agent for day-to-day supervision of care and coordination with physician services is a demanding and important one. Medical record personnel will interact frequently with this key professional who is on the "front lines" continually in matters of direct patient care.

Nursing personnel will include a mix of registered nurses, licensed practical nurses, and nurse aides. The designation of professional credential in documentation is important. A variety of other professional health care providers renders service in the long term care facility; these include activities therapist, occupational therapist, physical therapist, podiatrist, dentist, dietician, pharmacist, and social service. When the facility is relatively small, many of these practitioners will provide services on a contractual basis. Medical record personnel need to be aware of the names and credential designation of each of these practitioners.

Medical record personnel will include a credentialed practitioner, either in a line position as an employee of the facility or as a staff position by means of a consulting arrangement. There must be designated responsibility for the day-to-day operation of the medical record service which is provided by an employee of the facility. The chief executive officer has this overall responsibility, and normally the medical record personnel report to the chief executive officer in terms of line authority.

THE BASIC LONG TERM CARE RECORD

Each patient in a long term care facility must have an individual health record. Health records should be simple, realistic, and flexible but should also be detailed enough to contribute to patient care and treatment. A health record should contain complete information about the patient's illness and his treatment. Events should be recorded in the order in which they occur.

Such complete chronological recording justifies the diagnosis and proves that the condition warrants the treatment and the end result. The information is sufficiently detailed as to provide a basis for reimbursement by the various private and public funding agencies.

The following items are typically included in a health record for long term care facilities which participate in the Medicare-Medicaid programs, comply with state licensure regulations, and participate in Joint Commission accreditation:

1. Identification and financial data: Medicare number, Medicaid number, health insurance number, and responsible party for billing.

2. Transfer and related medical information from previous health care settings: reason for placement, summary by referring physician, copy of hospital discharge summary or summation of patient's medical problems, diagnoses, and physical examination.

3. Admission evaluation: attending physician, nursing service, dietary, activities, social service, and appropriate rehabilitative therapies.

4. Patient care plan: interdisciplinary plan reflecting each major discipline involved in patient's treatment.

5. Discharge plan: statement of potential for rehabilitation, alternate plans for maintenance of functional level if patient is placed for "balance of life" because he is no longer able to live independently.

6. Physician orders: treatment, tests, medication, diets, restraints, and restrictions.

7. Pharmacy consultation review of physician orders and medications given.

8. Progress notes: physician, podiatrist, dentist, nursing staff, consultant, and other professional personnel.

9. Physician discharge summary.

10. Miscellaneous: any and all reports as they apply to the particular case:

- Admission agreement and consent for care
- Patient rights acknowledgment
- Legal papers
- Health aids, personal property and valuables list
- Release of information forms
- Death certificate copy, release of body, and autopsy report

Minimum requirements for health record documentation will be discussed at greater length below. Individual state regulations should be checked for additional specifications related to medical record information. In some states, licensing regulations are more stringent than federal requirements.

IDENTIFICATION DATA

Information listed in the identification section of the record varies in different situations but should include enough data to positively identify each patient. Examples of entries which may be collected are listed below. Items which may change should be kept current with the changes posted in the patient's medical record in a highly visible place, e.g., the face sheet. These items are preceded by an asterisk.

- Patient's name, including aliases and nicknames
- Facility number
- *Address
- *Telephone number
- *Age
- Date of birth
- Place of birth
- Citizenship
- Social Security number
- Sex
- *Marital status
- *Nearest of kin or responsible agent
- *Address and telephone number of nearest of kin or responsible agent

- Father's name
- Mother's maiden name
- Usual occupation

IDENTIFICATION AND SUMMARY SHEET

To be completed by admitting clerk:

Family Name	First Name			Home Phone	File No.
Usual Address				Sex M F / Marital Status M S W D Sep.	Social Security No.
Age	Birth Date	Birthplace	Citizen	How Long at Usual Address?	Military Service Branch Years
Usual Occupation	Kind of Business or Industry		Employer's Address and Phone No.		
Name of Husband, Wife or Responsible Agent			Address		
Name of Father			Maiden Name of Mother		
Notify in Case of Emergency	Relationship		Address		Phone No.
Church Affiliation	Name of Clergyman		Address and Phone of Clergyman		
Welfare No.	Alien Reg. No.	Medicare No.	Insurance		
Previous Hospitalization	Hosp. No.	Dates	Diagnosis		
Admitted from	Referred by		Admission Date and Hour		
Physician	Address				Phone No.
Dentist	Address				Phone No.
Discharged To			Discharge Date and Hour		

Items below to be completed by physician:

ADMITTING DIAGNOSIS:

DIAGNOSES OF CONDITIONS ARISING LATER:

FINAL DIAGNOSIS:

CONDITION ON DISCHARGE:

SIGNATURE OF PHYSICIAN

FORM NH-128 PHYSICIANS' RECORD CO., BERWYN, ILLINOIS - PRINTED IN U.S.A. IDENTIFICATION AND SUMMARY SHEET

Form courtesy of Physicians' Record Company

FIG. 1 – IDENTIFICATION AND SUMMARY SHEET

- Religious preference
- Clergyman and address
- Mortuary preference

- Military service
- Insurance
- Medicare number
- Medicaid number
- Date of admission
- Time of admission
- Admitted from
- Referred by
- Attending physician
- Dentist
- Other information needed to satisfy state requirements

A combined identification and summary sheet is displayed in Figure 1. When this type of form is used, the physician is responsible for writing the final diagnosis and condition of the patient or prognosis at discharge. The attending physician's signature may be requested if the facility desires verification of physician entries directly on the identification and summary sheet. It should be noted that such a summary sheet does not replace the formal discharge summary which constitutes a separate document. The date and time of discharge as well as the place to which the patient was discharged should be filled in by medical record personnel.

TRANSFER OR REFERRAL STATEMENT

Long term care facilities need basic facts about each patient in order to provide appropriate care. These facts may be obtained from the transfer or referral form (Figures 2 and 3). When a patient is admitted to the facility, this form should accompany the patient; if it is not immediately available, this form should be requested immediately from the referring hospital, physician, or other facility. The transfer or referral form should state the reason for admission, the diagnosis, current medical information, and the patient's rehabilitative potential. The physician should also certify that the patient requires either skilled or intermediate care and for what time period such care is anticipated.

Additional items that this statement should contain are:

- Identification data from the summary sheet of the record

- Name of transferring institution
- Name of receiving institution
- Date of transfer

PATIENT INFORMATION AND
TRANSFER FORM

Name_____
         (LAST)   (FIRST)
                      Social
Age_____Sex_____Religion_____Security No._____
                                   (PREFIX)   (NUMBER)

Public Aid Number_____Medicare Number_____   Date of Transfer_____

Relative or
Guardian_____   Transferred to_____
                              (RELATION)   HOSP. NURSING HOME AGENCY

Relative or Guardian's
Address_____Tel._____   Address_____

                                                  Clinic
From_____Admission_____   Appt._____

Address_____   Date and Time_____

Marital Status M☐ S☐ W☐ D☐ Sep. ☐   _____
                                                  (ATTACH CLINIC OR MEDICAL APPOINTMENT CARD)
Address of Patient
Prior to Hospitalization_____

Physician in Charge   Will this Physician care for Patient
at Time of Transfer_____M.D.   after Admission to Nursing Home?_____

II. MAJOR DIAGNOSES   DIET, DRUGS, AND OTHER THERAPY
                                              at Time of Discharge

(Check if present)
Disabilities   Incontinence
  Amputation   Bladder
  Paralysis   Bowel
  Contracture   Saliva
  Decub. Ulcer   Activity Tolerance Limitations
Impairments   None   Moderate   Severe
  Mentality   Patient knows diagnosis?
  Speech
  Hearing
  Vision
  Sensation

IMPORTANT MEDICAL INFORMATION
(State allergies if any)

                                          Chest X-ray   date_____result_____
                                          C. B. C.   date_____result_____
                                          Serology   date_____result_____
                                          Urinalysis   date_____result_____

SUGGESTIONS FOR COMPLETING FORM
1. The purpose of this form is to insure continuity of care in transfer from hospital to home or home to hospital.
2. The form is not intended to supply information of long-term nature.
3. Original should accompany patient with transfer. Carbon retained in patient's record.

          Signature of Physician or Nurse_____Date_____
FORM A-450   PHYSICIANS' RECORD CO., BERWYN, ILLINOIS.   PRINTED IN U.S.A.

Form courtesy of Physicians' Record Company

FIG. 2 – PATIENT TRANSFER FORM (front)

- Hospital diagnoses/hospital number
- Nurses' report
  This includes patient attitudes, behavior, interests, func-

tional abilities (activities of daily living), unusual treatments, nursing care problems (likes and dislikes), nutrition, current medications and when last given, condition

III. PATIENT INFORMATION

SELF-CARE STATUS
(Check level of ability. Write S in space if needs supervision only. Draw line across if inapplicable.)

	Independent	Needs Assistance	Unable to do	
Bed Activity				Turns
				Sits
Personal Hygiene				Face, Hair, Arms
				Trunk & Perineum
				Lower Extremities
				Bladder Program
				Bowel Program
Dressing				Upper Extremities
				Trunk
				Lower Extremities
				Appliance, Splint
Feeding				
Transfer				Sitting
				Standing
				Tub
				Toilet
Locomotion				Wheelchair
				Walking
				Stairs

BED Low____ Mattress: Firm____ Reg.____
Other ________
Side Rails: Yes____ No____

BEHAVIOR
Alcoholic____ Belligerent____ Noisy____
Senile____ Suspicious____ Withdrawn____
May Wander____

MENTAL STATUS
Alert____ Forgetful____ Confused____

COMMUNICATION ABILITY	Yes	No
Can speak		
Can write		
Understands speaking		
Understands writing		
Understands gestures		
Understands English		

If no, state language spoken:____

DIET
Regular____ Low Salt____ Diabetic____
Bland____ Low Residue____

PATIENT USES
Appliance____ Catheter____ Colostomy____
Cane____ Crutches____ Prosthesis____
Walker____ Chair____

OTHER EQUIPMENT ____

ADDITIONAL PERTINENT INFORMATION
(Explain necessary details of care, diagnosis, medications, treatments, prognosis, teaching, habits, preferences, etc. Therapists and social workers add signature and title to notes.)

It is expected that the recipient's condition within the next 6 months will improve____
remain static____ deteriorate____

Rehabilitation potential: Is the recipient at his maximum level of functioning? Yes____ No____
If not, what improvements are expected in his functional capacity and self-care ability?
(a) Level of function to be attained____
(b) Length of time it is expected to take to arrive at this____

IV. SOCIAL INFORMATION (Adjustment to disability, emotional support from family, motivation for self-care, socializing ability, financial plan, family health problem, etc.)

SOCIAL ACTIVITIES
Encourage group____ individual____
within____ outside____ home.

Transport: Ambulance____ Car____
Car for handicapped____ Bus____

Social Welfare Agencies Active____ Signature____ Title:____ Date:____

Form courtesy of Physicians' Record Company

FIG. 3 – PATIENT TRANSFER FORM (back of Fig.2)

on transfer, and chest x-ray data and findings.

- Physicians' report
  This includes the reason for admission, order of medica-

tions, treatment, diet and activities, significant laboratory and x-ray findings, diagnoses, prognosis, and a brief summary of treatment.

Automatic transfer of patient information from a hospital to a long term care facility is often achieved by a transfer agreement which has been previously signed by both the hospital and the long term care facility. Once this agreement is in effect, the referring institution sends pertinent patient information directly to the facility receiving the patient. The transfer or referral form, copies of the hospital discharge summary, history and physical examination, chest x-ray, and other relevant reports accompany the patient to the long term care facility.

Patients may also be transferred from the long term care facility to other health facilities. Depending on the type of care required, patients may be transferred to an acute care hospital, another long term care facility, an ambulatory care center, or to a home care agency. The type of facility receiving the patient will determine the amount and type of information required. A copy of the transfer form is retained in the facility's medical record for the patient; the original accompanies the patient.

ADMITTING EVALUATION

An admitting evaluation is performed on every patient as soon as he is admitted to the long term care facility. The attending physician examines the patient and records an admission history and physical examination in the health record. Nursing service, dietary, patient activity department, and social service personnel visit the patient, make their assessment and enter their initial assessment of the patient's condition. If therapy orders are received on admission, the appropriate therapists will also begin evaluating the patient's needs.

History and Physical Examination

Included in the attending physician's admitting evaluation (Figures 4 and 5) are the medical and social history, physical examination, and treatment plan. The physician should date and sign the entire report. These data elements are the same as those required for acute care records (See Chapter 3). Some items that have an orientation specific to long term care are discussed here.

Reason for Admission – A concise statement of those conditions or circumstances which resulted in the patient's placement in the long term care facility. It will become the basis for the de-

Form courtesy of Physicians' Record Company

Fɪɢ. 4 – Aᴅᴍɪᴛᴛɪɴɢ Eᴠᴀʟᴜᴀᴛɪᴏɴ (front)

velopment of further statements which determine the level of care needed, as in skilled level or intermediate level care.

Social History – A description of the social environment of the patient, including where the patient lives, his friends, his occupation, and his family relationships and dependence on those relationships. This segment of the patient's record is typically

ADMITTING EVALUATION (Cont.)
PHYSICAL EXAMINATION

Family Name   First Name   File No.

General: Age_____Height_____Weight_____BP_____Communicable Diseases: ☐ Yes ☐ No

Skin:_____

Head & Neck:_____

Chest:_____

Heart:_____

Lungs:_____

Abdomen:_____

Genitourinary:_____

Musculoskeletal:_____

Neurological:_____

TREATMENT PLAN

Date_____   SIGNATURE OF PHYSICIAN

(NH-206 BACK)

Form courtesy of Physicians' Record Company

FIG. 5 – ADMITTING EVALUATION (back of FIG. 4)

compiled by social service staff and is often the basis for the discharge plan or for a plan to have the patient remain in the facility for the "balance of life."

History and Physical Examination – To be performed and recorded by the physician within 48 hours after admission. A copy of a physical examination completed within five days prior to admission is acceptable under certain conditions. If a hospital or private physician examination completed within five days prior to admission is used, signed and dated notations of changes in the patient's condition must be entered in the record by the attending physician. According to various regulations and standards, an annual physical examination by the physician must be completed.

This annual examination should include all items listed in the original examination, including significant changes in the patient's condition and any change in treatment plan. A reminder file can be used to help ensure the timely scheduling of annual physical exams. This reminder file is organized by date and used to remind record personnel of examinations or treatment updates which are due. It is useful to correlate this reminder file with that maintained by nursing service which usually schedules the examinations.

PATIENT CARE PLAN

This interdisciplinary plan emphasizes the interrelationship of each aspect of patient care. It is the working tool that provides a total care plan with input from each discipline involved in the care. It flows from the physician care plan with each health care professional contributing his unique skills toward fostering patient progress. The plan of care includes an assessment, statement of goals, identification of specific activities or strategies to achieve the goals, periodic assessment of goal attainment, and periodic update. The total patient care plan is composed when a patient is admitted to a facility (Figure 6). It is reviewed and revised periodically as the goals are reached or as the patient's rehabilitative status changes. The contents of this care plan bear directly on the designation of level of care to be provided under the Medicare classifications of skilled or intermediate care. This plan of care provides a basis for later medical care evaluation concerning both the quality of care and the general pattern of care given in the institution. In this respect, it may be considered the backbone of the medical record for a patient. From it most other patient care activities flow. Changes in the patient care plan may be easily summarized at

ADMISSION DATE________ LAST P.C.P./R.C.P. CONF. DATE________ NEXT P.C.P./R.C.P. CONF. DATE________

CURRENT DIAGNOSES:________

PERTINENT MEDICATIONS:________

PERTINENT TREATMENTS:________

ALLERGIES:________

PROBLEMS AND THEIR NUMBER WHICH ARE RESOLVED:________

PROBLEMS	DATE FIRST OCCURRED	NURSING	DIETARY	SOCIAL SERVICE	ACTIVITIES	REHAB. THERAPY	SHORT TERM GOALS	ACH'D DATE
Signature of Team Member & Date Completing this Care Plan____								

LONG TERM GOALS:________ DISCHARGE PLAN:________

PATIENT RESIDENT INFORMED OF PLAN YES ☐ NO ☐ IF NOT, REASON:________ REHAB. POTENTIAL ☐ GOOD ☐ FAIR ☐ POOR ☐ NONE

Form courtesy of Physicians' Record Company

FIG. 6 – PATIENT CARE PLAN

the time of patient discharge to provide a substantial portion of the discharge summary, showing either attainment of the goals established at admission, or changes in patient status which required modifications in those goals.

Discharge Plan

While the interdisciplinary patient care plan maps out the goals and activities for the overall treatment of the patient, a more specific document focuses on the discharge plan. This plan is begun at the time of admission giving a general assessment of expectations for discharge, e.g., return to family care after a period of convalescence. In some situations where there is no alternative for care of the patient, there may be no active discharge plan as such, other than maintenance of patient's level of functioning and provision of care and comfort for "balance of life." This realistic assessment is made and so stated. The details of the situation which entail such placement are spelled out.

In those instances where discharge is actively anticipated, the discharge plan is refined as the date and circumstances of discharge become specific. This discharge plan will focus on aftercare for the patient. Frequently this assessment and detailed planning is done through contract with a community agency such as a home health agency or similar social service group.

When the patient is ready for discharge, a copy of the discharge plan is given to the parties responsible for the individual's aftercare. The summary includes information about the current diagnosis, rehabilitation potential, and the course of treatment followed in the facility. Pertinent social information is helpful. Physician's orders are relayed to those rendering postdischarge care, as well as any instructions and self-care techniques taught the patient.

Orders

The physician should write, date, and sign orders covering medications, tests, treatments, restrictions, restraints, and diet for each patient. Because a long term care facility frequently has a variety of attending physicians who visit the patients either on a routine basis (usually monthly) or in an emergency visit, oral orders are somewhat common. State licensure regulations should be reviewed for the specifics concerning who may record an order given orally and the time frame within which such an order must be signed. In general, the following parameters are common.

Medication orders: These may be recorded by a licensed nurse, a registered pharmacist, or physician assistant. These must be signed within 48 hours by the prescribing/attending physician. To facilitate this process, such an order may be mailed to the physician, signature obtained, form returned, and filed on the appropriate order form.

Orders for specific therapies: A licensed physical therapist may record orders as they relate to physical therapy modalities and treatment. As with other oral orders, these must be signed as soon as possible after origination but no later than seven days.

Orders for specific treatments: A licensed nurse or physician assistant may record oral orders and act upon them. These oral orders must be signed as soon as possible after origination but no later than seven days.

With all oral orders, the entry should be immediately recorded on the patient's medical record by the person who received the order. This individual should sign and date the order. The professional designation of the receiver should be indicated, e.g., RN, RPT, etc.

Physician orders are initiated at various stages in the care of the patient.

(a) At the time of admission.

(b) At the time of any change in patient status.

(c) At the time of periodic review, at least every 30 days for the first 90 days following admission. In certain circumstances, intermediate level patients may be placed on an alternating schedule of 60-day intervals. The *Conditions of Participation* and interpretive guidelines provide further guidance on this matter. In all other circumstances, there is a 30-day periodic review requirement.

In any case, drugs should be ordered for a specified length of time by the physician and this should be noted on the order. Automatic stop orders for restricted medications are a routine procedure and should be delineated in the *Patient Care Policy Manual.*

Under an automatic stop system, all medications such as narcotics, sedatives, stimulants, antibiotics, tranquilizers, and anticoagulants must be discontinued after seven days or a time specified by the facility, unless ordered for a specifically longer time. When the stop order goes into effect, the staff should notify the physician that the drugs are being discontinued. No prescriptions can be refilled or ordered without a written authorization (new order) from the attending physician.

Devices used in patient care and treatment considered as "restraints" require written medical prescription. As with highly restricted medications, automatic stop orders on restraints should be routine and apply in all cases. State regulations for long term care facilities define the nature of restraints, the manner of application, the time frames for their use, and other circumstances relating to their use. The patient care policy should reflect these provisions. Whether or not a state regulation exists concerning these restraints, an automatic stop system is commonly provided so that any device of a restrictive nature must be discontinued after a limited time period and cannot be reemployed without a new written prescription by the responsible physician.

At the time of temporary or permanent discharge from the facility, a specific order must be written and signed prior to the discharge, leave, or transfer of the patient.

PHARMACY CONSULTATION REVIEW

The drug regimen of each patient is reviewed monthly by a qualified pharmacist. The findings of this review are documented in the record as well as reported to the medical director and chief executive officer. This review focuses on potential drug interactions, discrepancies in medications ordered versus given, and details relating to suggested changes in the pattern of medication. For example, if an item is ordered repeatedly but is not given to the patient for well-documented reasons, this would be called to the attention of the physician. The pharmacist's note may be included in the physician's order section, or it may constitute a separate drug regimen form. In either case, the entry is dated and signed by the pharmacist making the review.

PROGRESS NOTES

Progress notes consist of statements about each patient's progress as noted by various professional staff members. They give a chronological report of the patient's situation and include statements about reactions to treatment, general attitudes affecting treatment, and notations of any change in condition. They may be written by the physician, nurse, physician assistant, or any health professional providing care to the patient. All progress notes should be dated and signed. The provider of care, in signing the note, should also indicate his professional specialty.

Physician's Notes

Patients in a skilled nursing facility should be visited by their physicians a minimum of every 30 days, unless the alternate visit schedule is adopted. Intermediate care patients must be visited at least every 60 days. Each visit must be documented with a progress note by the attending physician.

Nurses' Notes

These are frequently maintained as a separate section in the medical record. These notes begin with a comprehensive statement concerning the general condition of the patient upon admission, including any pertinent history information, vital signs, mobility, skin condition and presence/absence of decubiti, attitude, mental status, and other specific signs and symptoms potentially requiring treatment. Periodic entries are made throughout the course of treatment, usually every month, with each nursing shift summarizing observations. Nurses' notes are written when any nonroutine event occurs, such as an incident, a particularly significant family interaction, notification of physician of patient status change, or patient refusal of food or medication.

Nurses' notes are limited to meaningful observations. Areas typically included are appetite, weight changes, attitude and mental status, ability to communicate, mobility, elimination, and ability to perform activities of daily living. Notation should be made of visits from physicians, friends, and family. Unusual signs and symptoms, actions taken, and the patient's response to treatment are also entered in these notes. All notes are dated and signed with the nurse's name and professional designation.

Rehabilitative nursing services must be provided routinely to patients requiring such services, and the results of this care should be readily available in the health record. Examples of rehabilitative nursing entries include the patient's ability to change positions, activities when out of bed, degree of self-care, and success of self-care instruction. An individual's progress in adjusting to disabilities or prosthetic devices should also be noted.

Drug reactions, any apparent change in the condition of the patient, any accident, and the date and time of these occurrences should be noted and signed. All medicines and treatments given should be recorded on the patient's record by a licensed nurse. Drugs to be administered "as needed" (PRN medications) should be charted as to time and date given, the reason for administration, and the result. After a drug has been discontinued or the patient has been discharged, the remaining portion of the drug should be accounted for on the health record. A notation should be made in the nurses' progress note that the medication has been destroyed, given to the patient if specified in physician's orders, or returned to the pharmacy. Such inclusions provide clarity of information and protect the patient as well as the facility.

Special forms may be used for recording vital signs (temperature, pulse, and respiration), blood pressure readings, intake and output, weight, medication and treatments, activities of daily living, and use of restraints.

Rehabilitative Services Notes

Specialized rehabilitative services such as physical therapy, occupational therapy, and speech therapy are provided upon physician order. These services are provided to patients requiring assistance in returning to their maximum level of functioning. A written plan of rehabilitative care is entered in the patient's record based on the interdisciplinary patient care plan. Reports on the patient's progress are communicated by the therapist to the attending physician at appropriate intervals and made part of the permanent medical record.

SOCIAL SERVICE REPORTS

The psychosocial aspect of patient care is assessed through regular interaction by the social service staff. If there is no permanent staff employed by the facility, such services may be provided through a contractual agreement.

Social service assessment begins in some instances before patient admission through a preadmission assessment to determine proper placement of the patient. If the preadmission assessment leads to formal admission to the facility, these preadmission notes become part of the medical record. For those applicants who are processed through the preadmission stage but are not admitted, the documentation of preadmission is maintained for the length of time any business record is kept. One reason for maintaining such preadmission assessments is to show compliance with the Civil Rights Act which prohibits discrimination. The reason for nonadmission to a facility should be clearly stated in such preadmission assessments.

The social service staff participates in the development of the interdisciplinary patient care plan, makes periodic entries and updates of the social service aspects of the patient and family interaction, and summarizes such findings, usually on a quarterly basis.

At the time of discharge planning, the social service staff may coordinate community services and/or alternate placement of the patient. Such processes are documented in the discharge plan.

SPECIAL REPORTS

Laboratory, radiographic, and other testing services are provided to patients upon written order of the physician. Reports of tests done during the patient's stay should be dated, signed, and placed in the record. The physician should be notified of test results as they are received.

DIAGNOSES

Admitting diagnoses should be recorded on the patient's health record at the time of admission, usually on the identification and summary sheet. Any diagnosis made during the stay in the health facility should be added to the patient's record and dated by the physician as he makes these diagnoses. If room is provided on the identification and summary sheet, subsequent diagnoses may be recorded here. Final diagnoses must be entered on the health record by the attending physician at the time of discharge from the long term care facility.

PHYSICIAN DISCHARGE SUMMARY

A discharge summary, including final diagnosis and prognosis, is required for all patients. It is to be completed by the physician promptly after the discharge. This summary generally includes admitting and final diagnoses, course of treatment, prognosis, and condition on discharge. The physician's signature completes this report.

MISCELLANEOUS REPORTS

Forms containing information of an administrative nature are often filed at the end of the record when the patient is discharged. During the patient's stay in the facility, certain items are maintained in an administrative file, usually kept in the business office. This administrative file will contain the following items.

- Legal papers, including commitment papers, guardianship, power of attorney, etc.
- The admission agreement or financial agreement between the facility and the patient or his responsible agent. In some states it may be necessary to have a consent to care form signed by the patient before certain treatments can be implemented. This is a legal protection for the facility.
- A health aids/property and valuables list should enumerate articles retained by the patient in the room and those held for safekeeping by administration. Such items as eyeglasses, dentures, and prostheses should be noted.
- Releases include many types. Release from responsibility for leave of absence should be signed by the patient or the person legally responsible for him. This protects the facility in case of accident and prevents possible false claims. Release from responsibility for discharge should be signed when the patient wishes to leave against medical advice. Consent for autopsy as well as release of the body to the

mortician should be signed by the nearest of kin. These consents legally protect the facility.

- A written authorization for the release of information should be signed by the patient or his legal representative before the facility gives information to an insurance company, attorney, or anyone asking for data about the patient. This written authorization should be filed with the record with an indication of material released under its provisions.

- In case of death, a copy of the death certificate may be kept as part of the health record if it is available. When an autopsy is performed, a copy of this report should become a part of the record.

- Patient's rights acknowledgment enumerates the patient's rights during his stay. A patient must be informed of his rights at the time of admission and there should be written evidence of this. A printed form containing the rights may be signed by the patient and placed in the record as proof of his being informed of these rights.

ACCIDENT/INCIDENT REPORTS

Unusual incidents or occurrences involving residents should be recorded in the nurses' notes and reported immediately to the chief executive officer or director of nursing services. Complete information on findings and treatment is collected, including the names of witnesses. Anything out of the ordinary, such as a fall from bed, administration of a wrong drug, or an accident involving a visitor should be reported on special accident or incident report forms (Figure 7). Such reports are used for administrative purposes only and should not be filed in the medical record. They are most often kept in a separate file in the chief executive officer's or medical director's office. Although this report is not filed in the patient's medical record, the information contained on it should correlate with the information recorded in the nurse's note, the physician's progress note (if any), or any other practitioner's entry.

ARRANGEMENT OF THE HEALTH RECORD

The arrangement of the record should meet the needs of the long term care facility. Most facilities use the source-oriented format, although problem-oriented recording lends itself well to the process of patient care planning since it is easy to follow the progress of one problem when scanning the health record.

INCIDENT AND ACCIDENT REPORT

"An Incident is any happening which is not consistent with the routine operation of the hospital or the routine care of a particular patient. It may be an accident or a situation which might result in an accident."

Person Involved	MALE ☐ FEMALE ☐ Nursing Unit_____
(Last Name, First Name, Middle Initial)	Name of First Person to See Incident or Accident

Date of Incident | Time of Incident A.M. P.M. | Exact Location of Incident Patient's Room ☐ Corridor ☐ Bathroom ☐ Dining Room ☐ Other (Specify)

PATIENT ☐ Patient's Condition Before Incident:
Ambulatory ☐ Assistive Device ☐ Wheelchair ☐ Safety Belt: Yes ☐ No ☐ Bedfast ☐
Alert ☐ Confused ☐ Disoriented ☐ Sedated ☐ Agitated ☐ Other (Specify)
Were Bed Rails Present YES ☐ NO ☐ UP ☐ DOWN ☐ | Was Height of Bed Adjustable YES ☐ NO ☐ UP ☐ DOWN ☐

EMPLOYEE ☐ Department | Job Title
Remained on Duty: YES ☐ NO ☐ | Assigned Shift: FIRST ☐ SECOND ☐ THIRD ☐

VISITOR ☐ Home Address | Home Phone

OTHER (Specify) ☐ Occupation | Reason for Presence at This Facility

Property Involved ☐ Equipment Involved ☐ Describe: | Repairs Requested YES ☐ NO ☐ | Was person authorized to be at location of incident: YES ☐ NO ☐

Describe Exactly What Happened: Why it Happened: What Causes Were. If any Injury, State Part of Body Injured. If Property or Equipment Damaged, Describe Damage.

Was Person Involved Seen by a Physician YES ☐ NO ☐ | When | Where | Physician's Name

Was First Aid Administered and/or Examination Given: YES ☐ NO ☐ | When | Place Administered | By Whom

Was Person Involved Taken to Hospital YES ☐ NO ☐ | When | Where Taken | By Whom

Indicate on Diagram Location of Injury

Right · Left   Left · Right

TYPE OF INJURY | PHYSICIAN STATEMENT, TREATMENT, RECOMMENDATIONS:
1. Laceration ☐
2. Hematoma ☐
3. Abrasion ☐
4. Contusion ☐
5. Strain ☐
6. Puncture ☐
7. Scratch ☐
8. Illness ☐
9. Other (Specify) ☐
10. None Apparent ☐

PHYSICIAN SIGNATURE | DATE

Name, Address & Phone No. of Witness(es)

Corrective Action:

Date of Report	Signature and Title of Person Preparing Report	Department Head Signature	Administrative Signature

Prepare in Duplicate (No Carbon Paper Necessary)

Form courtesy of Physicians' Record Company

FIG. 7 – INCIDENT AND ACCIDENT REPORT

Because many of the patient's needs are chronic, undifferentiated conditions rather than diagnoses, the use of the broader concept of problem/condition fosters attention to all aspects of patient care.

While the patient is in the facility, the record should be arranged for the convenience of the physicians, nurses, and other health care personnel. The sequence of documents should be spelled out in the facility's *Patient Care Manual* so consistency of practice is maintained. If the order of the record during the patient's stay is different from the final arrangement for permanent filing, the sequence may be rearranged at the time of final review. If the record retention schedule indicates record destruction after an approved time limit and if there is no activity associated with the records of discharged patients, it may be useful to arrange the record at discharge in the order that permits easy retrieval of information to be kept permanently, followed by all material which will be destroyed. This eliminates a detailed purging of the chart at the time of record destruction. The following is one example of a sequence of closed records:

- Identification and summary sheet
- Physician's discharge summary
- Transfer or referral statement
- History and physical examination
- Patient care plan
- Orders
- Pharmacy consultation reports
- Progress notes
- Nurses' notes
- Special rehabilitative service notes
- Laboratory and radiographic reports
- Discharge plan
- Miscellaneous papers

RECORDING TECHNIQUES

Notes should be brief but should communicate effectively to all staff members. Facts should be used rather than opinions. Prompt recording of all pertinent observations in the patient's record is the most reliable means of good communication between the physician and the staff. Each person involved in patient care needs current information about what others at the facility are doing, how the patient is reacting to treatment, his progress, and what treatment changes, if any, are recommended. The nursing service may use any simple technique for collecting information, such as temporary daily assignment cards (Figure 8) to check off routine items and significant occurrences. Information from these cards should then be entered on the patient's health record and the cards destroyed. Although the patient's total care plan has replaced the nursing care plan card in most facilities, it may still be used in some settings as a work sheet and is not a part of the permanent health record. When the patient is discharged, the card may be destroyed, all pertinent information having been recorded in the permanent record.

DAILY ASSIGNMENT CARD									
NAME AND ROOM	Bath T S B	Mouth Care	Fed	Up	Temp.	Pulse	Resp.	Turned	
BROWN. M	10	T	X		X	98	35	20	
JONES. J.	12	S	X		X	99	95	25	
SMITH, T	14	B	X	X		100	98	30	X
FIELD, O	16	S	X		X				
BEST, T.	18	S	X		X				
GREEN, M.	20	T	X		X				

FORM NH-165   PHYSICIANS RECORD CO., BERWYN, ILLINOIS
                     PRINTED IN U.S.A.

Form courtesy of Physicians' Record Company

FIG. 8 – DAILY ASSIGNMENT CARD

REVIEWING THE HEALTH RECORD

Medical record personnel in the long term care facility should develop procedures for the quantitative review of records while the patients are in the health care facility. This consists of checking that the required reports and signatures have been included in each record according to the prescribed time frames. Because the length of stay for long term care patients often extends to years, the system for review of records should focus on each stage of patient care so timely documentation is fostered. Time frames for such review are as follows: admission period, monthly review, quarterly review, annual review, special analysis at time of temporary transfer and return, and discharge review. Figures 9 and 10 are forms which reflect this continuous chart analysis; when a section is completed, for example admission, no further review of these documents is required.

If information or a signature is missing, reminders should be given to the appropriate staff member whose responsibility it is to enter the documentation or sign the information in the rec-

MEDICAL RECORD QUANTITATIVE ANALYSIS

PATIENT_____ DOB_____

ATTENDING PHYSICIAN_____ ADMISSION DATE_____

ADMITTED FROM_____

ADMISSION REVIEW – at end of first full week

	YES	NO	N/A	C O M M E N T
Complete Patient Identification				
Transfer Information Received				
Patient's Rights Acknowledged				
Consent to Treatment				
Power of Attorney Noted				
Patient Care Plan				
Discharge Plan				
Current Medical Findings				
Admission Diagnosis				
Physician Orders				
Physical Examination				
Chest X-Ray				
CBC and Urinalysis				

Form courtesy of Physicians' Record Company

FIG. 9 – QUANTITATIVE ANALYSIS REVIEW FORM (front)

ord. Members of the medical staff are responsible for review of records for quality of care. Medical record personnel can assist the physicians in this qualitative review by summarizing periodically the patterns of chart deficiencies and by making available summaries of the various legal and accrediting requirements for documentation.

PATIENT NAME_____

MONTHLY REVIEW

FILL IN MONTH AND YEAR								
Progress Notes Dated and Signed								
Physician Orders Dated and Signed								
Drug Regimen Review								
Nurses' Notes								
Use of Restraints								
Reason for PRN Meds.								
Unusual Incidents								
Dated and Signed								
Discharge Plan Updated								
Patient Care Plan Updated								

PERIODIC REVIEW as needed

Social Service Notes								
Rehabilitative Service Notes								
Diagnostic Service Reports								
Transfer to and from								
Dates_____								
Transfer to_____								
Information Sent/Received								

Date of Discharge_____   DISCHARGE REVIEW

Final Diagnosis	☐ Yes	☐ No	
Discharge Summary	☐ Yes	☐ No	
Death Certificate	☐ Not Applicable	☐ Yes	☐ No
Release of Body Receipt	☐ Not Applicable	☐ Yes	☐ No
Postmortem Summary	☐ Not Applicable	☐ Yes	☐ No

Form courtesy of Physicians' Record Company

FIG. 10 – QUANTITATIVE ANALYSIS REVIEW FORM (back of Fig. 9)

HEALTH RECORD FORMS

Chapter 9 "Forms Design and Control" gives principles of forms development for medical record documentation. These principles are as applicable to the long term care facility as to any other health care facility. One point of emphasis in forms development for the long term care facility involves quantity: because the patient population is relatively low (frequently under 100 beds per facility), large quantities of forms printed at one time could result in waste should some revision be necessary. A balance is needed between the cost saving gained by having a large quantity printed at one time and the usage rate over a one or two-year period.

FILING SYSTEMS

A filing system is necessary to protect records and to facilitate their location. An effective filing system for long term care records should enable one to identify a patient's record, to locate it quickly, and to retrieve it from any location in the facility. Because of the long period of stay, patient records will remain for weeks, months, and even years at the nurses' station until the time of discharge. Consequently, many basic principles of filing systems apply both to the inpatient records (e.g., charge-out system) as well as to the closed records which are processed for permanent filing upon discharge. The system should be that which does the job best; but whatever method is chosen, all parts of the record should be kept in one place as a unit.

This principle, filing all records in one place as a unit, has particular application in situations where a voluminous record is debriefed or thinned out. When material is removed from the active portion of the chart of an inpatient, the portion which is removed should be kept in the same location as the primary material. Thus, an active portion of the chart, for example, the current year's documentation, will remain in the in-house folder or chart holder; the debriefed portion will be marked as such and kept in a locked file at the nurses' station. At the time of discharge, both sections of the chart will be merged again. This same principle, one record in one location, applies to multiple charts for the same patient, as in the situation of a patient who has more than one admission to the facility.

ALPHABETIC VERSUS NUMERIC FILING

The records of patients who have been discharged may be filed either in alphabetic or numeric order. Alphabetic filing is suitable for a very small facility or one having a low patient turnover rate. In this system, the record is filed by last name, first name, and middle name *in strict alphabetical order.*

In large facilities or in those with short patient stay, numerical filing is recommended. In this system, the record is filed *in strict numerical sequence* by patient number.

In using the numerical filing method, a number must be assigned to the patient at the time of admission. Numbers in sequence are given to patients as they are admitted unless a unit numbering system is used. With the unit system, a number is assigned in sequence when a patient is first admitted, but for each readmission, that same number is used again. For example, a patient admitted for the first time might receive the number 127. If he is discharged from the facility and later readmitted, he would again be assigned number 127. His index card contains the unit number plus all dates of admission and readmission. This enables all records to be filed together.

In facilities not using the unit system, a new number is issued for each admission and readmission of a patient. The records created during each of these stays would be filed numerically but separately in the file.

A variation known as the serial-unit method of filing is sometimes used in long term care facilities where a new number is issued each time the patient is admitted, but records of previous admissions are always moved forward to the latest number. In situations where a new number is needed for each admission because of the needs of some related system, e.g., outside pharmacy contractual service needing a new number for each admission, this serial-unit system of filing fosters the unit record while meeting the needs of other components of the health care delivery system.

During the patient's stay, his record is kept at the nurses' station or in an area accessible to those making the notations. Section dividers are useful in designating each portion of the record, thus speeding the retrieval of specific information. While the patient is in the facility, the record may become too bulky for storage in the primary record holder. As noted earlier in this discussion, certain sections are moved to a secondary folder, marked accordingly in both the primary and secondary folders, with the secondary folder retained in an immediately accessible area.

Permanent storage of the records is facilitated through the use of file folders. Because activity levels for discharged records are relatively low, a lightweight folder is acceptable. See Chapter 10 for further discussion of filing methods and materials.

RETENTION OF RECORDS

Health records should be kept by the facility as long as required under the statute of limitations or state record-retention regulations. The licensure regulations for long term care facilities usually specify the retention period for a given state. The statute of limitations sets a time limit on initiating lawsuits involving patients and their treatment in the health facility. The time limit varies among states and for different types of lawsuits.

In the absence of a state or other regulation, the federal *Conditions of Participation* regulations apply for those facilities which treat Medicare/Medicaid patients; the retention period in these regulations is five years from the date of discharge, or, in the case of a minor, three years after the patient becomes of age under state law.

Review of pertinent state regulations, federal *Conditions of Participation*, and accrediting standards, coupled with a review of record usage after discharge, provides the chief executive officer and the medical record practitioner a sound basis for the development of a record retention schedule specific to the facility. When records are destroyed after the required retention period, basic information is retained permanently, including patient name, DOB, admission and discharge dates, names of responsible physicians, diagnoses and operations, operative reports and pathology reports if any, and discharge resume. Notice that records have been destroyed according to the retention/destruction policy is filed with the governing board so there is a formal, permanent record of this approved practice.

INDEXES

Just as in hospitals, indexes and registers are used in long term care facilities to locate information for a variety of purposes. They give summary information and lead to locating the health record. A patient index, a disease index, and admission and discharge registers are normally maintained in long term care facilities. The development and maintenance of indexes and registers are discussed fully in Chapter 13.

With records of long term care facility patients, the decision to assign detailed codes to the various diagnoses is based on the volume and frequency both of disease entities and on the use of the indexed material. When there is a low turnover rate in the facility, coupled with a small patient population and relatively few chronic disease entities, coding may not be necessary. An index of diseases can be maintained in conjunction with coding or merely by keeping a listing according to stated diagnoses and conditions.

DATA COLLECTION

The physician and members of the patient care and administrative staff of the long term care facility collect information needed for making decisions and judgments about services provided to patients and for furnishing information required by standard-setting and licensing agencies. Medical record personnel should routinely abstract data from health records of discharged and deceased patients and, as needed, from the inpatient records.

The following statistics have been found useful for meeting the needs of the long term care facility management: inpatient census, percentage of occupancy, length of stay, and death rate. The length of stay may be further refined in order to reflect those relatively short stays (a few months) as compared to the more typical length of stay which involves years. In facilities where there is a mix of relatively short convalescent and/or respite stay along with "balance of life" stay, such a differentiation provides more meaningful data. Where there is a pattern of transfer to and from acute care facilities for medical episodes, these patient movements may also be part of the statistical profile needed by management.

Statistics should be gathered in a uniform way using standard definitions. These standard definitions should be agreed upon in advance to permit comparisons among similar facilities. Data collection should be reviewed from time to time to weed out obsolete material and add new data if needed. Definitions for terminology used in many health care facilities are found in the *Glossary of Hospital Terms* published by the American

Medical Record Association. Chapter 14 of this text provides additional discussion of basic statistics and manner of compilation.

PATIENT MOVEMENTS

All events such as admissions, discharges, temporary hospital transfers, temporary leaves, including absence against medical advice, and deaths should be reported on the daily census report. Statistics on patient movements should be detailed for each patient care unit of the facility. Each day that the patient is on a temporary leave or temporary hospital transfer, his name must appear on the report. This daily census report should also include the number of patients present each day. A monthly tabulation of these figures is compiled providing a basis for further statistical computations.

UTILIZATION REVIEW

The objective of the utilization review function is to maintain high quality patient care and utilize the appropriate level of health care at the proper time at an acceptable cost. Utilization review is required for Medicare and Medicaid patients by the *Conditions of Participation: Skilled Nursing Facilities.* These standards designate two areas of focus for such studies: medical care evaluation studies relating to the pattern of care provided by the facility and review of extended duration cases. The studies relating to patterns of care may include all patients in the facility regardless of payment source. The review of extended duration stays is mandated for those patients who receive Medicare/Medicaid benefits.

The facility should develop a written utilization review plan which includes a specific committee to carry out the designated functions, a process for review of individual cases for extended duration, a system for the carrying out of studies concerning overall patterns of care, and procedures to carry out the necessary follow-up actions resulting from such reviews.

The medical record documentation in each patient record is the primary basis of evaluation for individual and patterned studies. There must be sufficient data in the records, with appropriate time frames, to support the rationale for extended stay. For the chronic, long stay patient, this continued review is as detailed as for a relatively short stay patient. For this reason, there can be no letdown in the quality of documentation simply because the patient has entered a lengthy episode of care, possibly involving a year or more.

Both the regulatory agencies and the accrediting bodies have detailed material concerning utilization review committee function and processes. These materials provide a facility with a pattern which can be adopted to meet its needs for medical care evaluation processes.

RELEASE OF INFORMATION

The patient health record, part of the doctor-patient relationship, is considered a confidential document. All employees of the facility are responsible for assuring that no unauthorized person ever takes any of these records out of the file, reads, copies, or otherwise tampers with them. Some individuals are authorized to access this information, and medical record personnel should be ready to make it available to them. Since legal requirements and restrictions about release of medical information vary from state to state, the facility should have a local attorney outline basic rules to follow. Many component state associations of the American Medical Record Association have compiled handbooks for the release of information for their respective states; these resources are available from such professional groups. Using the pertinent legal advice and related professional association material, the administrative staff, including the medical record practitioner, should develop a policy on the release of information for the facility. Chapter 17 of this text provides a detailed review of pertinent points, including record ownership, disclosure of information, court subpoena and/or deposition processes, and patient access.

Two areas in the practice of release of information in the long term care facility deserve particular attention. The first is the processing of information when a patient is being transferred from the facility for continuing care. In these instances, AMRA's position statement on "Confidentiality of Patient Health Information" specifies that a release is not necessary since the information is being released to another health care provider currently involved in the care of the patient. The transfer form should be completed to go with the patient. The second point, also associated with the transfer of patients from one facility to another, involves specificity of authorization. The facility will have requested, with authorization, materials from health care facilities which have treated the patient in the past. When material is released from the present facility's record, the only material which it is empowered to release is that generated during the course of treatment at the facility. In other words, there should be no rerelease of information obtained from previous settings. The patient's authorization covers only the record as generated in the course of treatment at each specific facility. Should another facility need such prior information, it is its duty to obtain the necessary consent of the patient and to set in motion the necessary procedures for obtaining such material.

SUMMARY

Because medical records are so important to the successful operation and management of long term care facilities, an appropriate record system should be developed for each facility. While plans can draw on the experiences of hospitals, clinics and other specialized facilities, individualized systems are advisable so specific needs are met. This chapter has defined the minimum standards for long term care records. In addition to studying this material, those engaged in maintaining medical records in a long term care facility are advised to read other chapters pertinent to specific areas of medical record science.

STUDY QUESTIONS

1. Differentiate among the following terms: life care center, skilled nursing facility, and convalescent care.
2. State the legal, regulatory, and accrediting agencies. Which ones are mandatory? Which are voluntary?
3. Indicate the key content for the following:
    a. transfer or referral statement
    b. physician's admitting evaluation
    c. total patient care plan
    d. nurses' progress notes
    e. physician discharge summary
4. Delineate the time frame for various elements of medical record documentation in terms of
    a. admission processes
    b. monthly and/or periodic activities

c. patient transfer to or from the facility

d. discharge processes

5. State the general purpose of utilization review and delineate two major functions of such review.

REFERENCES

Accreditation Manual for Long Term Care Facilities, 1981 Edition. Joint Commission on Accreditation of Hospitals.

"Confidentiality of Patient Health Information." A Position Statement of the American Medical Record Association. American Medical Record Association, 1981.

Consulting: Another Dimension, Part I – Principles of Consulting. American Medical Record Association, 1977.

Consulting: Another Dimension, Part II – Long Term Care. American Medical Record Association, 1979.

Developing Policies and Procedures for Long Term Care Institutions. American Hospital Association, 1975.

FINNEGAN, RITA. *ICD-9-CM Coding for Long Term Care: Learner's Manual*. Chicago, Illinois: AMRA, 1980.

——. *ICD-9-CM Coding for Long Term Care Personnel: Instructor's Manual*. Chicago, Illinois: AMRA, 1980.

"Long Term Health Care: Minimum Data Set." Report of the National Committee on Vital and Health Statistics. Hyattsville, Maryland: National Center for Health Statistics, 1980 (DHHS No. PHS 80-1158).

LOWE, MARY ANN. *Patient Care Plans in Long Term Care Facilities*. Ypsilanti, Michigan: Nursing Home Publishing Associates, 1983.

Modified Problem Oriented Medical Records in the Long Term Care Facility. American Medical Record Association, 1975.

Nursing Care Requirements in the States of the Union. Milwaukee, Wisconsin: National Geriatrics Society, 1983.

Quest for Quality: A Self-Appraisal Guide for Long Term Care Facilities. Washington, D.C.: American Health Care Association, 1982.

U.S. Department of Health and Human Services, Social Security Administration, "Subpart K: Conditions of Participation – Skilled Nursing Facilities."

chapter *6*

MENTAL HEALTH RECORDS

HISTORY OF MENTAL HEALTH CARE IN THE UNITED STATES

Mental health care was almost nonexistent in the United States until the early 19th century. One of the earliest pioneers was Dorothea Dix, who worked hard to improve the lot of mental health patients and the facilities in which they were housed. It was due to her persistence that the government enacted federal legislation which resulted in granting states land upon which mental hospitals could be built. These institutions, many of which are still in existence, served the population for many decades.

Almost one hundred years later, in 1916, the National Institute of Mental Health (NIMH) was created as an agency of the Federal Government. Studies at that time and later pointed up the fact that existing facilities were used mostly for holding the mentally ill or treating individuals in crisis situations, and that the great majority of patients needed more active care.

A major study entitled "Action for Mental Health" was published in 1960 and resulted in the passage of the Community Mental Health Centers Act of 1963. Its goal was to establish multiservice programs which would meet different and multiple needs of mental health patients. Several hundred Community Mental Health Centers have been established which provide treatment for mental illness in all of its various forms. These centers can be free-standing, under one roof, under several roofs, be connected with a hospital, or variations of these.

Public Law 94-63, passed July 29, 1975, is known as the "Special Health Revenue Sharing Act of 1975" and contains amendments to previous acts involving such areas as Health Revenue Sharing and Community Mental Health Centers. The amendments cover many items and relate specifically to services offered, comprehensive mental health services, and reimbursement.

Title XVIII of the Social Security Act provides payment for medical services in mental health facilities for persons over age 65 or under age 18. Title XIX provides assistance to states (at their discretion) for their mental health care programs. Both of these acts bring into focus reimbursement, Utilization Review, and the *Conditions of Participation for Hospitals.* Thus, it is concern for the mentally ill and the influences of legislation that have brought about the emphasis on the need for better care of patients and documentation of that care.

The first set of JCAH standards for psychiatric programs was published in 1972. Over the next several years, special standards were developed and published for child and adolescent psychiatric programs, for alcohol and drug abuse rehabilitation programs, and for programs treating the developmentally disabled.

With the movement in the late 1970s toward one set of standards for facilities providing multiprograms, standards for adult psychiatric, child and adolescent, and alcoholism and drug abuse programs were combined into one manual called the *Consolidated Standards Manual* (CSM). The latest edition of this manual now includes standards for mentally retarded and developmentally disabled programs as well. Effective October, 1987, all facilities which provide psychiatric care and are licensed as a hospital will be required to be surveyed under the *Accreditation Manual for Hospitals* (AMH). Standards for psychiatric programs have been incorporated into the AMH in those areas where the needs are different. Facilities which provide psychiatric care but are not licensed as a hospital such as free-standing alcoholism and drug abuse rehabilitation programs and community mental health centers will continue to be surveyed under the CSM. Psychiatric facilities licensed as a hospital have the option of being surveyed under either CSM or AMH standards until October, 1987.

Although there are certain characteristics which are unique to mental health records, general medical record documentation requirements and record-keeping practices are applicable. In the mental health care facility, the medical record practitioner will be responsible for many of the same activities that take place in the acute care general hospital. He should be familiar with the requirements for utilization review and patient care evaluation, the JCAH standards, and state licensing requirements. In addition, he should be prepared to provide appropriate service to the medical staff in its committee activities and to the clinical staff in its clinical charting activities. The medical record practitioner will also be responsible for the general administration of the medical record department.

In this chapter, the special types of record documentation that are required will be discussed. Emphasis will also be placed on record-keeping practices that are of more significance in mental health facilities than in acute care facilities. Much of the information presented regarding documentation requirements is based on the JCAH's *Consolidated Standards Manual for Child, Adolescent, and Adult Psychiatric, Alcoholism, and Drug Abuse Facilities and Facilities Serving the Mentally Retarded/ Developmentally Disabled*. The medical record practitioner should have access to these standards as well as the Medicare *Conditions of Participation*. The state mental health code should also be available for review of state documentation and record-keeping requirements.

CONTENT OF MENTAL HEALTH RECORDS

According to the American Psychiatric Association, the mental health record should document the evaluation, treatment, and course of the patient's illness. It also provides a means of communication between physician and other staff members contributing to the patient's care. The mental health record is also a basic source of information for study and evaluation of the care rendered and for reimbursement by third-party payers. The mental health record should contain all pertinent clinical information, which at a minimum should consist of:

- identification data
- source of referral
- reason for referral
- patient's legal status
- all appropriate consents for admission, treatment, evaluation, and aftercare

- admitting psychiatric diagnosis
- psychiatric history
- record of the complete assessment, including the complaints of others regarding the patient as well as the patient's comments
- medical history, report of physical examination, and record of all medication prescribed
- provisional diagnoses based upon assessment which includes intercurrent diseases as well as the psychiatric diagnoses
- written individualized treatment plan
- documentation of the course of treatment and all evaluations and examinations
- multidisciplinary progress notes related to the goals and objectives outlined in the treatment plan
- appropriate documentation related to special treatment procedures
- updates to the treatment plan as a result of the contained assessments detailed in the progress notes
- multidisciplinary case conferences and consultation notes which include date of conference or consultation, recommendations made, and actions taken
- information on any unusual occurrences such as: treatment complications, accidents or injuries to the patient, morbidity, death of a patient, procedures that place the patient at risk or cause unusual pain
- correspondence related to the patient, including all letters and dated notations of telephone conversations relevant to the patient's treatment
- discharge or termination summary
- plan for follow-up care and documentation of its implementation
- individualized aftercare or post treatment plan

ASSESSING THE PATIENT

Each program should conduct a complete assessment of each patient. Assessment is the process of gathering and ordering of facts about a patient by means of interviewing the patient and significant others, observing the patient, performing physical and mental examinations of the patient, and conducting other diagnostic tests. The purpose of the assessment is to identify the patient's needs during the current course of treatment and to serve as a basis for development of the patient's individualized treatment plan. The assessment should include identification of physical, emotional, behavioral, social, recreational, legal, vocational, and nutritional needs.

PHYSICAL ASSESSMENT

The physical assessment should include a medical, alcohol and drug history, and an appropriate laboratory workup. In inpatient programs, a physical examination must be completed within 24 hours of admission. In other types of programs, the need for a physical examination is determined by the physician; and the rationale for not conducting a complete examination must be documented. In programs serving children, adolescents, and mentally retarded/developmentally disabled patients, motor development and functioning; speech, language and hearing functioning; visual functioning; and the patient's immunization status must also be assessed.

EMOTIONAL AND BEHAVIORAL ASSESSMENT

An emotional or behavioral assessment should be completed and documented in the patient's record. The following items should be included:

- history and previous emotional, behavioral, and substance-abuse problems and treatment;
- the patient's current emotional and behavioral functioning;
- a direct psychiatric evaluation, when indicated;
- a mental status examination appropriate to the age of the patient, when indicated;
- psychological assessments, when indicated; and
- other functional evaluations of language, self-care, and social affective and visual-motor functioning, when indicated.

SOCIAL ASSESSMENT

The social assessment should include information related to the patient's environment and home; religion; childhood history; military service history; financial status; the social, peer group, and environmental setting from which the patient comes; and the patient's family circumstances including the family constellation and current living situation.

RECREATIONAL ASSESSMENT

An activities assessment should include information relating to the patient's skills, talents, aptitudes, and interests.

LEGAL ASSESSMENT

A legal assessment is not always conducted, but when appropriate it should include a legal history and a discussion to determine if the patient's legal situation will affect the patient's progress in treatment. If it is determined that it will, it should be included in the patient's problems to be addressed.

VOCATIONAL ASSESSMENT

A vocational assessment is not always conducted, but when appropriate it should include a vocational history, educational history which includes academic and vocational training, and a discussion with the patient regarding his past work experiences, attitudes toward work, and possibilities for future education, training, and employment.

NUTRITIONAL ASSESSMENT

A nutritional assessment is not always conducted, but when appropriate it should be documented. Patients being treated for eating disorders or patients having physical conditions which require special diets should have a nutritional assessment.

OTHER ASSESSMENTS

In addition to the initial assessments just described, there are circumstances which arise during the course of the patient's treatment which require special assessment. Examples of these are:

- − prior to the implementation of seclusion
- − prior to the application of restraints
- − prior to the use of electroconvulsive therapy
- − after a therapeutic pass

Documentation requirements for these and others are discussed in the Special Therapies section of this chapter.

Results of all assessments conducted should be documented in the patient's mental health record. They should reflect the fundamental needs of the patient and should include appropriate multidisciplinary clinical input. Assessments serve as the foundation for the development of the patient's individualized treatment plan.

TREATMENT PLAN

The JCAH requires that each patient have a documented plan of treatment. The AMH standards do not define the elements of the plan, however, the CSM standards describe in very specific terms what should be the content of a treatment plan and the frequency of documentation. Medicare also requires an individualized treatment plan in its *Conditions of Participation for Psychiatric Facilities.*

CONTENT OF THE TREATMENT PLAN

Goals and Objectives: The treatment plan should contain specific goals which the patient must achieve and which are based upon the patient's need as derived from the initial assessments. The treatment plan should also contain specific objectives which relate to the goals and should include expected achievement dates. These should be written in measurable terms in order to assess the patient's progress in attaining them. Setting goals and objectives in measurable terms (1) assures that each patient has an individualized treatment plan; (2) requires specific action which leaves little room for guessing; (3) communicates the same goal expectation to all staff members who work with the patient; and (4) enables those involved in the ongoing treatment of the patient, or other qualified personnel, to determine what treatment is being carried out.

Treatment Modalities: The treatment plan should describe the services, activities, and programs planned for the patient; should specify the staff members assigned to carry out the planned treatment; and should specify the frequency of the treatment modalities.

FREQUENCY OF DOCUMENTATION

Inpatient, Residential, and Partial-Day Programs: A *preliminary* treatment plan should be developed upon admission based upon the intake assessment. An *initial* treatment plan should be developed within 72 hours of admission based upon the assessments conducted within that time frame. This plan is used to implement immediate treatment. If the patient's stay exceeds 10 days, a *master* plan should be developed by the multidisciplinary treatment team based upon the comprehensive assessments of the patient's needs. This master plan should be reviewed within 40 days of admission and every 60 days thereafter for the first year of treatment and then every 3 months. All reviews should be conducted more frequently if clinically indicated, and all plans should be updated as needed.

Outpatient Programs: An *initial* treatment plan should be developed at intake based upon assessment of the patient's presenting problems, physical health, emotional status, and behavioral status. If the number of patient visits is more than 10, a *master* plan should be developed and should be based upon a comprehensive assessment of the patient's needs. This master plan should be reviewed and updated as needed every 20 visits or every six months, whichever comes first.

Programs Treating the Mentally Retarded/Developmentally Disabled: Requirements for preliminary, initial, and master treatment plans, and review and update of the master plan are identical to those for residential programs. In addition, when a patient has attained majority or is emancipated, there should be documentation that the treatment plan was reviewed by a multidisciplinary treatment team and that the following were considered:

- civil and legal rights; and
- the need for the patient to remain in the program.

OTHER REQUIREMENTS

The patient should be involved in the development of his treatment plan, and this should be documented in the patient's

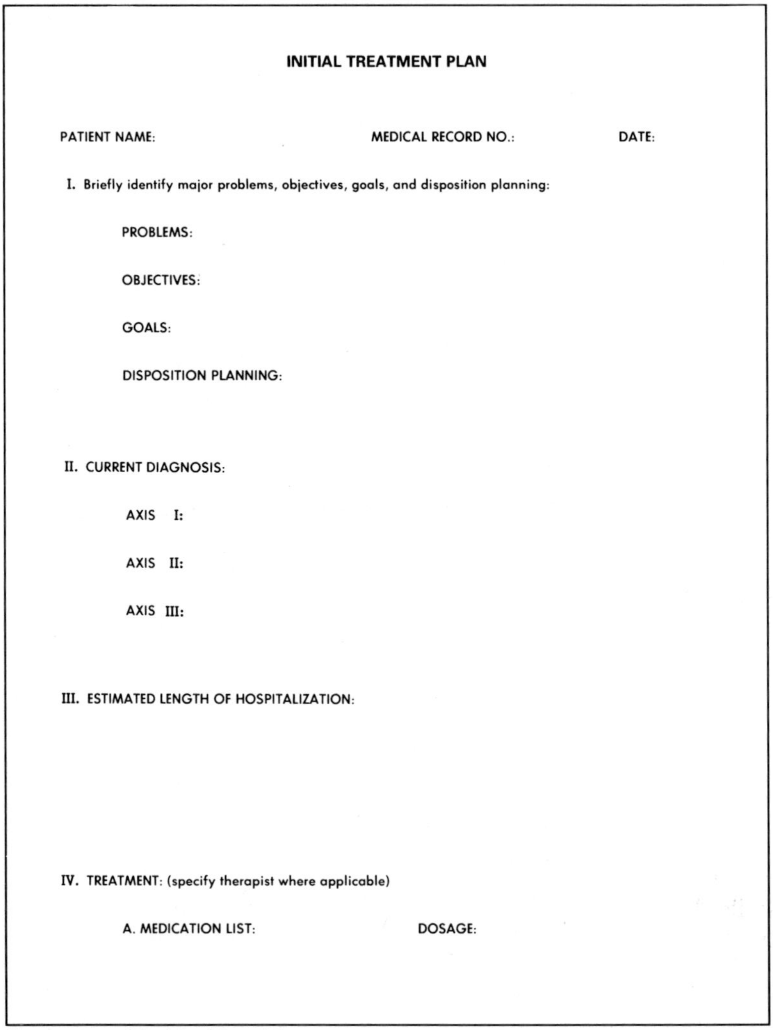

INITIAL TREATMENT PLAN

PATIENT NAME: MEDICAL RECORD NO.: DATE:

I. Briefly identify major problems, objectives, goals, and disposition planning:

PROBLEMS:

OBJECTIVES:

GOALS:

DISPOSITION PLANNING:

II. CURRENT DIAGNOSIS:

AXIS I:

AXIS II:

AXIS III:

III. ESTIMATED LENGTH OF HOSPITALIZATION:

IV. TREATMENT: (specify therapist where applicable)

A. MEDICATION LIST: DOSAGE:

Form courtesy of Physicians' Record Company

FIG. 1 – INITIAL TREATMENT PLAN (front)

record. The family or significant others should also be involved in the treatment plan, and this, too, should be documented.

In reviewing the patient's mental health record, one should

be able to determine from the treatment plan (1) what is being treated; (2) what treatments are being used; (3) the goals of treatment; and (4) who is responsible for carrying out the vari-

```
B. ☐ MEDICAL WORKUP:
      ☐ PHYSICAL EXAM:
      ☐ LABORATORY/X-RAY:
      ☐ OTHER:

C. ☐ PSYCHOLOGICAL TESTING:

D. ☐ SPECIAL PROCEDURES AND/OR CONSULTATIONS:

E. ☐ SCHOOL OR EDUCATIONAL EVALUATION:

F. ☐ SOCIAL WORK: (i.e., special evaluation, disposition planning, etc.)
      _____
      _____
      _____
      _____

G. ☐ ACTIVITIES THERAPY: (include goals and objectives)
      _____
      _____
      _____
      _____

H. ☐ NURSING CARE: (include goals and objectives)
      _____
      _____
      _____
      _____

I. ☐ THERAPY:
      1. INDIVIDUAL: ☐ Brief  ☐ Full Sessions____times per wk. with_____
      2. GROUP:_____times per wk. with_____
      3. FAMILY:_____times per wk. with_____

DATE:_____         SIGNATURE:_____
```

Form courtesy of Physicians' Record Company

FIG. 2 – INITIAL TREATMENT PLAN (back of Fig. 1)

ous treatments. The treatment plan should also clearly state the criteria, written in measurable terms, for termination of treatment services. (See sample forms in Figures 1, 2, 3, and 4.)

PROGRESS NOTES

Documentation of the patient's progress should be contained in the patient's mental health record. The progress notes are

---

MASTER TREATMENT PLAN

WEEK __1__

PATIENT NAME:_____ DATE:_____

TREATMENT TEAM:
Psychiatrist: Primary Nurse:
Social Worker: Activities Therapist:
Educational Liaison: Dietary Consultant:
CD Counselor:

FORMULATION:

DIAGNOSIS: AXIS   I:
                AXIS II:
                AXIS III:

NEEDS ASSESSMENT AND TREATMENT METHODS: (Emotional, Behavioral, Medical, Family, Social, Educational, Vocational, Activity.)

EXPECTED DATES OF ACHIEVEMENT

I. GOAL:
          OBJECTIVES:

  TREATMENT METHODS — Frequency — Person or Discipline Responsible:

II. GOAL:
          OBJECTIVES:

  TREATMENT METHODS — Frequency - Person or Discipline Responsible:

                    (Continue goals and objectives if applicable.)

DIAGNOSTIC QUESTIONS AND PROCEDURES: (Include specific unresolved diagnostic problems and techniques to be utilized to refine these.)

                                    _____
                                              SIGNATURE

Form courtesy of Physicians' Record Company

FIG. 3 – MASTER TREATMENT PLAN

considered to be part of the treatment plan. The progress notes should include documentation of implementation of the treatment plan, treatments provided, and the patient's response to that treatment. Also, revisions and updating of the treatment plan should be documented in the progress notes.

Progress notes are used to review the progress of the patient

---

REVISION OF MASTER TREATMENT PLAN

WEEK_____

PATIENT NAME:_____ DATE:_____

TREATMENT TEAM:
Psychiatrist: Primary Nurse:
Social Worker: Activities Therapist:
Educational Liaison: Dietary Consultant:
CD Counselor:

FORMULATION:

DIAGNOSIS: AXIS   I:
           AXIS II:
           AXIS III:

NEEDS ASSESSMENT AND TREATMENT METHODS:

EXPECTED DATES OF ACHIEVEMENT (New)

I. GOAL:
        OBJECTIVES:

   STATUS IN ACHIEVING GOAL AND OBJECTIVES:
   TREATMENT METHODS – Frequency – Person or Discipline Responsible:

EXPECTED DATES OF ACHIEVEMENT (New)

II. GOAL:
        OBJECTIVES:

   STATUS IN ACHIEVING GOAL AND OBJECTIVES:
   TREATMENT METHODS – Frequency - Person or Discipline Responsible:
                       (Continue goals and objectives if applicable.)
DIAGNOSTIC QUESTIONS AND PROCEDURES: (Include specific unresolved diagnostic problems and techniques to be utilized to refine these.)

DISCHARGE PLANNING: (Need for continued hospitalization, expected length of stay, aftercare planning.)
        METHOD:
PATIENT AND FAMILY PARTICIPATION IN AND RESPONSE TO THE TREATMENT PLAN:

_____
                    ATTENDING PSYCHIATRIST

Form courtesy of Physicians' Record Company

FIG. 4 – REVISION OF MASTER TREATMENT PLAN

in multidisciplinary case conferences. Records of these conferences are documented in the progress notes or on special forms designed for that purpose. Notations should include persons in attendance. All entries should be properly dated and signed.

DISCHARGE SUMMARY AND PLANS FOR AFTERCARE

The discharge summary and plans for aftercare are also included in the patient's record as part of the treatment plan. The discharge summary should be completed and filed in the patient's record within 15 days of discharge. The discharge summary should include a clinical resume that summarizes the following:

- results of the initial assessment and admitting diagnosis
- significant findings
- course and progress of the patient with regard to each identified clinical problem
- clinical course of the patient's treatment
- final assessment including the general observations and understanding of the patient's condition initially, during treatment, and at discharge
- recommendations and arrangements for further treatment including prescribed medications and aftercare
- planning for and securing of living arrangements for the mentally retarded/developmentally disabled patient appropriate to the individual's level of functioning
- final primary and secondary diagnoses

When appropriate, a written aftercare plan that provides reasonable assurance of continued care shall be developed with the participation of the patient, and when indicated, the family, or guardian.

SPECIAL THERAPIES

Mental health care facilities sometimes utilize procedures not generally found in the acute care hospital setting. Examples of special procedures are use of restraints, seclusion, psychosurgery, electroconvulsive therapy, the use of unusual medications or experimental drugs, therapeutic passes, and behavior modification techniques.

When it becomes necessary or desirable to treat a patient utilizing special procedures, the rationale for its use and the clinical indications must be clearly stated in the patient's record. The record should also contain evidence that indications for the special procedure have been reviewed by the head of the professional staff, or other appropriate persons, prior to implementation.

SECLUSION AND RESTRAINT

If a patient is to be placed in seclusion or in restraints, the physician must first conduct a clinical assessment of the patient. This must be documented in the patient's record and should include the clinical justifications for the use of seclusion and/or restraint and a summary of what less-restrictive intervention was tried without success necessitating seclusion and/or restraint. A written order must also be entered in the record prior to restraint or seclusion, and it shall be time limited and shall not exceed 24 hours. In an emergency, restraint or seclusion may be utilized by trained, clinically privileged staff. However, the assessment and order for the use of emergency restraint or seclusion, which must be documented in the record, may not exceed one hour. The physician staff member's oral order shall be required if restraint or seclusion is to be continued. It is further required that staff members provide appropriate attention to these patients at 15-minute intervals. This should also be documented in the patient's mental health record. It is important to remember that restraint or seclusion requires clinical justification and should be used only to prevent a patient from injuring himself, others, or from causing serious damage to the facility. Seclusion might also be used to prevent *serious* disruption of the therapeutic environment. Seclusion and restraint should never be implemented as punishment or for the convenience of the staff. It is generally recommended that seclusion should be considered as a viable treatment procedure before restraints. Seclusion, without the use of restraints, is a less restrictive alternative to restraints which also incorporates seclusion for the safety of the restrained patient. All use of seclusion and restraint should be reported, on a daily basis, to the head of the professional staff; and he or his designee should review each case and investigate unusual or possibly unwarranted patterns of utilization.

ECT AND OTHER THERAPIES

Electroconvulsive therapy, psychosurgery, behavior modification procedures that use painful stimuli, and the use of experimental or unusual drugs require the written informed consent of the patient or appropriate legally responsible person before the procedure can be carried out. The consents are to be made part of the patient's record. Consents for any of these procedures may be withdrawn, verbally or in writing, at any time.

Therapeutic passes are an important treatment modality for mental health patients. Therapeutic passes are used to assess the patient's ability to function outside of the safe and secure hospital environment, to assess the patient's ability to appropriately respond to daily activities and stimuli, to augment the patient's treatment plan by providing for enhancement of socialization and to foster a sense of freedom and self-determination. They are also used to allow the patient an opportunity at resuming role responsibility and to foster repair of ruptured or difficult family relationships. Therapeutic passes should be well documented in the patient's record. Documentation should include the justification for the therapeutic pass and the patient's response to the therapeutic pass. The proper use of therapeutic passes in relation to the patient's treatment plan may prevent premature discharge and the necessity of a readmission to continue treatment.

Behavior modification programs based on point systems, token economies, and/or level systems are becoming popular in the treatment of adolescent patients. These programs are usually very specific in relation to the patient's behavior and progress in the program. The patient's record should document the patient's progress within the program and in relation to his illness.

Patient's rights are becoming an important issue in the treatment of mental health patients. It is extremely important that the patient's medical record document any denials of patient's rights. Documentation should include the "good cause" for denial and the restoration of the right(s) when good cause no longer exists.

The medical record practitioner needs to be aware of any state laws which may place further constraints on the use of these types of procedures. He should be fully informed of state requirements for consents and other documentation. The mental health code of a particular state is usually a good source for this type of information.

RECORD DOCUMENTATION

PROBLEM-ORIENTED VERSUS GOAL-ORIENTED VERSUS SOURCE-ORIENTED

Problem-oriented, goal-oriented, source-oriented, or a combination of one or more of these documentation systems may be useful in mental health facilities. Source-oriented is probably the least favorable of the three. In the source-oriented record, information relevant to any one of a patient's problems, or goals, is scattered at random in admission notes, social histories, progress notes, nurses' notes, or in x-ray and laboratory reports. The record becomes bulky, is unorganized, and, as a result, retrieval of vital information is both difficult and frustrating. Communication among treatment team members is hampered, and ultimately patient care is negatively affected.

| 3-11 Shift: | Patient attended all activities throughout shift. Behavior was appropriate and she appeared in good spirits. She appeared sullen and sat alone in the corner of the patient lounge following the multifamily group. She did not interact with the other patients in the discussion of the TV show being watched and appeared to be reading a magazine instead. At 11 P.M. the patient was observed scratching at right wrist with a staple. She refused to talk about it at first, but then admitted she was "angry with my mom because she didn't show up for family group — I hate her." Scratches are superficial, area cleansed and doctor notified. Patient is on close observation with 15-min. checks and staff is working with her on discussing feelings rather than acting them out. |

FIG. 5 – SOURCE-ORIENTED (NARRATIVE) PROGRESS NOTE

In a goal-oriented and problem-oriented approach, problems are identified and numbered. Treatment plans identify the problems by number, and specific goals are decided upon. Plans of

---

Example A: Same as Example B but incorporating steps in treatment plan.

3-12-85   Goal #2: Dealing with angry feelings.

Observation (O): Joe related in group how he used anger to distance himself from others. He said that he could never talk with his parents as they never listened to him, and this made him feel helpless. "Lashing out" then made him feel better. Joe stated he is willing to work on this in group therapy.

Plan (P): Joe will undergo the "insult-compliment" exercise in the next group psychotherapy session and will give group members feedback on this experience.

3-19-85   G: Dealing with angry feelings.

O: Joe has shared with the other group members his historical and current pattern in dealing with anger. He is able to apply his insights in the group and appears to be trying out new behaviors regarding the expressions of his negative emotions. Group members gave him very supportive and insightful feedback. While somewhat defensive initially, Joe heard and responded well to the feedback.

P: Joe will relate at least five negative emotions to various group members relative to group members' behavior by 3-26-85.

FIG. 6 – GOAL-ORIENTED PROGRESS NOTE

action for each of the problems are established and related to the various disciplines. This allows members of the multidisciplinary team to document in relation to problems, goals, or both. In mental health, documentation related to the patient's strengths, program participation, and daily functioning are important in assessing the patient's need for continued treatment, the effectiveness of the treatment plan, and the progress of treatment. All members of the team participate in monitoring and documenting the patient's progress in the treatment plans and progress notes. It is important for the record to document the patient's response to treatment in relation to the various disciplines involved. Patients may be responding in one area and not another. Examples of the various documentation systems can be found in Figures 5, 6, 7, and 8.

Example B: Simple Format

3-12-85   Goal #2: Will deal more effectively with angry feelings and upsetting emotions.
Movement Toward Goal (MTG): Joe related in group how he used anger to distance himself from others. He said that he could never talk with his parents as they never listened to him, and this made him feel helpless. "Lashing out" then made him feel better. Joe stated he is willing to work on this in group therapy.

3-18-85   Goal #2: Dealing with angry feelings.
MTG: Joe has shared with the other group members his historical and current pattern in dealing with anger. He is able to apply his insights in the group and appears to be trying out new behaviors regarding the expressions of his negative emotions. Group members gave him very supportive and insightful feedback. While somewhat defensive initially, Joe heard and responded well to the feedback.

FIG. 7 – GOAL-ORIENTED PROGRESS NOTE

Problem #1: Self-Mutilative Behavior

S: "I don't want to talk about it – leave me alone."

O: Observed to be scratching at R. wrist with staple from magazine at 11 P.M. Three superficial 1-inch scratches on inner aspect of R. wrist with little bleeding. Area cleansed with soap and water. Patient affect: angry and sullen and refused to discuss incident. After 15 minutes 1:1 was able to state anger that mother did not show up for multifamily group tonight. Talked about feeling let down by mother and was able to contract that she would notify staff if she felt upset again.

A: Angry and hurt at mother. Feels that she doesn't get enough attention from mother and that mother doesn't care about her. Acting out rage by hurting self. Does not appear to be actively suicidal at present. Continues to show poor impulse control and difficulty expressing self with words.

P: Avoid secondary gains for scratching behavior. Matter-of-fact approach. Focus her to discuss what she was feeling before incident. Reinforce self-disclosure. 15-min. checks. Watch for infection and keep scratches clean.

FIG. 8 – PROBLEM-ORIENTED PROGRESS NOTE

REVIEW PROCESS

The medical record practitioner should assume responsibility for review of patient records. In an inpatient acute care psychiatric facility, this review should be conducted at least weekly while the patient is hospitalized. In an outpatient or partial-day program, this review should be conducted at least monthly. In a residential or long term psychiatric setting, this review should be conducted at least quarterly. A final review should take place within one working day of the patient's discharge. The focus of review is on quantity, timeliness, and quality of clinical documentation.

The medical record practitioner should develop a form to assist in the review process. The form should list all items that are to be checked. When in the process of developing the list, refer to the facility's medical staff bylaws, rules, and regulations; the JCAH standards under which the facility is accredited; and the Medicare *Conditions of Participation* for medical record documentation requirements. The state's mental health code should also be consulted. Also, any other special quality assurance documentation requirements of the mental health facility can be included on the chart review.

RELEASE OF INFORMATION

The medical record practitioner is responsible for the development of policies and procedures which safeguard the patient's right to privacy. The policies and procedures developed should specify the conditions under which information may be disclosed, who may release information under various circumstances, and the procedures for releasing information from the patient's medical record.

The policies and procedures for the release of confidential patient information must take into consideration the applicable state laws, JCAH requirements, and the federal regulations related to alcohol and drug abuse patients. It is recommended that all policies and procedures be developed to meet the most stringent laws or regulations which might apply to patient information within the facility. Policies and procedures which differ for different types of patients may make it possible to breach patient confidentiality simply by notifying a requestor that a more stringent requirement exists for a particular patient.

Federal regulations pertaining to the confidentiality of alcohol and drug abuse records are found in Title 42, Part 2 of the Federal Regulations. The Federal Regulations are very specific and stringent in regard to the release of confidential patient information.

CONSENTS

All consents for release of information are to be made part of the patient's record. The date the information was actually released, and the person who released the information should also be included in the record.

When developing policies and procedures for release of information and consent forms for the mental health facility, the medical record practitioner should consult the mental health code of the state in which he practices. State requirements and/or state mental health requirements are sometimes beyond the standards of the JCAH and regulations of the federal government. It is also important to be familiar with which laws, rules, and regulations pertaining to the release of confidential patient medical records exempt psychiatric and/or substance abuse records for those specific provisions and requirements.

Many states have developed laws related to access to the medical record by the patient or his authorized representative. It is important that these laws be carefully reviewed to determine the extent to which they apply to psychiatric and/or substance abuse records. Specific policies and procedures should be developed for implementing patient access requirements to psychiatric and substance abuse records or portions of general acute records that include psychiatric or substance abuse information.

In addition to written procedures for release of information, the medical record practitioner is responsible for the security of the mental health records. Policies should be developed indicating who, within the facility, has access to records and under what conditions access is allowed. For example, there should be a policy which states that only those members of the treatment team *involved* in the care and treatment of the patient should have access to the patient's medical records. Records should be stored in locked filing cabinets or secured filing areas. When records are removed from the files, a referencing system should permit location of the mental health record at any time. Records removed from the files should be removed only to other secured areas or should be returned to the permanent file area at the end of each day.

The JCAH requires that mental health records be retained at least five years from the date the case is officially closed. However, the medical record practitioner should also check the state mental health code for state record-retention requirements. For example, some states require that records be kept for a specified number of years after competency has been established, and most states require that the records of minors be kept at least until one year after that minor has reached the age of majority.

In Chapter 17 the contents of a valid consent form for the release of medical information are delineated.

SUMMARY

In this specialty area of patient care there have been profound changes taking place in the care of the mentally ill, especially in the last two decades. New treatment methods require fresh approaches to clinical record documentation. Psychiatric hospitals face continued pressure to cut costs while continuing to provide quality care. More and more third-party payers, surveying agencies, and other patient care reviewers are demanding access to patient information. Medical record practitioners practicing in mental health facilities have the opportunity to apply their skills in meeting these new challenges and to develop more efficient ways of documenting patient mental health care.

STUDY QUESTIONS

1. What are the minimum data requirements for mental health records?
2. What elements are included in the complete assessment of the mental health patient?
3. What are the elements of an individualized treatment plan? How frequently is documentation required?
4. When a patient is placed in seclusion, what data must be recorded in the patient's record?

5. Explain the differences between source-oriented, problem-oriented, and goal-oriented documentation.
6. What is the focus of record review of mental health records? What is the frequency of review in the various settings?
7. What does the JCAH require for a consent to be valid in a mental health facility? How does this differ from the Federal Regulations for alcohol and drug abuse patients?

REFERENCES

Accreditation Manual for Hospitals, 1985. Joint Commission on Accreditation of Hospitals, 1984.

Confidentiality for Alcohol and Drug Abuse Records. Title 42, Part 2 of the Federal Regulations.

Consolidated Standards Manual/85 for Child, Adolescent, and Adult Psychiatric, Alcoholism, and Drug Abuse Facilities and Facilities Serving the Mentally Retarded/Developmentally Disabled. Joint Commission on Accreditation of Hospitals, 1984.

Individual Treatment Planning for Psychiatric Patients. National Institutes of Mental Health, 1978.

chapter 7

HOSPITAL ORGANIZATION – AN OVERVIEW

ORGANIZATIONAL STRUCTURE

THE HOSPITAL DEFINED

A hospital has been defined in the *Glossary of Hospital Terms* as being:

> "A health care institution with an organized medical and professional staff, with permanent facilities that include inpatient beds, that provides medical, nursing, and other health-related services to patients."

In the organization of a hospital, especially of the voluntary type, there is a sharing of power in its operation, divided among its governing board, chief executive officer, and medical staff. This triad of forces has been dominant in the administration of hospitals for many years and, in all probability, will continue to be.

SINGLE HOSPITAL OWNERSHIP

This is the traditional kind of hospital that has flourished from the beginning of the 20th century. Its ownership might be the community, a church group, or the government at some level. It has been financed through local funding or by the sponsoring church or government, and often assisted greatly by endowments, gifts, and other funds obtained through public benefits and charities.

Because the costs of medical care have risen so fast in the past two decades that ordinary funding sources have not been adequate, hospitals have been forced to look for various means of cutting costs. Medicare's prospective payment system is an even stronger incentive to lower costs but still maintain quality health care. It is because of these pressures that many single ownership hospitals have joined forces with other hospitals in an effort to cut costs to remain in business.

MULTIHOSPITAL SYSTEMS

A multisystem has been defined as "two or more hospitals that are leased, sponsored, or contract-managed by a central organization." This organizational pattern provides a means of consolidating many resources, such as capital, services, and personnel. The impact has been shown to lower the costs of medical services. Management of this type will add a new dimension to the traditional pattern of hospital organization and administration; and it is predicted that by 1990, seven out of ten hospitals will participate in a multihospital system.

GOVERNING BOARD

The governing board, which is the ultimate authority in the institution, is made up of persons who are knowledgeable in their field and have a responsible standing in the community. In some instances governing boards include representatives of the medical staff, but this may not be legally possible in some states. Governing-board members are usually prominent business or professional persons who are willing to serve without remuneration for the good of the community.

The major responsibility of the governing body is to provide proper care of patients. This is done by selecting an efficient medical staff and administrator. The medical staff provides the medical services expected of the type of institution it serves, and the chief executive officer employs and directs the staff needed to maintain the hospital and its services.

ADMINISTRATOR/STAFF

The chief executive officer or hospital administrator is the manager of the hospital. He must be able to take the elements of manpower, material, technology, and capital, integrating them into a desired whole that is best for the hospital. His role is often that of a change agent, and his administrative responsibilities are extremely demanding. Although there are undergraduate programs in hospital administration, most are found in graduate schools of major universities across the United States and Canada. These programs consist of one or two years of full-time academic study and may include an administrative residency in a hospital or other health related organization.

The staff that is employed by the administrator may consist of many types and kinds of allied health professionals, nursing personnel, and support personnel. Their qualifications vary according to the facility's needs and patient care expectations. Figure 1 shows an organizational chart for a medium-sized hospital.

MEDICAL STAFF

The medical staff is probably the most indispensable element of the hospital's operation. Although the physicians who are staff members are not employees of the hospital, they depend upon the hospital to provide the working place that allows them to practice their profession. They are a very powerful part of the triad, and it is their unique relationship that makes hospital management and organization such a complex one.

Medical staffs are made up of fully licensed physicians and may even include other licensed individuals who are nonphysicians but are permitted to provide patient care services. Medical staff members must apply for privileges from the governing body; and their applications are evaluated on the basis of education, experience, ethics, competence, and physical health status. By this selection process, the governing body entrusts the direct care and treatment of patients to those practitioners who are deemed competent to provide high quality patient care. The medical staff, as a whole, is thus directly accountable to members of the governing body for its actions.

Additionally, there is another group of physicians practicing in the majority of hospitals, called the *house staff*. Most house staff physicians are graduates of medical schools who have been accepted to begin their medical practice as *interns* or their chosen specialty as *residents*. Internships usually last one year and

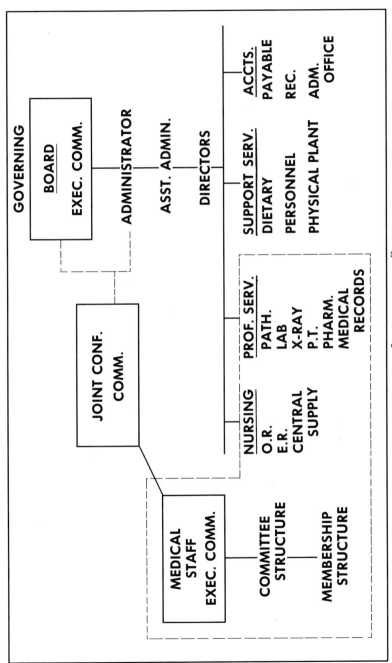

Fig. 1 – Hospital Organizational Chart

residencies from two to six years, depending on the specialty. Residents are usually licensed physicians, but interns will become licensed as soon as possible after graduation.

Hospitals in some locales may also utilize junior or senior medical students to perform physical examinations, take histories, and act as assistants in other capacities. Called externs, these students gain valuable clinical experience. House staff members are salaried members of the hospital staff. Their work, however, is closely supervised by members of the medical staff, which are responsible for their performance.

MEDICAL STAFF ORGANIZATION

The JCAH standards and state licensure laws require that every hospital has a single organized medical staff that has overall responsibility for the quality of professional services, as well as the responsibility of accounting, therefore, to the governing body. The JCAH further specifies that the medical staff has the following characteristics:

- It includes fully licensed physicians and may include other licensed individuals permitted by law and by the hospital to provide patient care services independently in the hospital.
- All its members have delineated clinical privileges that allow them to provide patient care services independently within the scope of their clinical privileges.
- All members of the medical staff and all others with individual clinical privileges are subject to medical staff and departmental bylaws, rules, regulations and review as part of the hospital quality assurance program.

The JCAH defines clinical privileges as permission to provide medical or other patient care services in the granting institution, within well-defined limits, based on the individual's professional license and his experience, competence, ability, and judgment. Clinical privileges are based on criteria established by the hospital.

The individual practitioners permitted to provide patient care services without direction or supervision vary from state to state. In some states, the state licensure act authorizes physical therapists and nurse practitioners to provide specified services without a physician's order. In other states, they are not regarded as independent practitioners.

In return for being given privileges to render treatment in a hospital within the scope of their clinical competence, members of the medical staff agree to provide quality medical care to their patients; to practice within the bylaws, rules, and regulations of the staff; and to contribute their time and expertise to assist in performing the administrative functions of the medical staff.

BYLAWS, RULES, AND REGULATIONS

The medical staff or any other organized group must have principles and policies by which it functions. Bylaws describe the who, what, when, where, and how the game is to be played. Medical staff bylaws are the mutually agreed upon principles and policies by which each medical staff member understands his rights and responsibilities. Medical staff bylaws have legal standing and are accepted by the courts as a basis for legal decisions. Rules and regulations outline the mechanisms and the details implementing the principles contained in the bylaws.

The bylaws, rules, and regulations adopted by the medical staff require approval from the governing body.

The JCAH specifies that provisions for at least the following are to be included in medical staff bylaws:

- A medical staff Executive Committee empowered to act for the medical staff in intervals between medical staff meetings with its function, size, composition, and selection procedures defined.
- Hearing and appellate review mechanisms for medical staff members and applicants for privileges.
- Mechanisms for corrective action including indications and procedures for suspension of an individual's medical staff membership.
- Description of the medical staff organization including categories of membership, officer positions including the method for selecting officers, their qualifications, responsibilities and tenure, and the conditions and mechanisms for removing officers from their position.
- Requirements for frequency of meetings and for attendance.

- A mechanism for assuring effective communications among the medical staff, hospital administration, and governing body.
- A mechanism for adopting and amending the bylaws, rules, regulations, and policies of the medical staff.
- An agreement requiring each individual with clinical privileges to provide for continuous patient care.
- Medical staff representation and participation in any hospital deliberation affecting the discharge of medical staff responsibilities.

Medical staff appointments must be made through a mechanism approved and implemented by the medical staff and the governing body in accordance with the provisions of the medical staff bylaws, rules, and regulations. Each applicant for membership must be oriented to the bylaws, rules, regulations, and policies and agree in writing to abide by them.

Criteria specified in the bylaws are to be uniformly applied to all applicants for medical staff membership and constitute the basis for medical staff appointment or reappointment. Criteria ordinarily include: evidence of current licensure, relevant training and/or experience, current competence, and health status. Other factors which also may be evaluated include: the ability of the hospital to provide adequate facilities and supportive services for the applicant and his patients; patient care needs for additional staff members with the applicant's skill and training; current evidence of adequate professional liability insurance, and the geographic location of the applicant.

In addition to making recommendations on individuals allowed to practice in a facility, recommendations on privilege delineation are required to define the scope of their practice. The JCAH allows considerable flexibility in the approach used to delineate clinical privileges. Hospitals may use specialty board certification; systems involving classification or categorization of privileges with the scope of each level well defined; or assign privileges related to an individual's experience in categories of treatment areas or procedures, as reflected in treatment results and the conclusions drawn from quality assurance activities.

In considering reappointments to the medical staff, hospitals under the prospective payment system are scrutinizing the clinical practice of each staff member for its effect on reimbursement.

The courts have established that the hospital, as an institution, may be held liable for harm caused by failure to properly assess the qualifications and performance of physicians rendering services to patients; and the hospital must undertake some type of intervention in care when necessary.

MEDICAL STAFF OFFICERS

The bylaws provide a mechanism to elect officers of the medical staff including generally a president, vice-president, immediate past president and secretary-treasurer to conduct the necessary hospital medical staff activities. In some institutions the title chief of staff is used instead of president, while in other institutions there may be a salaried chief of staff or medical director responsible for a wide variety of medicoadministrative duties, and a president of the medical staff who is responsible primarily for presiding at staff meetings, appointing medical staff committees, and communicating the views of the staff to the administration and governing board. Several officers usually represent the medical staff on the Joint Conference Committee.

MEMBERSHIP CATEGORIES

Many hospitals maintain several categories of medical staff membership for which applicants may apply:
- Active staff deliver most of the medical services in the hospital and perform all significant organizational and administrative duties pertaining to the medical staff.
- Associate staff are members who are being considered for advancement to the active medical staff.
- Consulting staff are highly qualified practitioners who are available as consultants when needed to improve patient care.
- Courtesy staff are given the privilege to admit an occasional patient to the hospital.
- Honorary staff are former members honored with emeritus positions or other outstanding practitioners whom the medical staff desires to honor.

MEDICAL STAFF DEPARTMENTS

In smaller hospitals, the medical staff is composed of relatively few physicians and specialty representatives, thus, there is no need to divide the staff into departments. Large medical staffs with many specialists may find it more effective in rendering quality patient care to maintain several departments. These departments or services usually represent clinical specialties such as Medicine, Surgery, Obstetrics-Gynecology in a medium-sized facility; while a large teaching hospital may also have departments for many subspecialties such as Urology, Cardiology and Ophthalmology.

A departmentalized medical staff has chairmen heading each service who are responsible for assuring the implementation of a planned and systematic process for monitoring and evaluating the quality and appropriateness of patient care and the performance of all individuals with clinical privileges in the department. The JCAH requires clinical departments to meet monthly to consider the findings of these ongoing monitoring and evaluation activities.

MEDICAL STAFF COMMITTEES

The medical staff framework established in the bylaws, rules, and regulations usually identifies several committees through which the responsibilities of the medical staff will be accomplished. As a minimum, there must be an **Executive Committee** which acts for the medical staff between staff meetings. In small facilities the medical staff as a whole may serve as the Executive Committee. This committee should meet monthly and maintain a permanent record of its proceedings and actions. It is responsible for coordinating the activities and general policies of the various clinical departments, making recommendations to the governing body on appointments to medical staff membership and delineating clinical privileges for each eligible individual, and organizing and reviewing mechanisms for quality assurance activities. The Executive Committee receives and acts on reports and recommendations from medical staff committees and clinical departments. The chief executive officer attends each Executive Committee meeting as an exofficio member.

Many hospitals have multiple committees with assigned charges. Common among them is the **Credentials Committee,** which is responsible for evaluating applicants for medical staff membership, making recommendations for initial appointments to the Executive Committee, conducting a regular review of each staff member's performance, and making recommendations regarding reappointments and hospital privileges.

Another common committee is the **Joint Conference Committee,** which serves as a medicoadministrative liaison between the governing body, the chief executive officer, and the medical staff. By providing an opportunity for interchange of information and discussion, the committee promotes mutual understanding of each other's problems and activities. Thus the broad experience, knowledge, and responsibility of both groups can be utilized before major decisions are made.

In many facilities the review of medical records is performed by a separate medical staff committee, generally titled the **Medical Record Committee.** In other facilities the ongoing evaluation of medical records may be designated as a responsibility of the entire staff, or of the Executive Committee. Regardless of the mechanism used, the medical staff is responsible for the maintenance of medical records that meet required standards for promptness, completeness, and clinical pertinence.

The following functions and responsibilities are usually assigned to the committee responsible for medical record review:

- Review of records for timely completion, clinical pertinence, overall adequacy for use in quality assessment activities, and, when necessary, as medicolegal documents.
- Review of records, including the results of all tests and therapies given, to assure they reflect the condition and progress of the patients.
- Determination of the format of the complete medical record, the forms used in the record, and the use of electronic data processing and storage systems for medical record purposes.

The medical record practitioner must take an active role in helping the medical staff comply with the JCAH's requirements for medical record review. He will work closely with the committee chairman to prepare agendas for interesting committee meetings which must be held at least quarterly. For each meeting, the medical record practitioner should prepare summary information regarding the timely completion of medical records. Medical record staff members may also screen medical records to present those which do not meet documentation criteria for committee review. These selected cases would vary from month to month so that all types are eventually scrutinized. The committee then analyzes them carefully, and, in addition, checks a representative sample of those which the medical record practitioner has accepted as adequate. These may be records chosen at random from the discharges, or they may be specific types of cases. In addition to reviewing the records of discharged patients, this committee should periodically perform an on-the-spot scanning of current inpatient records for completeness. This review is done on the patient units with the findings reported at Medical Record Committee meetings.

The medical staff responsibility for medical record review goes beyond the inpatient record. Ambulatory care medical records must also be reviewed, and Figures 2 and 3 illustrate how outpatient surgery might be audited. Information in these records must be complete and sufficiently detailed to facilitate continuity of care. If the hospital administers a home health care program, these records should also receive routine scrutiny.

Special review of emergency service records should be performed regularly by the Medical Record Committee to evaluate documentation of emergency patient care. Records of deaths occurring within 24 hours after admission to the emergency service should receive particular attention. Review of emergency records in disaster or riot situations is also indicated.

A Medical Record Committee cannot operate efficiently without rules and regulations. When these are approved and enforced by the medical staff, the completion of medical records becomes as automatic as other routine duties. While the staff, through its Medical Record Committee, makes the regulations, the medical record practitioner can, by using tact and diplomacy, secure the fullest cooperation in obtaining regulations that will smooth the path and assist in simplifying the work. The success of the medical record director will depend upon an ability to inspire record consciousness in the members of the medical staff. The physician's interest and cooperation makes the record worthy of preservation and later use.

The medical staff bylaws must provide sufficient authority for the Medical Record Committee to reject substandard records, pass judgment on the quality of clinical entries, enforce staff rules regarding delinquent records, and in every way promote

Total Records Reviewed: 20 Minor OPD Surgical Procedures (not performed under general anesthesia)
Period: January, 1985

REVIEW CRITERIA	RESPONSIBILITY	# COMPLIANCE	% COMPLIANCE
Documentation of:			
1. Reason for visit	Nursing	20	100
2. Physical findings	Nursing	20	100
3. Diagnostic and therapeutic orders	Medical Staff	20	100
4. Clinical observations	Medical Staff		
5. Reports of all procedures, tests, and results are present when compared with orders	Nursing	20	100
6. Diagnostic impression	Medical Staff	20	100
7. Discharge instructions or follow-up	Medical Staff	20	100
8. An accurate and complete description of the techniques and findings of every procedure performed shall be dictated or written immediately following the procedure by the surgeon who performed it.	Medical Staff	18	85
9. Pathology Report	Nursing	20	100
10. Signed Informed Consent	Nursing	20	100
11. Disposition of Patient	Medical Staff	20	100
12. All entries signed	Medical Staff	20	100

It is not necessary to obtain a signature each time a patient is seen in OPD. A current signature (within the last six months) on file is sufficient.

FIG. 2 – OUTPATIENT RECORD REVIEW

REVIEW CRITERIA	TOTAL DEFICIENCIES	MD	# DEFICIENCIES PER MD	# PATIENTS IN STUDY PER MD	% COMPLIANCE
8. An accurate and complete description of the techniques and findings of every procedure performed shall be dictated or written immediately following the procedure by the surgeon who performed it.	2	B	1	6	83%
		C	1	2	50%

FIG. 3 – MD DEFICIENCY ANALYSIS (back of Fig. 2)

and encourage the maintenance of high standards. Each physician has signed an agreement to abide by the bylaws when he joins the staff. Authority for disciplinary action of the individual physician is usually delegated by the governing body to the Executive Committee of the medical staff. Disciplinary action may take several forms such as:

- Temporary suspension of admission privileges.
- Temporary suspension of surgical or obstetrical privileges.
- Delay in promotion.
- Delay in expansion of privileges.
- Reduction in privileges.
- Downgrading in staff appointment.
- Requirement of mandatory consultation in specific categories not required of other staff members.
- Requirement of surgical or obstetrical assistance at operations or deliveries above general staff requirements.

The objective of such discipline is to impress the physician with the seriousness of the situation and to help him improve, not to damage him or his reputation in the community. Many hospitals have bylaw provisions whereby the medical record department notifies the admitting department when a staff member accumulates a specified number of delinquent records. Admission privileges are then refused for his patients until the records have been satisfactorily completed.

Other Committees

There are many other medical staff committees which may exist. In our medium-sized hospital shown in Figure 1, these might include Surgical, Tissue, Utilization Review, Pharmacy or Therapeutics, Infection, Emergency or Disaster, and Blood Bank. Each will have its own membership structure, goals, and objectives. But in a very small hospital with a limited number of staff members, one or two committees may serve the staff quite adequately.

MEDICAL STAFF OFFICE

In some hospitals, a medical record department staff member serves as medical staff secretary, responsible for maintaining the minutes of all medical staff committees and a credentials file for each staff member. This is a very appropriate responsibility for the medical record department, because the credentials file for each practitioner must include the results of staff monitoring and evaluation activities.

Other basic information which should be included in the credentials file of each practitioner includes: education, state licensure expiration date, previous practice, prior malpractice claim history, denial of medical staff privileges at other institutions, suspension or revocation of licensure, narcotic number, third-party payment program participation, reference letters, acknowledgment of Medicare fraud notice, and privileges granted with renewal dates.

Microcomputer support is very helpful in maintaining credentials files for a large staff because many items must be updated regularly, such as licensure expiration dates, Medicare statements, and privilege delineations. Continuing education attendance records for each practitioner may also be maintained via computer, for the JCAH standards specify that all individuals with delineated clinical privileges are to participate in continuing education.

Controls are necessary, however, to maintain such a system. Only medical staff office personnel can be authorized to enter data; all input data should have supporting documentation in the credentials file, and no documentation should be put into the file until it has been entered in the computer. In addition, access to credentials files must be strictly limited to authorized individuals. For this reason, the medical staff often prefers that a stand-alone microcomputer be used for credentialing files.

EVALUATION OF PATIENT CARE

The medical staff of a hospital has the delegated responsibility to oversee the quality of medical practice, and all individual staff members are accountable for the quality and appropriateness of care rendered to their patients. To accomplish this, the JCAH requires medical staff members to monitor clinical practice through regular reviews of certain functions: surgical case review, pharmacy and therapeutics function, medical record review, antibiotic usage, and blood usage. A small medical staff may elect to perform these functions as a whole or delegate this responsibility to the Executive Committee or a Quality Assurance Committee. In larger, departmentalized facilities, several committees may be established to monitor specific departments or services. All of these required monitoring activities may become a part of a hospital-wide quality assurance (QA) function, to which are added other dimensions of utilization review, risk management, concurrent and outcome reviews, problem identification, and problem resolution. Quality assurance is discussed further in Chapter 19. The ongoing evaluation of clinical records, however, is vital to the QA program because this review identifies good patient care and problem areas needing correction.

MEDICAL RECORD PRACTITIONER/ MEDICAL STAFF INTERFACE

In addition to working with medical record committee members in carrying out the committee's responsibilities, the medical record practitioner interfaces with the medical staff individually and collectively in many other ways:

- Assisting the medical staff in drawing up policies for medical record content/completion.
- Orienting house staff and new members of the attending staff to the hospital's record content and completion policies; manuals may be prepared for this purpose.
- Developing procedures to facilitate completion of incomplete records.
- Keeping physicians informed of the number of records requiring completion.
- Administering policies uniformly for completion of records.
- Providing timely transcription of reports for the medical record.
- Supplying data and assisting physicians in conducting research studies.
- Presenting educational programs for physicians on documentation requirements which impact on reimbursement.
- Making records available for the ongoing care of patients.
- Developing or revising medical record forms.

The medical record practitioner should take advantage of every opportunity to work with the medical staff and to serve on medical staff committees. Every contact provides an opportunity to display one's expertise in health care information processing. Cooperation among different groups comes about through communication with one another. The wise medical record practitioner, therefore, tries to communicate regularly with medical staff members individually and collectively.

Physicians often feel frustrated in the hospital setting which does not provide them the autonomy they are accustomed to in their own offices. In the hospital setting they are expected to comply with multiple requirements specified in the medical staff bylaws, rules, and regulations. Although an occasional physician may let his frustration show when confronted with a large number of incomplete records, the medical record practitioner who displays a cooperative attitude and directs a medical record department which serves the physician efficiently can develop a good working relationship with the medical staff and earn their respect for his expertise.

SUMMARY

While hospitals today are changing their patterns of ownership and administration, the authority and power to carry out their functions remain a three-pronged one of governing body, medical staff, and chief executive officer and staff. By far the most critical role is that played by the medical staff which holds the keys to good patient care. These keys include review functions of many kinds, ongoing evaluation of peers, and documentation production that is both medically and legally adequate.

The medical record practitioner is uniquely qualified and situated to be of assistance to both medical and administrative staffs.

STUDY QUESTIONS

1. Describe the organizational structure of a medium-sized general hospital.
2. Name several categories of medical staff membership and summarize the types of physicians each category encompasses.
3. Describe the purposes of the following medical staff committees: Executive; Credentials; Joint Conference.

4. Outline the functions and responsibilities of the medical staff committee which performs ongoing medical record review.

5. Summarize the role of the medical record professional with the medical staff.

REFERENCES

Accreditation Manual for Hospitals, 1985. Joint Commission on Accreditation of Hospitals. Chicago, Illinois, 1984.

Accreditation Requirements of the American Osteopathic Association. American Osteopathic Association. Chicago, Illinois. 1979.

An Analysis of the Revised Medical Staff Standards of the Joint Commission on Accreditation of Hospitals. Office of Legal and Regulation Affairs and American Academy of Hospital Attorneys. American Hospital Association. March, 1984.

BLANTON, WYNDHAM B. JR. "Understanding Differences Between Medical Staff and Administration." *The Hospital Medical Staff.* December, 1981.

EISELE, C. WESLEY, Editor. *The Medical Staff in the Modern Hospital.* New York, New York: McGraw-Hill, Blakiston Division, 1967.

FEINSTEIN, ALVIN R. "Quality of Data in the Medical Record." *Computers and Biomedical Research.* Vol. 1, 1970.

JCAH Monograph: Medical Staff Bylaws. Joint Commission on Accreditation of Hospitals, 1978.

KUSHMAN, LINDA. "A Medical Staff Credentialing Information System." *Hospital Topics.* Vol. 62, Jan./Feb., 1984.

RAKICH, JONATHON S., LONGEST, BEAUFORT B. JR., and O'DONNOVAN, THOMAS R. *Managing Health Care Organizations.* Philadelphia, Pennsylvania: W. B. Saunders, 1977.

THOMPSON, R. F., Coordinator. *Hospital Medical Staff Membership and Delineation of Clinical Privileges.* Oak Brook, Illinois: Hospital Research and Educational Foundation, 1977.

THOMPSON, RICHARD E. *Helping Hospital Trustees Understand Physicians.* Chicago, Illinois: American Hospital Press, 1979.

United States Department of Health and Human Services. *Conditions of Participation – Hospitals, and Conditions of Participation – Skilled Nursing Facilities.*

chapter *8*

THE MEDICAL RECORD –
MANAGEMENT OF CONTENT

The medical record is the permanent, legal document which must contain sufficient information to identify the patient, justify the diagnosis and treatment, and record the results. As such, it must be accurate and complete. But because documentation in the medical record is performed by a variety of health care providers – physicians, nurses, therapists, and others – and because it is performed as a secondary activity following the rendering of patient care, documentation may not always be as accurate or complete as necessary and desirable. A busy physician may inadvertently record a progress note in the wrong patient's medical record; a nurse may get a call to assist a patient and forget to record a medication given. Regular analysis of the documentation in the medical record should be performed to manage the content of the medical record so it fulfills its purposes of communicating patient care information; of serving as evidence of the patient's course of illness and treatment for various legal, reimbursement, and peer evaluation reviews; and of furnishing clinical data for administrative, research, and educational activities.

A health care facility's medical staff relies on the assistance of medical record practitioners for performing analysis of documentation in all medical records and notifying the appropriate individuals of omissions or inconsistencies which might make the medical record incomplete or inaccurate. These analyses may include different types of reviews and may be done at different times relative to the patient's occasion of service. Each health care facility decides on the type or types of analyses to be done according to their documentation needs and medical staff policies.

TYPES OF MEDICAL RECORD DOCUMENTATION ANALYSES

When medical record practitioners assist health care providers in identifying obvious areas that are incomplete or inaccurate, such as a missing signature on a progress note, a missing pathology report of tissue removed during surgery, or a pathology report describing Mrs. Smith's uterine cancer in Mr. Jones' medical record, the analysis is said to be quantitative. In quantitative analysis medical record practitioners use a list of recording requirements to identify deficiencies in medical record documentation. For example, the list would include "all entries must be dated and signed," "all tissues removed during surgery must have a pathology report," and "all forms must contain correct patient identification."

Medical record practitioners may also identify inconsistencies that may potentially identify documentation that is incomplete or inaccurate. This is qualitative analysis. Qualitative analysis applies a knowledge of disease process and the policies and standards established by the health care facility's administration and medical staff, and various licensing, accrediting, and certifying agencies to the review of medical record documentation. For instance, during qualitative analysis it might be noted that a complication has not been recorded on the face sheet or that the terms left and right have been interchanged. However, the health care provider makes the ultimate determination that documentation is incomplete or inaccurate, and the necessary additions or corrections. Qualitative analysis may also identify patterns in documentation where additions or corrections to specific medical records are not appropriate, but where subsequent improvement could be made through redesign of forms, educational activities, or other methods. Noting that one physician consistently fails to record a discharge progress note may be an example of such a pattern. This might be corrected by pointing out that the physician may be denied reimbursement for the visit to the patient on that day.

Quantitative and qualitative analyses should be distinguished from quality assurance. Quantitative and qualitative analyses are reviews of documentation in all medical records designed to provide assistance to health care providers in improving their documentation. The result of quantitative and qualitative analyses is completion of specific medical records by the health care provider and improved documentation practices. Quality assurance is a program performed by peer groups of health care providers designed to ensure that the health care delivered is optimal within the available resources of the health care facility and consistent with achievable goals. While quantitative and qualitative analyses may provide background information for focused studies of documentation problems as part of a quality assurance program, it is the peer group of health care providers that actually evaluates the specific problems and takes corrective action. It is the function of a quality assurance program to evaluate the quality of patient care and the effectiveness and efficiency with which the facility's resources are utilized. While complete and accurate documentation resulting from quantitative and qualitative analyses provides a more complete and accurate medical record from which to evaluate the quality of patient care, only the health care practitioners themselves can evaluate the care rendered. Figure 1 summarizes the characteristics of quantitative and qualitative medical record documentation analyses.

Medical record practitioners also perform a statistical analysis. This includes abstracting data from medical records for administrative and clinical decision making. Diagnostic and procedure data are coded and can be used to retrieve specific medical records for research purposes or to define and evaluate the health care facility's case mix. A uniform set of data is also abstracted from the medical record and transmitted to the business office for billing purposes. Statistical analysis utilizes an understanding of nomenclatures and classification systems, indexes and registers, and health care statistical methodology. These topics are discussed in greater detail in succeeding chapters.

The three types of analyses may be performed concurrently with the patient's occasion of service and/or retrospectively after the occasion of service has ended. In hospitals, analyses have traditionally been performed in the medical record department retrospectively upon termination of the hospitalization. This affords an opportunity to review the medical record as a whole, although it delays the completion or correction of documentation. In order to ensure that quality care is provided within the hospital's resources, concurrent analysis, performed on the nurses' station to identify omissions or discrepancies quickly be-

CHARACTERISTICS OF MEDICAL RECORD DOCUMENTATION ANALYSES

QUANTITATIVE ANALYSIS

- Identifies obvious areas that are incomplete or inaccurate.

- Uses a prescribed list of recording requirements.

- Applies knowledge of medical record content to the analysis.

- Performed by a person trained on the job.

- Result is a list of deficiencies which can be completed by the health care provider in the normal course of facility procedures.

QUALITATIVE ANALYSIS

- Identifies inconsistencies and omissions that may potentially be incomplete or inaccurate.

- Performed by application of general principles of documentation and/or specific criteria.

- Applies knowledge of medical record content, disease process, and policies and standards established by the facility administration and medical staff, and various licensing, accrediting, and certifying agencies to the analysis.

- Performed by credentialed medical record practitioner.

- Results include:

  1. A list of deficiencies which can be completed by the health care provider in the normal course of facility procedures.

  2. Identification of patterns of poor documentation practices for which improvement should be sought through individual discussion, referral to quality assurance program, or by educational means.

  3. Identification of potentially compensable events to be reported to the facility's risk management, quality assurance program, or legal counsel, as applicable, for further review.

FIG. 1 – MEDICAL RECORD DOCUMENTATION ANALYSES

fore they are compounded or misinterpreted, is becoming popular. Where once it was believed that concurrent analysis by medical record practitioners was costly to implement in terms of increases in personnel and materials for multiple sites and difficult due to space problems on the nurses' stations, hospitals are finding that the improved completion rates which result improve the flow of information to the business office and thereby improve cash flow.

Other benefits, such as improved utilization of resources, potentially improved patient care through timely and improved documentation, and decreased expenses in handling incomplete medical records, are less easy to quantify but are believed to accrue.

In long term care facilities, analyses have usually been performed during the patient's period of residency, although at monthly, semimonthly, and even quarterly intervals. Medical record practitioners or other administrative staff are beginning to perform more frequent analyses with an eye toward improving care and utilization of the facility's resources. Quantitative and qualitative analyses have rarely been performed by medical record practitioners in ambulatory care facilities or home health programs, although increased utilization of these services will increase the need for analyses of medical record documentation.

QUANTITATIVE ANALYSIS

DEFINITION

Quantitative analysis is a review of prescribed areas of the medical record for identifying specific deficiencies in recording. Because the analysis is specifically prescribed, it may be performed by specially trained clerical-level employees. The prescribed areas are usually set forth in a procedure developed jointly by the facility's credentialed medical record practitioner and health care providers in accordance with the facility's medical staff bylaws and administrative policies, and the standards of its licensing, accrediting, and certifying agencies. Each facility develops its own procedure, thus there are many variations. For instance, in some facilities the procedure may describe a review of only physician documentation, for it may be believed that nurses, therapists, and other provider groups are rarely named as parties to malpractice suits and thus their deficiencies are not as significant as those of physicians. In facilities where nonphysician providers have been involved in malpractice suits, or where documentation by these groups has been questioned in insurance audits or for other reasons, quantitative analysis may be performed on all documentation. Another common variation occurs in hospitals with computerized medical information systems. Since access to a computer is by a personal identification method (code, key, or physical attribute), facilities with computer systems may not require a written signature for authentication; and, therefore, quantitative analysis would not include a check for signatures.

PURPOSE

The purpose of quantitative analysis is primarily to identify obvious and routine omissions that can be easily corrected in the normal course of the hospital's procedures. This procedure makes the medical record more complete for reference in continuing patient care; for protecting the legal interests of the patient, physician, and hospital; and for meeting licensing, accrediting, and certifying requirements.

RESULTS

The result of quantitative analysis is identification of specific deficiencies. These deficiencies should be completed by the health care provider within a short time of their identification. The medical staff bylaws will specify a time frame for completion of medical records, which is in accordance with licensing, accrediting, and certifying agency requirements. Medical record department personnel may also aid in completing the medical record through assembling all medical record forms, through filing late reports, and by recording patient identification on forms which obviously belong to a particular medical record.

COMPONENTS OF QUANTITATIVE ANALYSIS

The basic components of quantitative analysis include a review of the medical record for:

1. correct patient identification on every form,
2. presence of all necessary reports,
3. required authentication on all entries, and
4. good recording practices.

Review for Identification

Whether performed concurrently or retrospectively, quantitative analysis will usually begin with the placement of the medical record forms in a prescribed order. This arrangement will aid in ensuring fast and easy retrieval of information from the medical record in subsequent patient care. It will also aid the analyst in checking for patient identification and missing reports. In assembling the forms, each page of the medical record, front and back, should be checked for the patient's identification, at least the patient's name and medical record number. Where missing, the page should be reviewed to determine that it does belong to the patient whose medical record is being analyzed and identification recorded. An advantage of performing quantitative analysis concurrently is that missing pages may be found more easily.

Review for Necessary Reports

There are certain reports that are common to all medical records, such as the reports of the medical history, physical examination, clinical observations (progress notes), and conclusions at termination of hospitalization (clinical resume and statement of final diagnoses and procedures). Other reports will be necessary depending on the patient's course in the hospital. If the patient had diagnostic tests, consultations, or surgery, reports of these procedures will be required. The procedure for quantitative analysis should specify which reports to check for, at what times, and under what circumstances. For instance, if a history and physical examination has not been performed within 24 hours of admission, this may be a deficiency which should be identified on concurrent analysis. If a physician dictates operative reports, and the report for a particular surgery is missing upon retrospective analysis, this would also be identified as a deficiency. It should be noted, however, that if a report of an action is missing because the action was not done, the report cannot be considered a deficiency that the health provider can add to the medical record. For instance, if there is no physician progress note on a given day because the physician did not visit the patient on that day, the physician should not be asked to write a progress note.

Review for Authentication

Quantitative analysis should also check that prescribed entries are authenticated. Authentication may be a signature, rubber stamp in sole possession of the owner, initials if identifiable within the medical record, or computer access code or key; and should include the professional title (MD, RN, etc.) of the author. An entry should not be signed by someone other than the author, although the facility may require countersignature of entries made by housestaff and students to demonstrate supervision by qualified professionals. Where countersignature is required, both the signature of the author and supervising professional should be included, as well as a note regarding the review of the entry, such as "reviewed," "concur with," or "carry out orders as noted."

Review for Recording Practices

Entries should also follow good recording practices. While quantitative analysis cannot solve problems of illegibility or incomplete content, it can aid in noting where entries are not dated, where errors have not been appropriately corrected, where there are skipped spaces that should be lined through to prevent subsequent tampering – particularly in progress notes and physician orders and where abbreviations have been used in the statement of final diagnoses and procedures. Error correction is a particularly important aspect of documentation. Alterations can easily raise questions of authenticity and negligence. When it is necessary to correct an error (such as when the health care provider has written in the wrong patient's medical record), the health care provider should be advised to draw a single line through each line of the error, add a note explaining the error (such as "wrong patient's medical record"), date and initial it, and then make the correct entry in chronological order indicating which entry it is replacing. If there is any doubt as to the subsequent admissability of the entry, it is a good practice to have a professional colleague witness the correction process.

By ensuring that all forms are present in the correct arrangement and that all entries are authenticated and reflect minimum standards of good recording practices, quantitative analysis is an important part of improving the accuracy and completeness of medical records.

QUALITATIVE ANALYSIS

DEFINITION

Qualitative analysis is a review of the content of medical record entries for inconsistencies and omissions which may signify that the medical record is inaccurate or incomplete. Such an analysis requires a knowledge of medical terminology, anatomy and physiology, fundamentals of disease processes, medical record content, and the standards of licensing, accrediting, and certifying agencies. It is usually performed by a qualified medical record practitioner.

PURPOSE

As is true of quantitative analysis, the purposes of qualitative analysis include making the medical record complete for reference in patient care, protecting legal interests, and meeting regulatory requirements. Because it is more in-depth than quantitative analysis, however, it serves these purposes more fully; and it also contributes background or supporting information for quality assurance and risk management activities. Qualitative analysis also assists in diagnosis and procedure-coding specificity and sequencing which is important for ongoing medical research, administrative studies and reimbursement.

RESULTS

The result of qualitative analysis may be identification of correctable deficiencies, patterns of poor documentation practices, and potentially compensable events. Many of the findings of qualitative analysis are deficiencies in specific medical record entries which the health care provider can correct. For example, an ophthalmologist may identify a cataract and its extraction as the final diagnosis and operation on the face sheet of a medical record. Upon qualitative analysis the history and physical examination report and the progress notes may reveal that the patient is being treated for insulin-dependent diabetes. The physician should be requested to list this condition on the face sheet as a comorbidity.

Some inconsistencies or omissions in documentation, however, cannot be verified after the fact, and, therefore, cannot be corrected. These are considered to be poor documentation practices which hopefully, upon identification, can be improved upon in subsequent documentation. For instance, in performing a physical examination, a physician may actually examine every body system but may record information about only those systems which are abnormal. This practice may result in no direct harm to any patient. However, there may be a time when the medical record is used as evidence in court, and the physician may be questioned about the evaluation and normalcy of those body systems about which there is no documentation.

Inconsistencies or omissions in documentation may also reflect actual patient care practice problems which are potentially compensable events – an occurrence that has resulted in harm to the patient and that may possibly expose the facility and/or provider to professional or general liability claims and may require the facility and/or provider to pay damages to the person harmed. In a classic case where the physician ordered "watch condition of toes" of a young patient with a fractured tibia, omission of entries reflected lack of observation. A suit for negligence followed when irreversible ischemia required amputation.

Where qualitative analysis identifies patterns of poor documentation or potentially compensable events, neither of which can be corrected after the fact, the documenting health care provider should be made aware of the faulty documentation and offered assistance or suggestions for future improvement. It should never be suggested that the documentation be rewritten, as such entries are alterations and will not stand up under scrutiny. In all cases, raising the issue of improving documentation practices with a health care provider must be done with diplomacy. The effectiveness of constructive criticism frequently depends on the rapport the medical record practitioner has with the health care provider. It may be necessary for the health care provider to perform a self-evaluation or to participate in a peer review of documentation so poor practices can be discovered by the offender or by peers. Providing educational reminders of good documentation practices or exhibiting classic instances of poor documentation and its results may also be helpful in improving documentation.

COMPONENTS OF QUALITATIVE ANALYSIS

Qualitative analysis may be performed "free-style" by applying the general principles of good documentation to the review of the medical record content, or a set of documentation criteria may be developed and applied. Use of criteria is generally considered to be more objective and provides written backup, especially for detecting patterns of poor documentation. The components of qualitative analysis include a review of the medical record content (assuming the completion of quantitative analysis) for:

1. complete and consistent recording of diagnostic statements,
2. consistency in entries by all health care providers,
3. description and justification for the course of the patient's hospitalization,
4. recording of all necessary instances of informed consent,
5. application of good documentation practices, and
6. occurrence of a potentially compensable event.

Review for Complete and Consistent Diagnostic Statements

Diagnostic statements will be made throughout the medical record, each reflecting the level of understanding of the patient's medical condition at the time it is recorded. Upon admission there should be an admitting diagnosis stating the reason for admission. The result of the history and physical examination should document an impression or provisional diagnosis that generally must be confirmed through additional diagnostic studies. In certain cases, the impression or provisional diagnosis cannot be narrowed down to one diagnosis, but rather several possible diagnoses with similar symptoms must be further evaluated. This comparison is called a differential diagnosis, and frequently is stated as "rule out (one or more diagnoses)," or "(diagnosis 1) versus (diagnosis 2)." Prior to surgery, a preoperative diagnosis should be recorded in a preoperative progress note. This diagnosis is a statement of the reason for surgery or the expected findings upon surgery. A postoperative diagnosis, recorded in a postoperative progress note, states the clinical findings of the surgery. Both preoperative and postoperative diagnoses should be included in the operative report. A great difference in these diagnoses may be suggestive of inadequate diagnostic workup or other issues related to quality of care. A pathological diagnosis may be required to provide a definitive postoperative diagnosis. A pathological diagnosis is a description of the morphology, or cellular characteristics, of the tissue removed during surgery; whereas a clinical diagnosis describes the etiology (cause) and/or abnormal functioning of an organ or system, or the body as a whole.

Upon termination of the hospitalization, all final (clinical) diagnoses and procedures should be stated on the face sheet or in the discharge summary. The analyst should check this list to determine that it is complete, consistent with documentation, and in correct sequence. The final diagnoses will include the principal and primary diagnoses, any complications, and those comorbidities affecting the hospitalization. The principal diagnosis and primary diagnosis must be carefully distinguished because of differences in statistical and reimbursement reporting requirements. The *Uniform Hospital Discharge Data Set* (UHDDS), which establishes definitions for official hospital reporting, defines the principal diagnosis as "that condition established after study to be chiefly responsible for occasioning the admission of the patient to the hospital for care." The primary diagnosis is "the most important or significant condition of a patient in terms of its implications for the patient's health, medical care, and use of hospital resources." For example, a patient may have been admitted for hernia repair and upon diagnostic study it is discovered that the patient has an early cancer. Although the cancer may be more significant than the hernia and thus the primary diagnosis, the hernia is the principal diagnosis because it reflects the reason for admission. When reporting this case for reimbursement, the hospital may be required to sequence the principal diagnosis first if it is to be reimbursed by certain third-party payors, or may sequence the primary diagnosis first if it is to be reimbursed by other third-party payors.

Secondary diagnoses are complications and/or comorbidities. A complication is a condition arising during the hospitalization that modifies the course of the patient's illness or the medical care required. Some complications include decubitus ulcer, postoperative hemorrhage, adverse reaction to medication, hospital acquired infections, neurological deficits, surgical emphysema, and injuries (perforations and punctures during surgery, falls, etc.). A comorbidity is a condition existing at the time of hospitalization which has potential for affecting the course of illness or medical care provided. Comorbidities are active conditions for which the patient is receiving treatment or is being monitored, such as insulin-dependent diabetes mellitus or hypertension. Sometimes physicians list personal or family history of diagnoses, or status postprocedures as secondary diagnoses. When using the list of diagnoses for coding purposes, it is not necessary to code these statements unless they are significant to the hospitalization. For example, family history of a familial disease may be significant for a patient admitted to rule out the familial disease.

Procedures also need to be listed completely. Each health care facility should specifically identify procedures which are to be recorded on the admission/discharge record and/or discharge summary. Some health care facilities require physicians to record only procedures performed in the operating room. Other health care facilities require physicians to delineate, in addition, procedures such as bone marrow biopsies, cardiac catheterizations, blood transfusions, and CAT scans. As a minimum, most health care facilities require that all procedures influencing reimbursement be listed. For the prospective payment system, lists of "OR" and "non-OR" procedures have been issued.

When listing procedures they should also be sequenced with the principal procedure first. The principal procedure is "one which is performed for definitive treatment rather than one performed for diagnostic or exploratory purposes, or was necessary to take care of a complication. The principal procedure is that procedure most related to the principal diagnosis."

Review for Entry Consistency

Qualitative analysis includes a review of medical record entries for consistency. Consistency refers to agreement or harmony of parts one to another and to a whole. As has already been mentioned, diagnostic statements should be consistent from admission through discharge, that is, they should reflect progressively more information about the condition for which the patient was admitted. Where the primary diagnosis differs from the principal diagnosis, it may be that a condition has been found in its very early stages, which is advantageous for the patient and reflects a holistic approach to medical care. However, a difference may mean that the reason for admission was not documented correctly, or that there was inadequate workup prior to admission so hospital resources are possibly being used inappropriately, or that a potentially compensable event occurred during hospitalization. Diagnostic statements should also demonstrate consistency among the operative report, tissue report, diagnostic studies results, and consent forms. Differences here usually reflect poor documentation practices.

Other entries should also reflect consistency. Three common areas where inconsistency can result in miscommunication of patient care information are among progress notes written by different members of the health care team; among orders, medication records, and progress notes; and among admitting and discharge information recorded by different health care personnel. For instance, a nurse's progress note may indicate that the patient spiked a fever, while the physician may make no mention of the fever. Such inconsistency leaves open to question whether either the nurse or physician recorded correctly, and whether or not the physician evaluated the condition and decided to take no action.

Review for Description and Justification of Hospital Course

In addition to consistency, the medical record as a whole should also display specificity and thought processes. The medical record must describe and justify the course of the patient's hospitalization. The medical record, therefore, must document results of diagnostic studies, treatment, patient education, and patient location fully. "Test results normal," "patient doing well," and "patient given instructions" are examples of generalizations which describe nothing. The medical record should also display thought processes – the reasoning that leads to each decision, even if the decision is to take no action (as might have been the case in the previous example of the fever). This is especially important when there is a change in treatment plan. Not only should the alternate treatment be described, but the purpose for the new treatment, modification, or discontinuance should also be explained.

Review for Recording Informed Consent

Specificity and reasoning also apply to the recording of information regarding patient consent for treatment. Each hospital has a policy consistent with legal requirements on informed consent. The medical record practitioner must know this policy and apply it when performing qualitative analysis. Physicians should be encouraged to not merely comply with the policy, but to take care in recording all instances of informed consent, such as in description of possible side effects from medication when its administration does not normally require completion of a special "consent form."

Review for Documentation Practices

Other characteristics of documentation which are qualitatively analyzed include evidence of timely recording of entries, legibility, use of approved abbreviations throughout the content, and avoidance of extraneous remarks. The medical record should contain no unexplained time gaps. This is especially important in emergency situations where not only is there a tendency to document less due to lack of time, but increased risk for error, and subsequent scrutiny of entries for malpractice. Legibility refers to penmanship, use of ink for permanence of recording, and the careful completion of forms. Illegible entries and use of abbreviations not on the list of medical staff approved abbreviations are as useless as if nothing were recorded. Finally, while the medical record should reflect honest and candid statements, these should be recorded with caution. The medical record should never contain derogatory or critical comments. In the event such a comment is made, the author should either elect to let it stand, being aware of possible consequences, or treat it as an error (see previous discussion on error correction).

Review for Potentially Compensable Events

Finally, qualitative analysis should identify any potentially compensable events. Figure 2 displays a sample of some criteria which may be used in identifying potentially compensable events. The concept of identifying and analyzing "nonspecific clinical occurrences" originated with InterQual Incorporated, a consulting firm to health care providers, when consulting for the California Medical Insurance Feasibility Study (CMIF). The medical record should fully document an occurrence of harm to the patient.

SAMPLE CRITERIA FOR IDENTIFYING POTENTIALLY COMPENSABLE EVENTS UPON QUALITATIVE ANALYSIS

Medical Record No.:_____   Analyst:_____   Page 3 of 4

	YES	NO	DEFICIENCY/PROBLEM DESCRIPTION
QUALITATIVE ANALYSIS – SCREENING CRITERIA, CONT.			
Does the medical record contain appropriately signed authorizations and consents?			
a. For routine treatment			
b. For surgical procedures/hazardous treatment			
QUALITATIVE ANALYSIS – POTENTIALLY COMPENSABLE EVENTS			
Is this admission for complication or incomplete management of problem on previous admission to this hospital?			
Was there an unexplained transfer from a general care unit to a special care unit during this admission?			
Is there an infection not present on admission?			
Is there a neurological deficit present at discharge which was not present on admission?			
Did the patient suffer cardiac or respiratory arrest during this admission?			
Was the patient transferred to another acute care facility except for administrative reasons?			
Was a procedure cancelled or repeated due to improper preparation of patient, technician error, or equipment failure?			

FIG. 2 – IDENTIFYING POTENTIALLY COMPENSABLE EVENTS

INCOMPLETE MEDICAL RECORD CONTROL

The result of quantitative and qualitative analysis is the identification of specific deficiencies, patterns of poor documentation, and potentially compensable events.

INCOMPLETE/DELINQUENT MEDICAL RECORDS

Medical records with specific deficiencies that can be completed by a health care provider are termed incomplete medical records. Health care providers are notified of the incomplete medical records and are expected to complete them within a time specified in the medical staff bylaws. When an incomplete medical record has remained incomplete after the defined time for completion has expired, the incomplete medical record is referred to as a delinquent medical record. Frequently, health care facilities determine and monitor their "incomplete medical record rate" and their "delinquent medical record rate." The incomplete rate is the number of incomplete medical records over the number of discharges during the required completion period. For example, if a facility discharges 75 patients in the 30 days in which providers are given to complete their medical records, and 25 are incomplete, the incomplete rate for that period is 33 percent. The delinquent rate is calculated as the total number of delinquent medical records over the average number of discharges during a completion period. For example, if the hospital currently has 50 delinquent records in total, and it averages 75 discharges per period, its delinquent rate is 50 over 75 or 67 percent.

A delinquent rate of over 50 percent (representing more than a full period's discharges) is considered a serious problem. Of course, many factors influence how this rate is interpreted. If the incomplete rate is very high, one can expect a higher delinquent rate. The age of the delinquent medical records is also a factor. A 40 percent delinquent rate of medical records remaining incomplete for only two or three extra weeks may be more desirable than a delinquency rate of 20 percent representing medical records of several months delinquency. The type of delinquency is still another factor. Delinquencies due to missing history and physical examination reports or operative reports are more serious than delinquencies due to missing discharge summaries or signatures. The completion period will also affect the delinquency rate, especially when comparing rates across hospitals.

DEFICIENCY NOTIFICATION

Health care providers need to know they have incomplete medical records and what deficiencies they contain. When concurrent analysis identifies deficiencies, the deficiencies can be noted directly on the medical record, commonly by a form inserted within the medical record, adhesive tape or rubber stamp placed on the cover, a removable sticker placed directly on the medical record form containing the deficiency, or a combination of these. The next time the provider documents in the record, it is expected the deficiency will be corrected. When retrospective analysis is performed, or when deficiencies remain from concurrent analysis upon discharge, health care facilities have different ways of getting medical records completed. In some facilities health care providers are expected to routinely visit the medical record department to attend to record deficiencies. In other facilities, providers may be notified in writing that they have incomplete medical records and to visit the medical record department; or, in other facilities, to request the records to be brought to a specified location within the facility. Such notification may be a copy of the deficiency form or may be a standard notification announcement. In still other facilities, incomplete medical records may be held on the nursing station until they are completed; or they may be routinely brought to the provider's office within the facility. Medical records should not be removed from the facility for completion, as they are then not accessible for any emergency care required by the patient or for other purposes.

When performing retrospective analysis, specific deficiencies may be noted on the same type of form, tape, stamp, or sticker as described for concurrent identification of deficiencies. See Figure 3 for samples of such deficiency forms.

FILING OF INCOMPLETE MEDICAL RECORDS

When incomplete medical records are kept in the medical record department, they may be filed in one of three ways: in the permanent file, in a separate incomplete file by provider name, or in a separate incomplete file by medical record number. Each

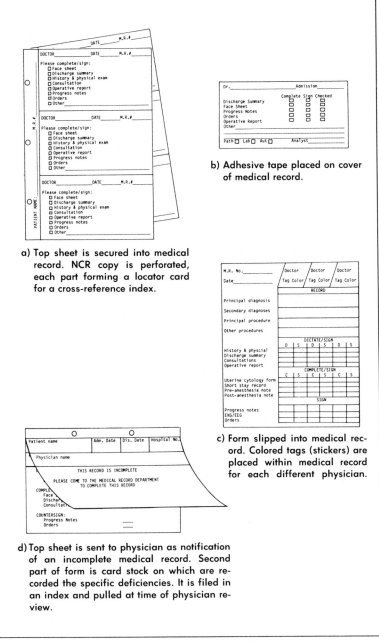

a) Top sheet is secured into medical record. NCR copy is perforated, each part forming a locator card for a cross-reference index.

b) Adhesive tape placed on cover of medical record.

c) Form slipped into medical record. Colored tags (stickers) are placed within medical record for each different physician.

d) Top sheet is sent to physician as notification of an incomplete medical record. Second part of form is card stock on which are recorded the specific deficiencies. It is filed in an index and pulled at time of physician review.

FIG. 3 – SAMPLE DEFICIENCY FORMS

way has advantages and disadvantages. Filing incomplete medical records in permanent files makes them less accessible to providers but saves retrieval time if the medical records are very active after discharge. This filing arrangement may be most appropriate for hospitals with ambulatory care services to which patients return after discharge. The means of filing which is most accessible to providers is in a separate file by provider name. The disadvantage of this approach is that when multiple providers, such as the attending physician, surgeon, consultant, and respiratory therapist, have deficiencies on the same medical record, a cross-reference system must be established. Filing incomplete medical records in a separate file by number is a compromise between filing them in a permanent file and separately by provider name.

Computerized incomplete systems can be very helpful for controlling all aspects of incomplete medical records. Once specific deficiencies are input into the computer (the procedure for which can be aided by computer prompts), several outputs can be generated. For instance, a printed list of deficiencies can be generated immediately, or later upon provider review. A series of notices to the provider of incomplete and delinquent medical records can be generated, as well as a composite list of provider's incomplete and delinquent records for department chairpersons. Statistics can also be computed, including not only the general incomplete and delinquent rates, but rates per provider, types of deficiencies, age of delinquent medical records, etc. The computer can also aid in medical record location, such as in situations where multiple providers have deficiencies on the same medical record.

FINAL CHART CHECK

When providers have worked on incomplete medical records, it is advisable to do a "final chart check," or "reanalysis" of these records to ensure that all deficiencies have been completed. It is extremely important that medical records be completed on a timely basis, for incomplete medical records affect the quality of patient care which can be rendered in a health care facility. Incomplete medical records also impact on the facility's licensure and accreditation status. For instance, the Joint Commission on Accreditation of Hospitals states that "substantial serious or sustained medical record deficiencies or delinquency may be the basis for a hospital's receiving less than the maximum accreditation status." In the event that a medical record remains incomplete after a health care provider has terminated his or her association with the facility, the facility policy should be followed for filing the record as incomplete. Usually, the medical record committee will review the record and write a note to the effect that it could not be completed due to the resignation or death of the responsible provider. No other provider should complete a record on a patient unfamiliar to him or her.

HANDLING INFORMATION ON DOCUMENTATION PRACTICES AND POTENTIALLY COMPENSABLE EVENTS

When the result of qualitative analysis is identification of poor documentation which cannot be completed or corrected after the fact, the medical record practitioner must be guided by the medical staff bylaws, hospital administration, and the AMRA Code of Ethics. Every situation may ultimately indicate a different action for solution. Frequently, patterns of poor documentation identify a need for more focused peer review by medical staff committees, including the medical record committee, tissue committee, quality assurance, etc. For instance, if it is noticed on qualitative analysis that a form for newborn physical exam reports routinely contains some omissions, it may be appropriate to advise the medical record committee to evaluate the form for possible revision. Another example occurs when it is noted that records completed by orthopedic and ophthalmology specialists rarely contain reports of gynecologic exams on female patients. Concerned that early signs of cancer may be going unnoticed, it could be recommended that the quality assurance program study this finding in more depth.

The provider may also be contacted directly about poor documentation practices. For instance, qualitative analysis may identify that one physician writes with an aqua-colored felt-tip pen which bleeds through the paper, obscuring the writing on the other side and not photocopying well. A sample may be shown to the provider and a request made to use another writing instrument.

General information about poor documentation practices may be distributed through a newsletter, bulletin board announcements, or in-service programs. For instance, information on sequencing of principal diagnoses and their impact on reimbursement may best be distributed by in-service programs. A newspaper clipping about a malpractice case in which poor documentation was a factor may be posted on a bulletin board or summarized in the facility's newsletter.

Finally, when a potentially compensable event has been identified, the facility's risk management, quality assurance program, or legal counsel, as applicable, should be notified. Early identification and analyses of these events to determine whether there is liability potential can result in timely and prudent efforts to minimize potential losses.

In handling any information on poor documentation and potentially compensable events, it is extremely important to maintain the confidentiality of the information. This information is sensitive, and only those authorized to handle such information should be provided with the information.

SUMMARY

Managing the content of the medical record through analysis of documentation is an important function of the medical record department in all health care facilities. By reviewing all medical records during or following an occasion of service for completeness and accuracy, the medical record practitioner makes a significant contribution to the health care facility. Completion of medical records and improved documentation result in improved communication among all health care providers, contributing to improved patient care. Other results of quantitative, qualitative, and statistical analyses provide a medical record which completely and accurately describes and justifies the services rendered to a patient for legal, reimbursement, peer evaluation, licensing/accreditation, and research/educational purposes. The nature of the analyses performed in any given health care facility depends on the policies and needs of the facility's medical staff and administration and on the demands of the facility's licensing, accrediting, and certifying agencies. There are as many variations as there are facilities, for each adopts the general procedures outlined in this chapter to its own unique situation.

STUDY QUESTIONS

1. What is the major purpose of (a) quantitative analysis, (b) qualitative analysis, and (c) statistical analysis?
2. What are three major differences between (a) quantitative and qualitative analyses and (b) quality assurance?
3. What are the advantages and disadvantages of concurrent and retrospective analyses?
4. How do analyses of medical record documentation differ among health care facilities?
5. What specific knowledge must an analyst possess in order to perform quantitative analysis?
6. What general characteristics of documentation does a person performing qualitative analysis look for in a medical record?
7. Distinguish between the following sets of terms:
   a. incomplete medical records/delinquent medical records
   b. deficiency/pattern of poor documentation/potentially compensable event.
8. Explain the various ways health care providers may (a) be notified of incomplete medical records, (b) be informed of deficiencies in specific medical records, and (c) have access to incomplete medical records.

REFERENCES

American Medical Record Association. *Glossary of Hospital Terms.* AMRA. Chicago, Illinois, 1983.

Care Communications. *The Record That Defends Its Friends.* Chicago, Illinois: Care Communications, Inc., 1979.

CURRAN, WILLIAM J., and SHAPIRO, E. DONALD. *Law, Medicine, and Forensic Science.* Boston, Massachusetts: Little, Brown & Co., 1970.

ESTRAND, NORMA A. "Record Monitoring with a Personal Computer." *Journal of the American Medical Record Association.* April, 1984.

FINNEGAN, RITA. *Data Quality and DRGs*. American Medical Record Association. Chicago, Illinois, 1983.

FLORA, C. ROSALIA. "Coordinating DRG Assignment Through Inpatient Record Analysis." *Journal of the American Medical Record Association*. August, 1984.

FREEMAN, TANYA J. "Setting the Stage for Improved Record Content." *Journal of the American Medical Record Association*. May, 1984.

InterQual, Inc. *Identifying and Analyzing Clinically-Related Occurrences*. InterQual, Inc., Chicago, Illinois, 1982.

Joint Commission on Accreditation of Hospitals. *1985 Accreditation Manual for Hospitals*. JCAH. Chicago, Illinois, 1984.

KESSLER, PAUL, and JOSEPH, ERIC D. *The Risk Management Primer*. Chicago, Illinois: Care Communications, Inc., 1981.

LEE, MARGARET P. "Concurrent Medical Record Analysis in a Community Hospital." *Journal of the American Medical Record Association*. June, 1984.

National Committee on Vital and Health Statistics. *Uniform Hospital Discharge Data, Minimum Data Set*. April, 1980.

Webster's New Collegiate Dictionary. Springfield, Massachusetts: G. and C. Merriam Company, 1977.

chapter 9

FORMS DESIGN AND CONTROL

Each hospital has the responsibility to provide medical record forms to fit its needs. Neither the American Hospital Association nor the Joint Commission on Accreditation of Hospitals recommends any specific medical record forms. In some communities, several hospitals have joined together and adopted basic medical record forms acceptable to the medical staffs of each hospital. This is helpful to the physician who practices in more than one hospital.

Thoughtful design of the forms which become part of the medical record will provide a more readable, useful, and less bulky record. Good forms can accomplish several purposes: (1) they can reduce writing time and avoid duplication of information and (2) standardize information that is provided. Well-designed forms are also easier to complete.

Responsibility for designing medical record forms is sometimes delegated to the hospital forms committee, which in some hospitals may be a subcommittee of the medical record committee. In others, the medical record committee may assume the responsibility for forms. The medical record practitioner should be an active member of any forms committee. Committee duties include the reviewing of new forms proposed by the medical staff, various hospital departments or persons, and revising and discontinuing forms no longer needed. The medical record practitioner assists the forms committee and hospital department by (1) making available the various requirements and statutes that may control the content of the form in a particular state; (2) being knowledgeable about rules governing forms design such as quality of paper, spacing, printing styles, logical sequence of material; and (3) collecting sample medical record forms to assist in developing the hospital forms. There should be a demonstrated need and reason for every item on the form.

REQUEST FOR NEW OR REVISED FORM

INSTRUCTIONS THIS FORM MUST BE COMPLETELY FILLED OUT AND FORWARDED TO FORMS CONTROL
ALL REQUESTS FOR NEW OR REVISED FORMS MUST HAVE A SAMPLE OR ROUGH DRAWING ATTACHED.

DATE

REQUEST FOR ☐ NEW FORM ☐ REVISED FORM | FORM TITLE | PRESENT FORM NO.

PURPOSE OF NEW OR REVISED FORM

WHAT PROMPTED THIS REQUEST?
☐ ORGANIZATION CHANGE ☐ PROCEDURE CHANGE ☐ TO IMPLEMENT ESTABLISHED PROCEDURE
☐ INTERNAL DEPT REQUIREMENT ☐ REQUEST OF ANOTHER DEPT ☐ MGMT ☐ GOVT, CUSTOMER OR OTHER REQMT

FORM PREPARED ☐ DAILY ☐ WEEKLY ☐ MONTHLY ☐ OTHER (EXPLAIN) ______

DATA ENTERED BY ☐ HAND ☐ TYPEWRITER ☐ OTHER (EXPLAIN) ______

FORM FILED BY ☐ DATE ☐ SUBJECT ☐ NUMBER

FORM FILED IN ☐ FOLDER ☐ BINDER ☐ OTHER (EXPLAIN) ______

FORM USED INTERNALLY ONLY ☐ YES ☐ NO

FORMS OBSOLETED

DATA TO BE ENTERED ON (GIVE FORM NOS)

DATA TO BE ENTERED FROM (GIVE FORM NOS)

DISTRIBUTION OF FORM

PART	PERSON OR DEPT RECEIVING COPY	REASON COPY IS REQUIRED
1		
2		
3		
4		
5		
6		

FORM PRENUMBERED ☐ YES (Give Reason) ☐ NO

START UP QTY | MONTHLY USE THEREAFTER | ANNUAL QTY

NEW EQUIPMENT REQUIRED

EXPECTED BENEFITS TO BE DERIVED FROM NEW OR REVISED FORM

EXPECTED DOLLAR SAVING $______PER YEAR

EFFECT ON CLERICAL WORKLOAD
WORKLOAD WILL BE: ☐ INCREASED______ HRS PER MONTH ☐ DECREASED______ HRS PER MONTH

REQUESTED BY | PLT & DEPT | APPROVED (Dept Head)

Courtesy Association for Systems Management

FIG. 1 – REQUEST FOR NEW OR REVISED FORM

The recording of items that "might be nice to have," or "may be needed someday," should be eliminated since the time required for recording is usually disproportionate to the value of the information. It is recommended that, when possible, the original copies be filed in the medical record, a legal document. Figure 1 illustrates a "Request for New or Revised Form." This form should be completed by the requester before embarking on a new or revised form design.

The principles set forth in the following paragraphs apply not only to forms used in patient medical records but also to those needed for internal usage within the facility.

FORMS ANALYSIS

A logical approach to forms analysis is to review all the forms used in a certain procedure. Using this selective approach not

---

BASIC FORMS ANALYSIS GUIDE
(Related to Procedure Being Reviewed)

A. STARTING POINTS	B. REASSESSMENT POINTS
1. NEED	
What justifies the existence of the forms based on what they accomplish? What other forms are used fully or partially that relate to or duplicate the information requested? What are the form deficiencies?	Is all the information needed? Is the cost justified? Can the forms or some of their items be: Eliminated? Simplified or Resequenced? Combined? Added? Is there a more efficient way or better source?
2. PERSONNEL	
Who needs the data? Who inputs the information? Who extracts or summarizes the information?	Can other staff (in the same or different departments) perform the tasks more efficiently? Can the forms be redesigned such as resequencing, to simplify entering and extracting?
3. PLACE	
Where are forms transcribed and processed? Where are the forms distributed? Where are the forms filed?	Can execution of forms be done better elsewhere? Can distribution be reduced by the reassignment of who writes or processes the forms? Does the design of the forms aid in filing, finding, storage, and disposition?
4. TIME	
When are the forms written and processed? When are the forms filed?	Are the forms processed in a logical sequence? Can peak loads be reduced by better scheduling of the forms flow? Can information needed from forms be requested during a slow period?
5. METHOD	
How are the forms written? How are the forms processed? How are the forms transmitted? How are the forms filed?	Can the writing method be improved? Can the routing or mailing method be improved? Have the forms been designed to use the most efficient office equipment?

NOTE: FOR ALL THE QUESTIONS POSED ABOVE, THERE SHOULD BE AN ANSWER TO "WHY?"

Fig. 2 – Basic Forms Analysis Guide

---

only makes the review easier to manage (fewer forms), but also helps those who are evaluating the forms to focus on the efficacy of the reporting mechanism. Forms within a procedure should have a similar purpose. See Figure 2 for a basic forms analysis guide.

Reviewers should understand the procedure so that their analyses can be complete. One needs to know the answers to the what, when, where, who, how, and why questions for each step of the procedures involving the form. One must determine what source documents are required to complete the form, and know how many copies are distributed.

The following sources should be checked to obtain background information related to procedures:

- Manuals, regulations, or directives which describe functional responsibilities and procedures that relate to the forms under study.
- Forms History File and the Forms Subject/Title File (see sections in this chapter which explain the contents and purposes of these files).
- Completed forms which will show the types of errors made in completing the forms.
- Organizational charts which show the relationships of the department responsible for the forms to other departments.

Some of the reasons which prompt an analysis of forms are:

- Existence of operational problems of backlogs, bottlenecks, unusual time lags, repetition, or numerous errors.
- Areas suggested by top management for potential savings and improvement.
- Suggestions made by the operating staff.

INTERVIEWING

During the analytical process, persons who are concerned with entering data on forms should be interviewed, as well as those concerned with extracting or summarizing data from them. There may also be a need to interview persons who must review, audit, transmit, or file the forms. This is especially true when there is more than one copy of the form prepared which involves different groups of people.

The responsibilities of the person being interviewed must be determined, as well as the role he assumes in relation to the form. The following questions are appropriate:

- Does the form exist solely or partly for his use?
- Which items are entered on the form, and which copies are prepared to satisfy his requirements?
- For what purposes does he need forms, items, or copies?

The interview should include a discussion of every processing step and the method of processing followed by each person while working with each form. Note of the supplies and equipment used should be made, as well as how frequently a person processes the form and the average amount of time spent on one process. Forms should be examined from which, or to which, information is copied as a part of preparing or using the form under study. Filled-in copies of all forms and copies of any related documents pertinent to the study should be collected. Make sure that all links of information are present. Write down any reminders needed to reconstruct the forms-processing procedure after the discussion is over.

FORMS APPRAISAL

For a series of forms used in the same procedure, in order to determine the number of times the same items appear on each of the forms, a "Data Frequency Chart," similar to the one shown in Figure 3, can be helpful. By developing such a chart, it may be possible to reduce the number of forms used in a department or throughout the organization.

The name of the procedure under review along with the date and the name of the person performing the analysis should appear on the chart. The title of each form related to the procedure should be written in the title section with its form number situated just below the title. One form should be analyzed at a time. Enter a description of each data item which appears on the first form on a separate line under the column headed "Data Items." Number each data item sequentially. Place a check mark ($\sqrt{}$) or an "x" under the title column on the data item line for the form undergoing analysis. When the second form used in the procedure is analyzed, some of the data items may have already been recorded (from the first form). If that is the case, do not record the data item description again, but place a check mark under the appropriate title column for the form being analyzed on the appropriate data item line. Record in the data item column for the second form a description of only those

DATA FREQUENCY CHART   Page_____of_____

Procedure: FORM TITLE

Date Reviewed_____

Analyzed By_____

Item No.	Data Items	No.	No.	No.	No.	No.	No.	No.	No.	No.	Total Items

FIG. 3 – DATA FREQUENCY CHART

items which did not appear on the first form. Place check marks for the additional data items recorded from the second form in the appropriate title column. Follow the same procedures for all subsequent forms related to the procedure being analyzed.

When the posting has been completed for all forms used in the procedure, count the number of times the same item appears and record the total in the last column.

Following these steps, it can be determined if some of the forms can be combined or some data items or forms eliminated, as well as bringing to light other items which may be needed based upon procedure requirements.

QUANTITIES

In order to lay out the proper form design, it is important to know the quantity of forms to be ordered. This is because the methods of reproduction of the form govern the form design.

For example, if a 3-part form is being designed which will be used at the rate of 50 sets a month, it may be wise to use a padded form with pencil carbons to be inserted by the user. Should the usage rate be several hundred per month, it might be more efficient to design the form as a carbon-interleaved snap out. If the snap-out form is to be ordered at a rate of only a thousand at a time, an edge-glued stub might be specified. The reason for this is because the form would very likely be produced on a flatbed press, since the small quantity would not justify the preparation time required for a rotary press. An order of 10,000 forms, however, should be designed to run on a rotary press, utilizing an inside-glued stub.

Professional forms designers can aid greatly in developing the more complex forms, especially those used for computer output. However, one should have a working knowledge of various printing requirements so methods recommended by professionals can be understood.

It is usually sufficient to order a six-month to twelve-month supply of a form, depending on the discounts and the storage space available. If the form is subject to critical changes within a short period of time, one may wish to order a smaller supply.

A standard form should be used for stocking, printing, and ordering forms. Figure 4 shows a sample which may be used for this purpose.

LEAD TIME

Certain types of forms take longer to produce than others. Enough lead time (from the date the order is placed to the date of delivery) must be allowed to achieve the desired implementation date. Below are estimated time periods for the reproduction

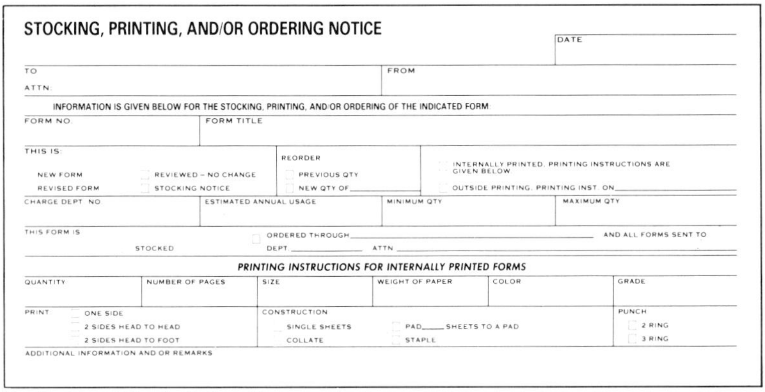

STOCKING, PRINTING, AND/OR ORDERING NOTICE

DATE

TO

FROM

ATTN:

INFORMATION IS GIVEN BELOW FOR THE STOCKING, PRINTING, AND/OR ORDERING OF THE INDICATED FORM:

FORM NO. | FORM TITLE

THIS IS:

NEW FORM

REVISED FORM

REVIEWED – NO CHANGE

STOCKING NOTICE

REORDER

PREVIOUS QTY

NEW QTY OF ____

INTERNALLY PRINTED, PRINTING INSTRUCTIONS ARE GIVEN BELOW

OUTSIDE PRINTING, PRINTING INST. ON ____

CHARGE DEPT. NO. | ESTIMATED ANNUAL USAGE | MINIMUM QTY | MAXIMUM QTY

THIS FORM IS

STOCKED

ORDERED THROUGH ____ AND ALL FORMS SENT TO

DEPT. ____ ATTN ____

PRINTING INSTRUCTIONS FOR INTERNALLY PRINTED FORMS

QUANTITY | NUMBER OF PAGES | SIZE | WEIGHT OF PAPER | COLOR | GRADE

PRINT: ONE SIDE; 2 SIDES HEAD TO HEAD; 2 SIDES HEAD TO FOOT

CONSTRUCTION: SINGLE SHEETS; COLLATE; PAD ____ SHEETS TO A PAD; STAPLE

PUNCH: 2 RING; 3 RING

ADDITIONAL INFORMATION AND OR REMARKS

Courtesy Association for Systems Management

FIG. 4 – STOCKING, PRINTING, AND/OR ORDERING NOTICE

of just a few types of forms. These estimates can vary based on locality and the season in which the forms are to be reproduced:

Single-part forms (up to 11″ x 17″)	2 to 3 weeks
Single-part forms (over 11″ x 17″)	3 to 4 weeks
Tags and envelopes	4 to 8 weeks
Carbon-interleaved snap-out forms	8 to 12 weeks
Continuous forms	10 to 15 weeks

DROP SHIPMENTS

Some printers will make arrangements to warehouse forms and make drop shipments as they are needed. This method enables one to take advantage of the lower cost per thousand that is available as the size of the order is increased. A good deal of foresight must be exercised to be assured that a heavily used form will be able to endure for a year or more without any changes in design or construction.

FORMS CONTROL

FORMS HISTORY FILE

The forms history file provides a complete picture of each form in the organization from its development to its current status. It should be arranged according to the numbering system used to identify forms which should be as simple as possible.

A forms history file can be set up by establishing a folder for each form and filing it by form number. Each folder should eventually contain the following:

- A copy of the current edition of the form and any previous editions.
- Drafts showing significant stages of development and pertinent correspondence.
- A copy of the directive authorizing use of the form.
- The original request for approval of the form and any requests for revisions indicating the names of all units using the form and the rate of use.
- Evidence relating to the official final approval for the printing or reproduction and issuance of the form.
- A record of all actions taken on the form, including a cross-reference to the subject/title file.

The forms history file should be periodically reviewed and updated. Folders on discontinued or obsolete forms should be removed from the active file on a timely basis, appropriately annotated, and placed in a separate discontinued history file for such time as required by the organization's records retention schedule.

FORMS SUBJECT/TITLE FILE

The forms subject/title file provides the means by which forms dealing with related subject matter are brought together. One copy of each form is classified by purpose and placed in a subject/title folder.

The main purposes of the subject/title file are to:

- Avoid the creation of a new form when an existing form could be revised to serve the need.
- Detect those forms which might be eliminated or which might be consolidated with similar forms.
- Identify forms which should be analyzed and redesigned for simplification and uniformity of format, nomenclature, item sequence, spacing, size, and so forth.

- Generate studies of forms in relation to the systems and procedures used.

The subject/title file is not an easy file to develop because of the many possible subject headings that could be assigned to some forms. However, one subject heading can be selected and forms filed under that heading, producing as many cross-reference cards as necessary to tie the subjects together and locate the form. It is the best type of control file to use when making an analysis of the organization's forms.

FORMS IDENTIFICATION

All forms should be appropriately titled and numbered. Form numbers should be issued sequentially and may be prefixed or suffixed by a code for the originating department or section. A numeric assignment for forms is the most flexible control method. However, alphabetical characters can be used or a combination of alpha-numeric characters. It is recommended that when a form is back printed (printed on both sides), or if the form comprises several pages, the primary form number (the sequential number) should have as its last character a lowercase alpha character, such as an "a" to represent the first page and a "b" to represent the reverse side of the form or the next page, and so forth.

For forms used in an automated environment, one may wish to identify each one by assigning the computer program number that will be receiving the data input. This can be easily accomplished through a coordinated effort between the Forms Control Department (or person) and the Data Processing Department.

Insofar as is possible, it is desirable to have most identifying data in the same place on all forms used by the institution. The following identifying items should be printed in the lower-left corner of the form or in any other corner dependent on the form design:

- Form Number (to include any prefixes or suffixes)
- Edition Date – Month and Year Originated or Revised
- Copyright Symbol (©) when applicable, with "Copyright" spelled out following the symbol
- Year Copyrighted (when applicable)
- Institution's Name (in full, or use the acceptable abbreviation or acronym)

As an example, the identifying line at the bottom (or at another suitable location) of the first form generated by the Jewish Hospital of Michigan would appear as follows if the following conditions existed: The form is new; it is back printed; the front side is being numbered; the originating department is Medical Records and has a code number of 10; and the edition date is January, 1985:

> 0001a-10 01/85 MRD © Copyright 1985 JHM
>
> or
>
> 0001a-10 01/85 MRD © Copyright 1985 Jewish Hospital of Michigan

If the same form was revised in March, 1985, the imprint would be as follows:

> 0001a-10 Rev. 03/85 MRD © Copyright 1985 JHM (or the full name)

Most forms used internally by hospitals are not copyrighted and, therefore, will not require the information related to the copyrighted materials on the identifying line.

Supersession notices adjacent to the new form number can be helpful, for example, "Replaces Form 0111, 06/84, which will not be used." Supersession notices are particularly advantageous during the first three or four years of a new or revitalized program when a large quantity of forms is revised, consolidated, and eliminated. Such notices also serve as guides to users and stockroom clerks in eliminating obsolete stocks and requisitioning current forms.

FORMS CONTROL REGISTER

A Forms Control Register is essential for the proper control of form numbers issued, as well as for other identifying information. It can be maintained either manually or by computer.

The following items with accompanying comments and instructions can be included on the Forms Control Register.

Column No.	Column Heading	Comments and Instructions
1	Form Number	Enter the next sequential number to be assigned.
2	Title	Enter the full title of the form. Do not abbreviate.
3	Form Size	Enter the form dimensions, i.e.: 8½" x 11".
4	Edition Date (Mo./Yr.)	Enter the month and year the form was sent to printer. This date should correspond with the date printed on the form even though the actual implementation date may take place later. This date represents the thinking at the time of the completed design. It is possible that changes may take place in the organization before implementation that will not be reflected on the form being published.
5	Revised Ed. Date(s)	Enter the month and year the form is revised. Allow enough space in this column for several dates. Different dates should be separated by a semicolon.
6	Originating Department	Enter the name of the department or section that initiated the form. The department name can be abbreviated.

FORMS DESIGN

A form should be designed to meet the requirements of the system for which it is to be used. The design should be clear and the form easy to complete to save on clerical labor and to increase office efficiency.

PRINCIPLES OF FORMS DESIGN

Five major components usually exist on all forms. They are as follows:

1. Heading – Includes the title and form number (not necessarily appearing together).

2. Introduction – Explains the purpose of the form. Sometimes the purpose is identified in the title.
3. Instructions – Includes items on how to fill in the form and what to do with the form.
4. Body – Consists of the grouped or sequenced items for the specified information desired.
5. Close – Space for approving signatures.

Design rules which should be followed are:
1. Study the purpose and use of the form and design it with the user in mind.
2. Design the form as simply as possible; omit unnecessary information and lines.
3. Include the title and form number on each form.
4. Use standardized sizes whenever possible.
5. Use standard terminology for wording instructions.
6. Arrange items in the proper sequence.
7. Preprint constant data to keep fill-in data to a minimum.
8. Allow adequate spacing for the method of fill in (manual or by machine).

TITLES AND SUBTITLES

The title of a form may appear in one of several places. Standard positions are: top left, center, top right, left or right bottom. In a vertical card file, for example, you may wish to put the title at the bottom of the form to reserve the top portion for fill-in data. In a visible file – you may wish the title at the top so that pertinent control information can be seen at the bottom.

A subtitle should be used when the main title needs further explanation or qualification.

When forms are to be completed by persons outside the organization, the company's name should be included in the title.

FORM NUMBERS

The lower-right margin or lower-left margin is the best location for the form number and edition date. In these locations, tearing into or obliterating the number is avoided if the form is stapled in the upper left corner. Form numbers will also be visible if the forms are bound at the top. Stocking of forms will also be facilitated by having form numbers at the bottom.

When a form consists of several separate pages or is back printed, the form number should appear on each page so if one page is separated from the others, it can be easily identified. It also assists in the proper collation of forms with multiple pages.

EDITION DATE

The edition date or publication date should appear on each form. This date assists the user in determining whether the current edition is being used and helps in the disposition of obsolete stocks. The edition date usually appears next to the form number.

PAGE IDENTIFICATION

When there are multiple pages of a form, page numbers should be assigned. The page number can be in a numerical or alphabetical sequence. The page number can be placed in the upper-right corner or lower-right corner of the form. This will help the printer in assembling the materials for printing and in collating following printing.

When designing a form which requires continuation sheets and the number of such pages is unknown to the user at the outset, each page should be provided with a space for page insertion, such as "Page_____of_____pages." The page number and total number of pages are entered in the blank spaces by the person completing the form.

INSTRUCTIONS

General instructions should be brief and placed at the top of the form. The user should be able to immediately determine how many copies are required; who should submit the form; and where, when, and to whom copies should be sent.

If more detailed instructions are required, the reverse side of the form can be used; however, a reference to this should be included in the general instruction section. Lengthy instructions can also be placed on the front of the form if there is enough space for data and instructions, on a separate sheet, or in a booklet. Instructions may also appear as an administrative directive prescribed by the organization. Instruction should not be placed among entry spaces because that gives the form a cluttered appearance and hinders completion.

WORKING AREA AND ARRANGEMENT

The working area is the part of the form that is devoted to the substantive work of the form. Careful consideration must be given to the arrangement of the information requested which includes proper grouping, sequencing, and aligning of the data. Consideration must also be given to margins, spacing, and methods by which the respondent will supply information.

Grouping. If different persons are to enter data on the same form, the data to be completed by each person should be grouped according to the sequence of processing steps involved.

Sequencing. After related items have been put together, they should be placed in a sequence which will eliminate any unnecessary writing motions and make it easy to transcribe information from the form. Numbering items makes reference easier and faster and also helps as a reference for detailed instructions. If an item has several parts, they may be identified by following the traditional number-letter outline system.

Aligning Data. Data on the form should be arranged to facilitate the flow of writing from left to right and from top to bottom. Items on the form can be aligned vertically for a minimum of tabular and marginal stops.

MARGINS

Reproduction facilities require margins as working space for sprocket holes which permit the mechanical gripping of paper during the printing process, and for trimming the paper when several copies of a form are printed on large sheets. Allow a minimum margin of $\frac{2}{6}$ inch at the top, $\frac{3}{6}$ inch at the bottom, and $\frac{3}{10}$ inch at the sides. If card stock is used, at least $\frac{1}{8}$ inch should be allowed as margin on all sides.

Obtain your printer's specifications for margins and when you wish the image for a form to extend to the edge of the paper or card. The latter process is called bleeding, and this style can result in increased handling costs.

SPACING

When designing a form where the data will be entered with a typewriter, follow these guidelines:

Horizontal Spacing: Allow $\frac{1}{12}$ inch for elite or $\frac{1}{10}$ inch for pica type. $\frac{1}{10}$ inch accommodates either elite or pica and allows for maximum entry space. Allow extra spacing, if desired, to prevent crowding.

Vertical Spacing: There are six vertical lines per inch on the standard typewriter, elite or pica. Allow $\frac{1}{6}$ inch, or its multiple, for each line of typing. If an executive typewriter is used, allow 5.28 vertical lines per inch.

Follow these guidelines for handwritten spacing:

Horizontal Spacing: Provide $\frac{1}{10}$ to $\frac{2}{12}$ inch per character.

Vertical Spacing: Provide $\frac{1}{4}$ inch to $\frac{2}{6}$ inch. When a box design is used, $\frac{2}{6}$ inch is required.

When a form can be filled in by hand or by typewriter, or a combination of both, determine the horizontal space by the hand fill-in requirements and the vertical space by typewriter requirements. The $\frac{2}{6}$-inch vertical spacing will accommodate either typewritten or handwritten entries.

BOX DESIGN

The box design is commonly used in forms design, because it increases available space on a form as much as 25 percent and it gives a form an attractive appearance.

Horizontal rules may extend from the left to the right margin depending on the data items to be included. The insertion of vertical rules creates the box and they should be aligned wherever possible to keep the number of typewriter tabular stops to a minimum. The typing position of each line should begin from a common left margin allowing the typewriter carriage to be returned to the same position.

Items of information, called "Printed Captions," are placed in the upper-left corner of the boxes allowing the captions to be visible when typing. A blank space reserved for future use to

be filled in by someone else should be labeled "Do not write in
the space," or "Leave Blank." It may also be designed showing
the department name responsible for entering information into

AMERICAN MEDICAL RECORD ASSOCIATION
875 North Michigan Avenue   Suite 1850, John Hancock Center
Chicago, Illinois 60611   (312) 787-2672

INDEPENDENT STUDY DIVISION

APPLICATION FOR ENROLLMENT

Information **MUST** be **TYPED**. (See reverse side of form for instructions.)

1. Check Program Applied For:
   __ ISM-General Study (In-Service)
   __ ISM-MRA-MRT Academic Program
   __ ISM-Continuing Education
   __ ISM-National Certifying Examination Candidates
   __ Health Record Management in Nursing Homes

4. Name (Last, First, M.I.)
5. Date of Birth

2. Check Specific Module(s) Applied For (ISM Programs Only):

1	5	9	13
2	6	10	14
3	7	11	15
4	8	12	16

6. Home Address (Street, Apt. No.)
7. City, State, Zip Code

3. Have you been enrolled in any AMRA Independent Study Program? Yes____ No____

8. Employer (Name of Facility)
9. Type of Facility
10. Home Telephone A.C.

11. Address Where Employed
12. City, State, Zip Code
13. Business Telephone A.C.

14. Present Job Title
15. No. Years Employed in Current Position
16. No. Hours Worked per Week
17. Typing Speed
w.p.m.

18. Name of High School
19. High School Address (Street, City, State, Zip Code)
20. Year Graduated

21. School in Which Currently Enrolled
22. School Address (Street, City, State, Zip Code)
23. Year of Study (encircle one)   1   2   3   4

24. Highest level of post secondary education (encircle one only):

No post secondary education . . . 0
Associate of Arts 1
Associate of Science 2

No degree, but college credits under
30 semester hrs. 45 quarter hrs. . . 3
No degree, but college credits over
30 semester hrs. 45 quarter hrs. . . 4

Bachelor's degree 5
Master's degree 6
Ph.D. (Doctor of Philosophy) . . 7

25a RRA? Yes____ No____
25b ART? Yes____ No____
(Enter I.D. No. below)

AMRA I.D. Number

26. **FOR AMRA-APPROVED MRA/MRT ACADEMIC PROGRAM STUDENTS ONLY** (To be completed by Program Director):

NOTICE: An Agreement must be on file between the student, Program Director, and academic institution as to the number of credits, if any, to be given by that institution after successful completion of module(s).

I verify that the above-named student has been accepted for enrollment in the medical record program at

(Name of University or College)

I also verify that an agreement is on file relating to the number of academic credit hours that will be granted upon the successful completion of Module(s)_____
(specify Module Nos.)

Name of Program Director (Please type)   Signature of Program Director   Date Signed

27. Payment Information

To Be Paid By (specify name below)

a. Registration Fee . . . . _____
b. Tuition . . . . _____
c. Amount Enclosed . . $ _____

28. **I verify that the education information as well as all other information provided above is true and accurate.**

Mail course material to (enter address):

Signature of Applicant   Date

FOR OFFICE USE ONLY

29. Date Received by Acct._____
30. Amount Received $_____
31. Processed by_____

32. Date Application Approved_____
33. Date Enrolled_____
34. Processed by_____

35. Registration Account No.

008-7 82 ISD ·· AMRA Copyright 1982

FIG. 5 – A SAMPLE BOX-DESIGN FORM

the blank section. See Figure 5 for a sample box-design form.

The following items summarize some of the things to avoid
in forms design, as well as listing attractive features which
should be considered in the final design of a form.

FEATURES TO AVOID IN FORMS DESIGN

- Heavy ruled lines.
- Lines that bleed off the edge.
- Narrow margins.
- Choppy layouts; crowded entries.
- Lack of symmetry; off balance.
- Mixture of design styles.
- Unconventional type styles or fonts.
- Type too large or too small.

ATTRACTIVE FEATURES

- Frequent use of hairline and double-hairline rules.
- Adequate margins at top, bottom, and sides.
- Occasional use of white space to keep the form from looking too busy.
- Neat arrangement of boxes with vertical line continuity to the extent possible.
- Careful selection of appropriate type sizes to suit each need.
- Artistic placement of company logo and other insignia.
- Occasional use of shading or reverse printing in place of rules.
- Restrained use of color, when available.
- Balanced design; symmetry, or a studied lack of symmetry.

SUMMARY

Each hospital has the responsibility to develop medical record forms to fit its needs. Responsibility for designing medical record forms is delegated to the hospital forms committee. Although a variety of styles of medical record forms are used in hospitals throughout the country, certain basic essentials must be included if the hospital is to maintain accreditation standards. Medical record forms will not of themselves guarantee accurate and adequate medical records. However, if forms provide for the recording of essential data and if the physician carefully records the information requested, accurate and adequate medical records will result.

STUDY QUESTIONS

1. What sources can be used to obtain background information for procedures related to a proposed form?
2. In basic forms analysis, what questions should be answered in the reassessment of a form?
3. What is the purpose of a "Data Frequency Chart" in forms appraisal?
4. Why should there be a "Forms History File"?
5. What are the five major parts of a form?
6. What features should be avoided in forms design?

REFERENCES

MAEDKE, WILMER O., ROBEK, MARY F., and BROWN, GERALD F. *Information and Records Management.* Beverly Hills, California: Glencoe Press, 1974, 449 pages.

MYERS, GIBBS, and JOYCE, JAMES M. *Forms Design and Management: Manual Computer.* Cleveland, Ohio: Assn. for Systems Management, 1978, 59 pages.

——— and MATTHIES, LESLIE H. "Forms Order Quantities." *Journal of Systems Management,* V35, No. 11, November, 1984, pp. 6-7.

———. "Esthetics in Forms Design." *Journal of Systems Management,* V35, No. 12, December, 1984, pp. 16-17.

chapter *10*

FILING METHODS, STORAGE, AND RETENTION

Normal daily operations in many areas of a health care institution can be severely hampered by poor management of records; therefore, it is imperative that the medical record practitioner establish systems and procedures for the efficient distribution and use of medical records throughout the facility. Efficiency in these functions is perhaps the most important single factor in establishing good rapport among other members and departments of the health care institution.

RECORD NUMBERING AND FILING SYSTEMS

Medical records in most health care institutions are filed numerically according to patients' admission numbers. In the past, some hospitals have filed records according to patients' names, discharge numbers, or diagnostic code numbers. Alphabetical filing by patient names is more cumbersome and subject to more error than numerical filing. Filing by discharge numbers and diagnostic code numbers generally proves to be unsatisfactory, because other important records or registers generated in the facility are concerned exclusively with admission numbers. For example, the patients' register and the number index are based on admission numbers. If a patient's index card is lost, his hospital admission number may be obtained from either of these sources, provided his name and admission date are known. But if his master patient index card shows a discharge number, the register and number index are of no assistance in locating this number. Record location then becomes extremely difficult.

There are several types of numbering and filing systems. Regardless of which of these systems is utilized, medical records requiring new numbers should have them assigned chronologically, and this number should be common to all departments of the hospital.

SERIAL NUMBERING

In serial numbering, the patient receives a new number each time he is admitted to or treated by the hospital. If he is registered three times, he acquires three different admission numbers. The patient Edward Brown is admitted to the hospital and receives the number 52783. When he returns for ambulatory care follow-up one week after discharge, he is registered under patient number 52829. If he is admitted to the hospital again the following year, he receives a third number such as 64287. All numbers assigned to a patient must be recorded on his card in the master patient index.

SERIAL FILING SYSTEM

Serial filing is a result of a serial numbering system. Because a new number is issued for each occasion of service, a medical record must accordingly be developed. This means the patient's medical records are filed in as many places in the file as the number of times the patient has been admitted to the facility and given another number.

UNIT NUMBERING

In unit numbering, the patient is assigned a patient number on his first admission which he retains for all subsequent admissions and treatments. With unit numbering, each time Edward Brown arrives at the hospital for treatment, documentation on his care will be compiled under the first number he was assigned – 52783.

UNIT FILING SYSTEM

Unit filing is a result of a unit numbering system. This numbering system provides a single record which is a composite of all data gathered on a given patient, whether as an inpatient, ambulatory care, or emergency patient. The patient's entire medical record is thus in one folder under one hospital number.

SERIAL-UNIT FILING ADAPTATION

This filing system is a synthesis of the serial and unit numbering systems. Each time the patient is registered, he receives a new hospital number; but his previous records are continually brought forward and filed under the latest issued number. If patient Edward Brown returned for an ambulatory care visit following discharge, he would receive number 52829; but his inpatient admission data, filed under 52783, would be brought forward to be filed with the notes made during his most recent visit. A unit record is thus created. When the older records are brought forward, an outguide must be left in the file where the old chart was pulled to indicate the new number under which the record is now filed. The empty chart folder marked with a referral to the new number is a satisfactory outguide.

OTHER ADAPTATIONS OF UNIT NUMBERING AND FILING SYSTEMS

The unit numbering and filing system is very popular with health facilities due to the ease of retrieving patient information when it is all filed in one place under one number. Two adaptations of unit numbering used in health care facilities are of particular note – social security numbering and family numbering.

Social Security Numbering – The use of social security numbers for patient identification is a very controversial subject. They are used effectively in Veterans Administration hospitals which receive assistance from the Social Security Administration for location of unknown numbers. But other health care facilities have used the social security number as a patient identifier with varied success. The American Hospital Association recommends that social security numbers not be used as the medical record numbering system.

When considering using the social security number as the patient's hospital registration number, it should be understood that the social security number is not a national identifier. There is no legal requirement that every U.S. resident have a social security number. There are certain federal and state laws that require an individual to have a social security number; however, where use of the number is not required by law, the person may refuse to provide the number.

It is an advantage to use the social security number to identify a patient, because it is unique to him and distinguishes him from any other patient in the facility. However, some individuals (mainly young people and newborns) do not have social security numbers and must be issued "pseudo numbers."

"Pseudo" social security numbers can be issued from a special bank or series used only for those patients admitted without social security numbers. The Veterans Administration issues pseudo numbers in a very interesting fashion.

Pseudo "social security" numbers are assigned to patients not possessing an actual number. Assignments are based on numerical designations for the patient's initials and utilization of the birth date for the balance of the number. The code for numerical assignment to the alphabet is as follows:

1 abc	5 mno	9 yz
2 def	6 pqr	0 used when
3 ghi	7 stu	no middle
4 jkl	8 vwx	initial

Thus, John Brown, born January 1, 1946, would be issued the following number:

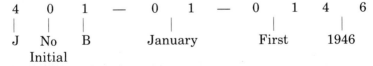

Other disadvantages to using this number include instances where patients have more than one social security number (in some cases patients have had five or more), and the fact that a nine-digit number is thought to be excessively long.

Planning for expansion of the medical record file area is difficult with the social security numbering system. Some areas of the file may fill up faster than other areas, since patients randomly arrive at the hospital thus requiring constant shifting of medical record folders to provide for an even distribution of the files.

Family Numbering – Another adaptation of unit numbering is the family numbering system. Family numbering usually consists of placing extra pairs of digits which signify placement of the individual in the household. These digits are usually placed immediately before the regularly assigned number. Prefix number pairs have a definite sequence and meaning, as follows:

01 = head of household (either mother or father)
02 = spouse
03
04 } Children or other family members
05 etc.

An illustration of this is shown below:

>   01 – 123456
>   /   /
>   head   family number (the same for all members of
>   of   that family)
>   household

>   02 – 123456
>   /
>   spouse

>   03 – 123456
>   etc.
>   /
>   children or
> other members

All patient information on one family is thus filed together by the family number. In the example above, the number 123456 provides a unit number for each family member and it groups these records of one family together for easy reference of related problems. This system is particularly helpful for neighborhood health centers and mental health centers utilizing family counseling techniques. One disadvantage of family numbering is the frequent change and reassignment of numbers as family composition changes, usually caused by marriage and divorce. Through divorce, a spouse may become head of another separate household. A child may become a spouse or head of a household through marriage. In these circumstances, not only does the individual prefix change, but a new household number must be assigned, resulting in an entirely new patient record.

ADVANTAGES AND DISADVANTAGES OF UNIT NUMBERING AND UNIT FILING

Some form of a unit numbering and filing system is recommended with the patient's records being centralized in a single

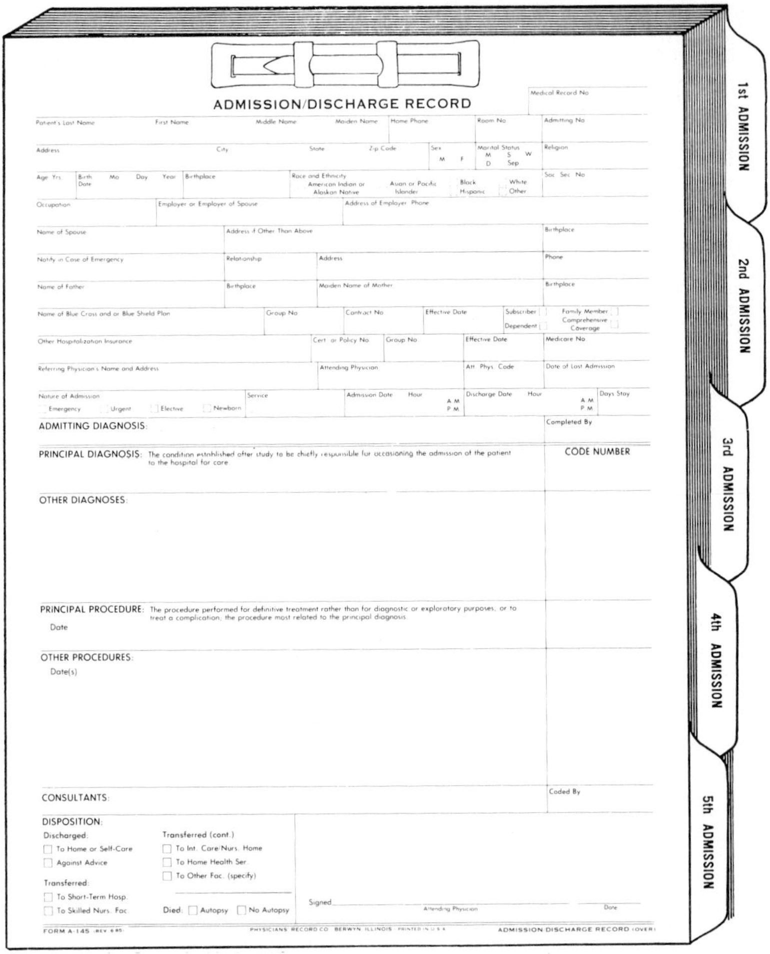

Form courtesy of Physicians' Record Company

Fig. 1 – File Folder with Two-Pronged Fastener and Chart Dividers

chart folder. This method provides the health care facility and medical staff personnel with a complete picture of the patient's medical history and therapy, and it eliminates the task of gathering separate parts of a patient's records to put together.

It also eliminates the task of bringing forward the older records to the new location and assigning them new registration numbers (serial-unit filing system). A fastener with two prongs may be used to bind the records of various admissions together. If, in addition, some method of tabbing or indexing (Figure 1) is used, it is possible to turn at once to any particular record in the group.

Multiple-volume records present a problem when a unit filing system is maintained. Records documenting multiple occasions of treatment may become so thick that additional folders are needed to house one complete medical record. In order to alert filing personnel and health care professionals using the record that a medical record is contained in several folders, it is wise to mark each folder with both the volume number and the total number of volumes. For example, the first folder can be labeled "Volume 1 of 2," the second folder "Volume 2 of 2," etc. It is important to remember that *all* folders on one patient must be relabeled whenever another volume is added to the set. The first folder labeled "Volume 1 of 2" would change to "Volume 1 of 3" as a third folder is added.

When a unit record is utilized, it is essential that those persons assigning registration numbers determine whether or not the patient has been previously treated by the facility. With the unit numbering system, the patient is not assigned another number if he has previously been registered. Occasionally a patient may mistakenly be assigned a new registration number. This error can be rectified by voiding the number on the most recent admission and filing the record under the first number issued to that patient.

In a manual system, the voided number is usually not reassigned to another new patient since it requires a great deal of clerical time to track the number and enter the new patient's name on the correct number index page. If numbers are computer generated, the task of tracking unused numbers is not difficult if the computer program is designed to reuse such numbers. The number of digits used in the registration number for both manual and automated systems should be adequate to cover anticipated growth in new admissions based on hospital projections over a specified time period.

FILE EXPANSION

Planning for file expansion is affected by the choice of a numbering system. It is necessary to leave 25 percent of the shelves open when using the unit numbering and filing system, because additional room is needed to allow for the expansion of the individual medical records. When using the serial-unit filing system which requires moving medical records forward, gaps may occur on the shelves as records are pulled. This is particularly apt to happen when readmission rates are high. With the serial numbering and filing system the shelves remain constant, expanding only at one end of the file as new numbers are assigned to patients.

PURGING OF FILES

Purging inactive records from the file is simple when using serial and serial-unit numbering and filing. The hospital number is an indicator of the age of the record: the lower the number, the older the record. With serial-unit numbering and filing, old records of patients who are readmitted are always moved forward and filed under a higher registration number. Those records which are not moved forward within a prescribed time period are designated inactive. With the serial system, old records (those with the lowest hospital numbers) are easily selected from the file shelves for inactive storage.

With the unit system, however, purging inactive records requires that the contents of each folder be individually inspected to determine the year of the last admission, ambulatory care visit, or emergency treatment; since the hospital number is not an indicator of record activity. Health care facilities that use unit numbering often mark the outside of each patient's folder with the year of most recent treatment activity to facilitate the purging process. This can also be accomplished by using pressure-sensitive color-coded tabs with the year preprinted on the tab. When this technique is used, one must be careful not to order more tabs than are needed for a specific year. If blank tabs are used, it will be necessary to have a table showing the color assignment for each year. Either method will prevent having to open each medical record folder to search and find the latest date of admission and/or treatment.

NUMBER SOURCES

A health facility usually creates its own bank of patient identification numbers, arbitrarily deciding the highest number of digits it wishes to use before starting over again with the number 1. It is difficult to remember or work with numbers containing more than 6 digits; although when terminal or middle digit filing is used, longer numbers can be easily handled because they are broken up into segments. This system will be described in greater detail later in the chapter. But for most health facilities, numbering from 000001 to 999999 will supply an ample number reservoir lasting many years. Starting a new number series for each year with a letter or number prefix (e.g., 85-456231 or A-456231) is not advisable, since an error in the prefix makes record retrieval extremely difficult.

Numbers which have not yet been assigned are usually held in a master control book or register by either the medical record department or patient registration area. The choice of where numbers are controlled depends on the needs of each facility and the procedures used to issue them. The responsibility for number allocation should be placed where the most accurate and trouble-free operation can be accomplished.

If a facility is automated, the computer program can control the issuance of numbers by automatically assigning the next sequential number to a new patient admission. The computer can also search and determine if the patient already has an assigned unit number.

If the medical record department retains responsibility for number control, large blocks of numbers (100, 200, or 500 consecutive numbers) are often issued to patient registration areas with a consistently high volume of new admissions. This practice reduces the amount of requests received by the medical record department for number assignment.

CHANGING FROM SERIAL TO UNIT NUMBERING

Changing from serial numbering (or a serial-unit filing system) to unit numbering and filing is easily accomplished by following the steps below.

1. Select a date to make the change, preferably the first day of the calendar or fiscal year.

2. Begin issuing unit numbers on the selected day. (The last unused serial number can be used to begin the unit system or an entirely new series, if desired.)

3. Assign readmitted patients a new unit number, bringing forward their previous records and filing them under the new number. Leave empty folders of the previous records in their original places in the file. Make a cross-reference on the folder to the new unit number.

4. Leave in the file under their original numbers all records of patients not readmitted. After a specified time, all medical records remaining in the original file area may easily be purged from the active file area and taken to inactive storage.

TYPES OF FILING

Straight Numeric

Numeric filing refers to the filing of records in exact chronological order according to registration number. Thus, consecutively numbered charts appear in sequence on the file shelves. For example, the following four medical records would be filed in consecutive order on a shelf: 465023, 465024, 465025, 465026. Obviously it is a simple matter to pull fifty consecutively numbered records from the file for study purposes or for inactive storage. Probably the greatest advantage of this type of filing system is the ease with which personnel are trained to work with it. This approach to filing has, however, certain inherent disadvantages. Because a clerk must consider all digits of the record number at one time when filing a record, it is easy to misfile. The greater the number of digits that must be recalled when filing, the greater the chance for error. Transposition of numbers is common: Record 465424 can be misfiled as Record 464524. A more serious drawback to straight numerical filing is that the heaviest filing activity is concentrated in the area of the file housing the medical records with the highest numbers (representing the newest or most recent records). Several clerks filing records at the same time in such areas are bound to get in each other's way.

Finally, quality control of filing is difficult with this system. Since clerks are usually filing in the area of the most current records, it is not feasible to fix responsibility for a section of the file to one clerk.

Terminal Digit

Terminal digit filing is a simple and accurate filing method which increases productivity of file clerks.

Usually a six-digit number is used and divided with a hyphen into three parts, each part normally containing two digits. The primary digits are the last two digits on the right-hand side of the number. The secondary digits are the middle two, and the tertiary digits are the first two on the left side of the number (Figure 2).

In a terminal digit file, there are 100 primary sections, ranging from 00 to 99. When filing, a clerk considers the primary digits first, taking the record to the corresponding primary section. Within each primary section, groups of records are matched according to secondary digits. After locating the correct secondary digit section, the clerk files in numerical order by the tertiary digits. In the file, the second tertiary digit changes with every record. Note the following sequences in a terminal digit file.

46-52-02	98-05-26	98-99-30
47-52-02	99-05-26	99-99-30
48-52-02	00-06-26	00-00-31
49-52-02	01-06-26	01-00-31

The terminal digit method of filing when using six numbers has been described, but adaptations can be made by using five, seven, or even the nine digits found in the social security number. With a five-digit number, one could break it into three sections, as follows:

1-23-45   0-00-01   etc.

With seven digits, the breakdown might be:

123-45-67   000-00-01

The nine digits in the social security number can be broken down in many ways, but one that is often used is to break the last group of four numbers into two sections, calling the last two digits the primary digits and the second pair the secondary digits. Then the remaining five digits are used for sequential filing. The following illustrates this method:

243 - 09 - 5228 becomes 24309 - 52 - 28

tertiary digits · secondary digits · primary digits

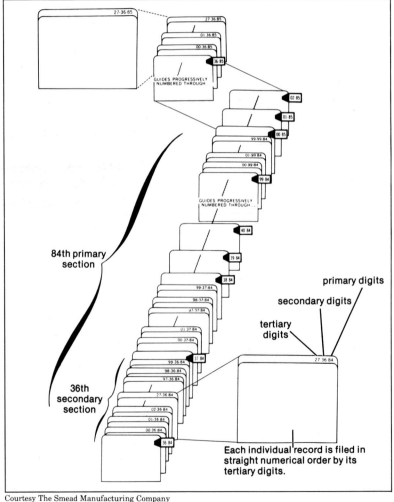

Courtesy The Smead Manufacturing Company

Fig. 2 –
HEALTH RECORD NUMBER 27 36 84 IS FILED IN THE 84TH PRIMARY SECTION, AND THE 36TH SECONDARY SECTION, BY ITS TERTIARY DIGITS, 27

The family numbering system, as described earlier in this chapter, consists of a six-digit family number and a two-digit prefix to identify each individual family member. Since all parts of a family's record are placed together in the file, the terminal digit application of 01-623472 would require that the records be filed by the last six digits.

01	—	62	34	72
head of household		tertiary digits	secondary digits	primary digits

The advantages of terminal digit filing are numerous. As new records are added to the file, their terminal digit numbers are equally distributed throughout the 100 primary sections. Only every 100th new medical record will be filed in the same primary section of the file. The implications of this "perfect" distribution are extensive. The congestion that results when several clerks file active records in the same area of the file is eliminated. Clerks may be assigned responsibility for certain sections of the file (e.g., when four clerks are filing, the first clerk can be responsible for terminal digit sections 00-24, the second for 25-49, the third for 50-74, and the fourth for 75-99). As registration numbers are still assigned in straight numerical order, the work is evenly distributed with each clerk having approximately the same number of active records in each section. Numbers 463719, 463720, and 463721 are assigned in strict sequence, but the records are filed in terminal digit sections "19," "20," and "21" respectively. Inactive records may be pulled from each terminal digit section as new records are added. In this way the volume of records in each primary section is controlled, and large gaps in the file which require backshifting of records are prevented. This volume control also simplifies file area planning.

Misfiles are substantially reduced with the use of terminal digit filing. Since the clerk is concerned with only one pair of digits at a time, the transposition of numbers is less likely to occur. Even if the tertiary digits are increased to three, e.g., 245-68-90, recalling three digits is easier than recalling seven. The use of preprinted, color-keyed folders is recommended. This further helps in the reduction of misfiles. The clerk is immediately alerted to a possible error if a folder with a yellow band is filed into a group of folders with dark green bands. Figure 3 is a table which shows colors associated with two-digit primary numbers and one-digit primary numbers which are available through some vendors.

TWO-DIGIT PRIMARY NUMBERS	ONE-DIGIT PRIMARY NUMBERS	COLORED BANDS
00-09	0	Purple
10-19	1	Yellow
20-29	2	Dark Green
30-39	3	Orange
40-49	4	Light Blue
50-59	5	Brown
60-69	6	Cerise
70-79	7	Light Green
80-89	8	Red
90-99	9	Dark Blue

Courtesy of Physicians' Record Company

FIG. 3 – COLORED BANDS FOR PRIMARY NUMBERS

The training period for new personnel is usually a little longer for a terminal digit system than for a straight numeric system, but most file clerks learn it in a few hours time. More units of shelving may be required initially, since expansion must be planned by equipping the total file area from the start. With straight numeric filing, additional shelving units can be added as existing shelves become filled.

Middle Digit

In middle digit filing, the clerk files according to pairs of digits as in the terminal digit method. However, the primary, secondary, and tertiary digits are in different positions. The *middle* pair of digits in a six-digit number are the primary digits; the digits on the left are the secondary digits; and the digits on the right are the tertiary digits.

56   –   78   –   96

secondary   primary   tertiary

Shown below are sample sequences from a middle digit file.

56-78-96	99-78-96
56-78-97	99-78-97
56-78-98	99-78-98
56-78-99	99-78-99
57-78-00	00-79-00
57-78-01	00-79-01

From the first 4 numbers listed in the samples, one can see that blocks of 100 charts (i.e., 56-78-00 through 56-78-99) would be filed in straight numerical order. This has several advantages: first, it is simple to pull up to 100 consecutively numbered charts for study purposes; second, conversion from a straight numerical system to a middle digit system is much simpler than conversion to a terminal digit system, for blocks of 100 charts pulled from a straight numerical file are in exact order for middle digit filing. Middle digit filing provides a more even distribution of records than straight numerical filing, although it does not equal the balance achieved by a terminal digit filing system. Clerks may be assigned responsibility for certain middle digit sections. As in terminal digit filing, the clerk is filing by pairs of digits rather than by six or seven digits; therefore, misfiles are reduced.

There are certain disadvantages to middle digit filing. Training is more involved than is training for straight numeric or terminal digit filing. Gaps result in the file when large groups of records are pulled for inactive storage. Middle digit filing does not lend itself well to numbers with more than six digits.

CONVERTING TO TERMINAL OR MIDDLE DIGIT FILING

Many hospitals start terminal digit filing at the beginning of a new year or when they move into a new file area. Instead of converting the past files into terminal digit, the medical records are brought forward to the terminal digit area as the patients are readmitted to the health care facility.

If the past files are to be converted, the problem is simplified if the department is also moving; because the conversion can take place simultaneously with the move. However, if the conversion takes place in the same area, everything must first be moved out before the area can be mapped out and section guides installed. When converting, all records must be sorted first according to the primary digits (terminal digit); secondly by the secondary digits; and lastly by the tertiary digits.

Conversion can be either a concerted effort for a number of people, or it can be spread over a period of time with regular personnel if properly planned in advance. If the latter method is used, the routine work must be kept flowing smoothly.

During the conversion two important tasks should also be accomplished:

1. Find misfiled records.
2. Account for all numbers that are not in the file (if unable to locate the record, an empty folder should be placed in the file with the notation that the medical record was missing as of the date of the move).

If time permits, it is beneficial to replace worn folders (if new color-coded folders are not being adopted). In addition, all names and hospital numbers may be checked with either the number index or the patients' register to ensure accuracy.

PHYSICAL FACILITIES IN THE FILE AREA

The medical record department must include sufficient space and equipment to store patients' records so they are easily accessible when requested. Adequate filing equipment, lighting, temperature control, supplies, and attention to safety in the file room all contribute to the productivity of filing clerks.

RECORD STORAGE EQUIPMENT

Open-shelf file units and five-drawer file cabinets are the most commonly used storage units for medical records. Open-shelf units are recommended over cabinets for the following reasons: (1) they are less expensive than file cabinets; (2) personnel can file or pull records faster because there is no opening or closing of drawers; and (3) most importantly, open shelves are space savers, accommodating more records in a given floor area, as well as requiring less aisle space. Thirty-six inches is recommended for aisles between units, although thirty inches is adequate when there is a critical shortage of floor space. When file cabinets are arranged in a single row, a three-foot aisle between rows is adequate. When the cabinets face each other, five-foot aisles are required to allow room for opening two face-to-face drawers.

File cabinets provide a somewhat neater filing area, and they protect records from dust and dirt. However, good housekeeping in an open-shelf filing area will alleviate the need to protect records from exposure to room dust and dirt.

When purchasing storage units, one must determine the number of linear filing inches provided by the units and the number of filing inches currently being used to store medical records. Then the projected linear filing inches required for the next five or ten years should be added. This sum divided by the number of linear filing inches available in a storage unit will determine the number of units to buy, assuming there is adequate space. The medical record department which currently uses 1,435 linear filing inches to store its medical records wants to buy new open-shelf filing units. Each of the shelves in a new five-shelf unit measures 33 linear filing inches. With five shelves per filing unit, the total filing inches in one shelving unit would be 165 linear filing inches.

> 33 inches per × 5 shelves in = 165 filing inches in
> shelf   each unit   each shelving unit

At present, 1,435 filing inches are required to store the medical records. It is estimated that an additional 300 filing inches should be added to allow for five-year expansion capabilities. Total filing inches required are 1,735. To determine the number of file shelving units to purchase, divide the required filing inches by the number of linear filing inches in each shelving unit.

> 1,735 filing inches ÷ 165 inches per = 10.5 shelving
>   shelving unit   units

In order to provide for all of the projected file space, a total of 11 shelving units should be purchased. If adequate space in the file area is a problem, ten file shelving units could be installed, but this would not provide for a full five years' expansion.

Shelving may be purchased with more than five shelves per unit, some as many as eight shelves high (Figure 4). Due consideration should be given to the fact that the higher the shelving, the more need there will be to provide step stools for the file clerks so that file numbers can be read accurately on the top shelves.

Pairs of units placed back to back in long rows are the most compact arrangement for storage units in the file area. Moveable file units on tracks are also available and should be consid-

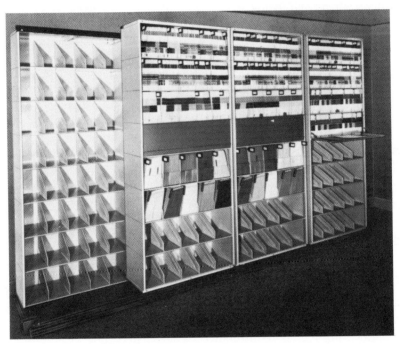

FIG. 4 – OPEN SHELVING

ered if storage space in the filing area is a problem. In addition to saving space over conventional file shelving units, moveable files increase operating efficiency; since the file area itself is more compact and personnel do not have to walk as far. Limited access to the file area may be a major disadvantage to some facilities with highly active files. As only one aisle is provided for several units of shelving, it is often impossible for two individuals to work in adjoining sections of the file. Medical record departments with one or two persons responsible for filing may find moveable files very beneficial to their efficient operation (Figure 5).

Automated filing systems have been developed which bring requested records to clerical personnel at the touch of a few buttons. The amount of clerical time and energy expended is greatly reduced with automation, but the cost of such systems proves very prohibitive to many health care facilities.

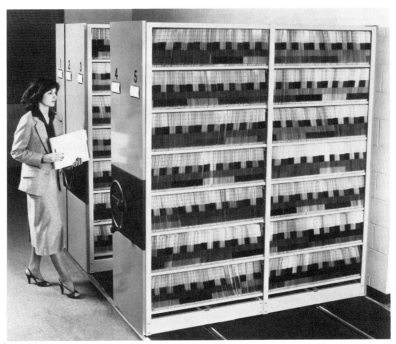

Courtesy Ames Color File

FIG. 5 – MOVEABLE FILES

GUIDING THE FILES

Guides should be placed throughout the files to expedite the filing and finding of records. The number of guides needed depends upon the thickness of the majority of the medical records in the file. For records of medium thickness, a guide for every fifty records is adequate. For very thick records, more guides are needed than for thin records. Active files generally require closer guiding than inactive files.

When purchasing guides, durability and visibility should be the primary concern. The tab or projection on the guide should project far enough beyond the records to ensure complete exposure of the numbers on the guide.

Usually two pairs of numbers appear on each guide in terminal and middle digit files. For example, guides for the primary digit section $\underline{00}$ might be as follows:
84

$$\frac{00}{84} \qquad \frac{01}{84} \qquad \frac{02}{84} \qquad \frac{03}{84}$$

Note that the top number on the guide is the secondary number, and the bottom number is the primary number. In a terminal digit file, the first record to appear behind guide 00 would be 00-00-84, followed by the record 01-00-84.

In the middle digit file, records 00-02-00 and 00-02-01 would be filed immediately behind the $\underline{00}$ guide.
02

To determine the total number of guides needed, the following formula may be used:

$$\frac{\text{Total number of records}}{\text{Number of records between guides}} = \begin{array}{c} \text{Total number of} \\ \text{guides} \end{array}$$

If the total number of records is not known, an estimate may be made by multiplying the filing inches by the average number of records per inch. Records on several shelves should be counted to determine the average number of records per inch.

Once the total number of terminal digit guides has been calculated, the number pattern on the guides can be determined. There are 100 primary sections in the file area from 00 to 99. If the total number of guides necessary for the filing area is 100, one guide per primary section would be sufficient. The pattern on the guide would read 00-00, 00-01, 00-02, etc. Two hundred total guides would result in 2 guides per primary section, with one at the beginning and one in the middle of each section.

00-00   00-01   00-02
50-00   50-01   50-02

Thus, to determine the pattern on terminal digit guides, divide the total number of guides by the 100 primary sections. This answer depicts the number of guides within each primary section, and these guides should be distributed evenly among the secondary numbers in that section.

Table for determining pattern of terminal digit guides:

TOTAL NUMBER OF GUIDES NEEDED		PRIMARY SECTIONS		GUIDES IN EACH PRIMARY SECTION	PATTERN ON GUIDES
10,000	÷	100	=	100	00 00 01 00 (every 100 numbers) 02 00 etc.
5,000	÷	100	=	50	00 00 02 00 (every 200 numbers) 04 00 etc.
2,000	÷	100 ·	=	20	00 00 05 00 (every 500 numbers) 10 00 etc.
1,000	÷	100	=	10	00 00 10 00 (every 1,000 numbers) 20 00 etc.
500	÷	100	=	5	00 00 20 00 (every 2,000 numbers) 40 00 etc.
400	÷	100	=	4	00 00 25 00 (every 2,500 numbers) 50 00 etc.
TOTAL NUMBER OF GUIDES NEEDED		PRIMARY SECTIONS		GUIDES IN EACH PRIMARY SECTION	PATTERN ON GUIDES

In a straight numerical filing system, guides must be continually changed. This is also true for middle digit filing. Because new hospital numbers are issued in chronological order, new guides must be placed in the file so as to reflect the numerical increase of the two left-hand digits of the hospital number. Similarly, as old records are permanently removed from the file, guides in affected sections of the file require change. Terminal digit guides, on the other hand, are more permanent; because their primary and secondary digits keep recurring as new hospital numbers are assigned to patients.

PROTECTIVE COVERS FOR RECORDS

In order to keep their parts intact and to protect the sheets from tearing and the effects of repeated handling, medical records should have protective covers. Some that are popular are chart covers, file folders, and large envelopes. For an additional small charge, chart covers can be equipped with fasteners which hold the sheets in place. These fasteners can be located at the top of the cover or on the left side as with books. The fold of the file folder should be scored or bellowed to allow for expansion (see Figure 6).

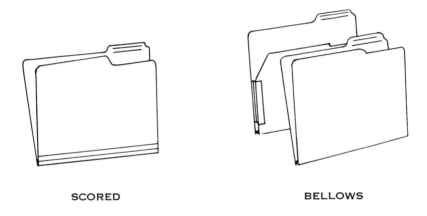

SCORED   BELLOWS

Fɪɢ. 6 – Fɪʟᴇ Fᴏʟᴅᴇʀs

Record folders may be purchased with preprinted numbers on the cover which provide a neat and legible appearance. The patient's name as well as the hospital number should appear on the folder or cover. A sequential list of years printed horizontally on the front right-hand side of the folder allows for checking the year of most recent admission and makes purging inactive records an easy process.

SAFETY

Safety factors are an important consideration in the filing area, and safety rules should be conspicuously posted. The prevention of falls is of prime importance, particularly when clerks are working with the upper shelves in open-shelf units. Skid-proof ladders are a wise investment. Work areas with table space should be interspersed throughout the files. There may be either pullout shelves in the record-storage unit or carts of some type to assist in processing records within the filing area. Adequate lighting reduces eyestrain. Proper conditioning of the air with regard to temperature, humidity, and dust control is essential for fire prevention and employee productivity.

ORGANIZATIONAL PATTERNS OF FILES

Storage and retention of medical records in a health care facility should facilitate the retrieval of requested records. There are two basic methods of filing records – centralized and decentralized.

CENTRALIZATION

Simply stated, centralized means that all materials and information about a patient are funneled into a single file held in a central location. In hospital applications, a centralized file usually means that the patient's inpatient, ambulatory care, and emergency records are filed in a single file in a central location.

DECENTRALIZATION

Decentralized files result when certain parts of a record are filed in another location away from the central file area. In hospitals this usually means the emergency record of a patient is filed where emergency records are stored, or ambulatory care records are filed in the ambulatory care area. This leaves only the inpatient records to be filed in a central file; and, of course, this could consist of one or more inpatient admissions. But even though a "unit" is made of several inpatient admissions for a patient, its placement in a filing system is not considered to be centralized; unless the emergency and ambulatory care records are included.

ADVANTAGES/DISADVANTAGES OF EACH

Centralization has many advantages, some of which are listed here:

- There is less duplication of effort with regard to creation, maintenance, and storage of records.
- There is less overall expenditure on space and equipment.
- A composite record containing all available information is of greater help to the health care team than one in which parts are scattered in several places.
- Procedures and policies for record activity are standardized.
- Personnel may become more proficient in various file room functions and procedures.
- Record control and security are easier to maintain.
- Supervision of file room personnel is more consistent.

However, in spite of the obvious advantages, circumstances often make it expedient to decentralize records, either temporarily or permanently. This may occur when clinic patients are being seen frequently on an outpatient basis; so it is easier and more efficient to store the record in the clinic, at least for the duration of the frequent patient visits. Another situation in which decentralization might be justified is when a health facility operates from several buildings or locales, and a decentralized record system would require far less transportation time and effort.

Other terms used for decentralization are "controlled/decentralized" (records are housed separately but controlled through uniform policies, procedures, methods, and forms) and "satellite" (records remain in a satellite location of active treatment, then are returned to central file area).

Whatever the reasons for decentralizing records or the terminology used to describe it, one should be sure that the methodology chosen is best for the health facility.

RECORD CONTROL

Regardless of whether files are centralized or decentralized, there must be centralization of authority over them. One person, logically the director of the medical record department, should be authorized to establish and maintain control over all filing procedures and record usage.

REQUISITIONS

Routine requests for records, as from ambulatory care clinics or physicians performing research, should be delivered to the medical record department by a specified time of day established by hospital administration or medical staff policy. An established time assists in determining staffing needs within the department. A common practice is to require that all routine requisitions for records be received in the department the afternoon before the day on which the records are needed. The exact time set for the deadline (noon or 4:00 P.M., for example) is dependent on (1) the volume of requests received daily and (2) the number of filing room personnel available to pull requisitioned records.

Patient care areas requesting records for scheduled appointments should bear the responsibility for filling out requisition slips which are readable and which have patients' names and hospital numbers filled in correctly. The medical record practitioner may, however, direct record personnel to make out requisition slips for physicians and administrative personnel.

Nonroutine requests for records such as those from the emergency department must be processed as quickly as possible by medical record personnel. Phone requests for records needed immediately (sometimes referred to as "STAT" requests or ASAP – as soon as possible) are acceptable; file clerks can make out the necessary requisitions for these requests. Personnel from the requesting department should, in most instances, be required to pick up the needed record in the medical record department.

The requisition slip is usually a three-part form (see Figure 7). The minimum amount of information which must be included on the slip is the patient's name and hospital number, the name of the requisitioning patient care area or person, and the date on which the record is needed.

One copy of the requisition slip is fastened to the medical record when it is pulled from the file. Another copy becomes the sign-out slip which is placed in an outguide and filed to replace the pulled medical record. The outguide and sign-out slip are removed from the file when the record is returned. Still another copy of the requisition slip may be sent to the department which

REQUISITION FOR MEDICAL RECORD

Name of Patient_____

Terminal
Digit No.

Date_____Time_____a.m.
p.m.

Out to_____

Location or Clinic_____

Form courtesy of Physicians' Record Company

FIG. 7 – REQUISITION FOR MEDICAL RECORD

made the request, or retained in the medical record department as a reference to those records which have been sent to other areas of the facility and not yet been returned. A small card file box may be used to house the *locator file* which contains copies of requisition slips for all patient records removed from the department. The locator file is arranged in numerical order by medical record number. When the patient's record is returned to the medical record department, this copy of the requisition slip is removed from the locator file and destroyed. If a medical record is not returned within the established time, the locator file provides a ready reference for reminding the requestor of the need for the record to be returned promptly to the medical record department. In large institutions in which scheduling of appointments is done with data processing equipment, the sign-out slip may be in the form of a punched card, a hardcopy printout from a machine, or a computerized record tracking system may be installed.

CHARGE-OUT SYSTEM

The *cardinal rule* in the file area is that *no record can be removed from file without being replaced by an outguide and/ or a requisition slip.* This rule applies not only to extra-departmental personnel but also to employees of the medical record department.

```
┌─────────────────────────────────────────┬──────────────────────┐
│                                          │                      │
│         COMMUNITY GENERAL                │                      │
│             HOSPITAL                     │                      │
│                                          │                      │
│    TRANSFER OF MEDICAL RECORD            │                      │
│                                          └──────────────────────┤
│                                                                 │
│   Date_____                                  │
│                                                                 │
│   From_____ │
│                                                                 │
│   To_____ │
│                                                                 │
│   For: Clinic Appt._____ Corres._____ Room No.____│
│                                                                 │
│   To Be Used By Dr._____ │
│                                                                 │
│        Please Send This Card to Medical Record Dept. Immediately│
│                                                                 │
└─────────────────────────────────────────────────────────────────┘
```

Form courtesy of Physicians' Record Company

FIG. 8 – TRANSFER NOTICE

An individual receiving a record should assume responsibility for returning it in good condition and at the designated time. Certain rules should be established with regard to the length of time a record may be kept out of file. It is wise to require that medical records be returned at the close of each day; so that if emergencies occur, records are available when needed. Records should never be removed from the facility except under subpoena or valid court order.

Physicians or other hospital personnel may sign out records from the department to take to a work area during the day, but all records must be returned to the department by closing time. If the same records will be needed again within several days, they may be temporarily stored in separate files within the medical record department.

Transfer of records from one signed-out location to another in the hospital requires the use of a transfer card or slip. Use of these eliminates the need for such records to be sent back to the medical record department before being forwarded to the second requesting party. Transfer notices are sent to the file area where they are placed in the outguide (see Figure 8).

OUTGUIDES

Outguides provide an important means of control over record usage. They are used to replace a folder that has been removed from the files. The guide remains in the files until the borrowed folder is returned and refiled. Folders or sign-out cards with pockets for storing requisition slips are popular for this purpose. The use of colored outguides is helpful to the clerk in spotting the correct location for refiling a record. Since outguides are used over and over again, sturdy construction is essential (see Figure 9).

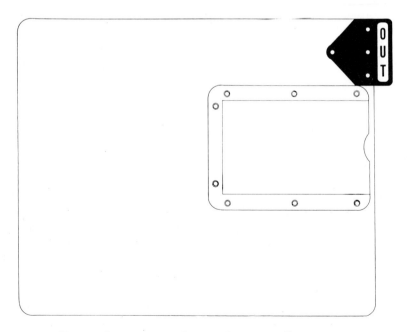

FIG. 9 – OUTGUIDE WITH PLASTIC POCKET FOR REQUISITION

AUTOMATED CHART LOCATION SYSTEM

A computerized chart location system is an ideal method of tracking medical records. Commonly the patient name, patient number, reason code, and user code are entered via a terminal to sign out a record to a user. The computer automatically records the date and time on each transaction. If the tracking system utilizes the same data base as the master patient index, the computer may automatically provide the patient's name when his number is entered; so only verification of the accuracy of the name is required. Bar codes representing the patient's number may also be used on each medical record to speed up the process of checking medical records in and out. To use bar codes, however, bar code labels must be placed on each record folder; and bar code readers (a wand passed over the bar code on the medical record) must be purchased. The remaining information required to complete each transaction is entered via the keyboard.

The installation of a computerized tracking system is highly recommended if the department's file activity justifies the expense. Such systems may be developed on inexpensive personal computers in smaller facilities or on mainframe computers in larger facilities. At a minimum, such a system should have the ability to perform the following functions: (1) inquire of chart location by medical record number, (2) check charts out by location, (3) check charts out by doctor, (4) check charts in, (5) display charts checked out by location, and (6) display charts checked out by doctor or requester number.

The location of medical records within the medical record department work flow is also facilitated by the installation of an automated system.

LOCATING MISFILES

Regardless of the number of record control systems used in the medical record department file area, occasionally a patient's record will be placed in the wrong location or will not be signed out correctly. Various techniques are available to assist a person in locating a medical record that has been misfiled. Among these techniques are:

1. Look for transpositions of the last two digits of the number, or of the hundreds or thousands digits. The number 46-37-82 may be filed as 46-37-<u>28</u> or 46-<u>73</u>-82.

2. Look for misfiles of "3" under "5" or "8" and vice versa; and of "7" or "8" under "9." The number "9" may be taken as a "7" if it is worn.

3. Check for a certain number in the hundred group just preceding or following the number, as 485 under 385 or 585, or under other similar combinations.

4. Check for transpositions of first and last numbers.

5. Check the folder just before and just after the one needed. It sometimes happens that a folder is put into another folder rather than between two folders.

COLOR CODING OF RECORD FOLDERS

Color coding refers to the use of color on folders to aid in the prevention of misfiles and in the location of misfiled records. Color bars in various positions around the edges of folders (known as blocking) create distinct patterns of color in various sections of the file. A break in the color pattern in a file section signals a misfiled record. Color coding is most effective when used in conjunction with terminal digit and middle digit filing, although workable color-coding systems can be used for straight numerical filing.

One approach to color coding in a terminal digit or middle digit file utilizes ten different colors to signify the first primary digits 0 through 9. Two color bars or blocks appearing in the same position can be used to signify each of the two primary digits. In this case the top color bar represents the left-hand digit of the primary set, and the bottom color bar represents the right-hand digit of the primary set. If brown is the color assigned to the digit 8 and green is the color assigned to the digit 4, a chart numbered 16 94 84 in a terminal digit file is color coded with a brown band on top, with a green band directly beneath it.

Additional color bars may be added to indicate secondary digits, and there are many combinations which can be used.

In setting up a color-coding system, it is generally advisable to limit coding with color to two or three digits. This ensures a simple, easy-to-learn system. Folders already color coded may be purchased from commercial firms, or employees of the medical record department may apply colored tape to the folders.

OTHER FILING RULES AND PROCEDURES

Some basic rules to aid in efficient handling of medical records include:

1. When records are returned to the medical record department, they should be sorted before being filed. This facilitates the finding of needed but unfiled records, and makes refiling easier.

2. Except for hospital personnel who have been instructed to use the file area during evening and nighttime hours, *only medical record department personnel should be authorized to handle records.* Physicians, hospital staff members, and personnel from other departments of the hospital should not be allowed to pull records from the permanent filing area. During the evening hours, emergency room personnel and supervising nurses should leave returned records at a designated place in the record area or in one specified location if the medical record department is closed.

3. Records with torn covers and those with loose papers should be repaired promptly to prevent further damage or loss of valuable information.

4. An audit of the files should be made periodically to locate misfiled records and check requisitions which indicate records have not been returned. Such an audit might promptly indicate that certain clinics or departments are holding records beyond the prescribed time limit. In such cases the medical record director will then investigate the situation and take any corrective measures indicated.

5. Medical records involving legal actions should not be stored in the general files; these can be filed in a locked file cabinet in the medical record director's office. However, outguides should be placed in the permanent file to indicate that these records are in a "special" file.

6. Filing-area personnel should be responsible for keeping the shelves neat and orderly. Disorderly files increase the likelihood of misfiles.

7. Medical records being processed or used by employees within the department should remain on desk tops or in specified files so they can be available at any time.

8. Written procedures for filing-area personnel are of assistance in their training and in maintaining control over the files.

9. Records which are voluminous should be separated into two or more volumes.

10. Loose laboratory slips, x-ray, and other reports received regularly for processing by the department should be date-stamped when received, and every effort should be made to incorporate them into the records as soon as possible. Reports not filed on the day received should at least be sorted in a way which will facilitate finding them when needed. Care should be taken to be sure such reports are in the correct section of the inpatient or outpatient portion of the record.

11. The person supervising the file area should keep a report of activities in the area. Items included in the report might include: number of requisitioned charts pulled each day, number of emergency calls, number of misfiles, or records which could not be found. Counts such as these provide useful information for planning work and for control over the files.

TRANSPORTATION OF RECORDS

There are several ways to transport records. In most hospitals, the majority of records are hand-carried from one point to another; therefore, medical record departments should establish specific delivery and pickup schedules for the different sections of the hospital. Frequency of delivery and pickup is dependent upon the amount of record activity. Medical record personnel cannot deliver individual records on short notice to requesting departments as a matter of routine. Unless otherwise provided, departments requesting a record for emergency use should dispatch one of their own employees to pick it up.

Some hospitals are equipped with pneumatic tube systems which rapidly transport single records to various departments. Strict rules regarding the use and maintenance of a tube system are essential. One of the drawbacks to such systems is the fact that tubes are often too small to contain a thick record.

Dumbwaiters, record elevators, and horizontal conveyors are often used to transport records. A patient registration area located directly above a medical record department can make good use of a dumbwaiter or elevator.

Technological innovations in the areas of microfilming and computer processing can be expected to speed up the transfer of patient data from one location to another.

MEDICAL RECORD RETENTION POLICIES

The medical record director who has ample space for storing medical records is indeed among the fortunate few in his profession. For most practitioners, there is a never-ending battle against overcrowded files.

The alert medical record professional has developed a formalized plan or record retention schedule for the automatic transfer of eligible records to inactive storage and later destruction of the medical record itself. This alleviates the problem of deciding what to do with the overcrowded files once a year.

The length of time a medical record is retained in active and inactive storage will greatly depend on the type of health care facility and the activity of the medical staff. In developing a record retention policy, a health care institution must be guided by its own patient care and research activities, taking into consideration the possibility of future legal actions by patients. Based on these factors, a decision should be made regarding the age of a record before it is placed in inactive or alternate medical record storage.

INACTIVE MEDICAL RECORDS

A definite plan for handling inactive records must be established in order to provide filing space for a continuously expanding active file. Practically speaking, the chief criterion for determining record inactivity is the amount of space available in the department for the efficient storage of newer medical records. In one department, records of discharges which are five years old may be designated as inactive; whereas in another department with an acute shortage of filing space, inactive records may be defined as records only one or two years old. If there is no more space for active record storage, an effort should be made to systematically retire older records to inactive status at the same rate as new records are being added.

Inactive records can be stored in another area of the facility; they can be microfilmed; they can be commercially stored; or they can be destroyed in compliance with record retention statutes.

Files for inactive records may be established in areas of the facility physically separate from the medical record department. As old records are removed from the active files, they should be replaced by transfer slips to the inactive files, or their location may be noted in the computerized tracking system. This will eliminate unnecessary searching.

Although microfilming is discussed in another chapter, it should be pointed out here that microfilmed records require only a minimum amount of storage space; so space can usually be found in the medical record department to house the film, thereby maintaining physically centralized active and inactive files.

A few hospitals have utilized commercial storage companies to house inactive records. These companies ordinarily make deliveries to the hospital upon request from the medical record department. When this method is employed, it is advisable to have a contract drawn up stipulating the arrangements made for storage and retrieval, especially the requirements for confidentiality of the records.

Several alternate approaches to conservation of filing space may be made. For example, nurses' notes from charts of very recent discharges may be microfilmed or stored in the inactive file, in this way increasing the amount of space in the active file for older records. This plan would be desirable in a hospital with a high readmission rate.

DESTRUCTION OF MEDICAL RECORDS

Although some small hospitals destroy inactive medical records by shredding or burning, most health care facilities microfilm medical records because they lack the storage space required to maintain medical records for recommended retention periods. In 1974 the American Medical Record Association and the American Hospital Association jointly endorsed a *Statement on the Preservation of Patient Medical Records in Health Care Institutions.* This publication is being revised but no substantive changes are foreseen. The 1974 version states:

Since a hospital or other health care institution is seldom requested to produce medical records older than ten (10) years for clinical, scientific, legal, or audit purposes, it is ordinarily sufficient to retain the medical records of cases ten (10) years after the most recent patient care usage in the absence of legal considerations. Accordingly, it is recommended that complete patient medical records in health care institutions usually be retained, either in the original or reproduced form, for a period of ten (10) years after the most recent patient care usage. After this period, such records may be destroyed unless destruction is specifically prohibited by statute, ordinance, regulation, or law, provided that the institution:

1. retains basic information such as dates of admission and discharge, names of responsible physicians, record of diagnoses and operations, operative reports, pathology reports, and discharge resumes for all records so destroyed;
2. retains complete medical records of minors for the period of minority plus the applicable statute of limitations as prescribed by statute in the state in which the health care institution is located;
3. retains complete medical records of patients under mental disability in like manner as those of patients under disability of minority; and
4. retains complete patient medical records for longer periods of time when requested in writing by one of the following:
   a. an attending or consultant physician of the patient,
   b. the patient or someone acting legally in his behalf, or
   c. legal counsel for a party having an interest affected by the patient medical records.

If the adoption of a record retention policy as suggested by this statement would reduce the previous period of retention by a health care institution, it is recommended that any new policy be developed with the full knowledge and participation of the medical staff, legal counsel for the institution, and any past or present liability insurance carrier affording coverage during any time in which the affected records were made.

In summary, the definition of inactivity with reference to medical records in a given hospital depends on (1) the amount of filing space available in the medical record department and (2) the yearly expansion rate of current files (number of filing inches needed for each year's records). In establishing a plan for the disposition of inactive records, one must consider (1) volume of research; (2) readmission rate for inpatients and outpatients; (3) statutes of limitation in the state in which the hospital is located; and (4) costs involved in microfilming, inactive storage, and destruction of records.

MISCELLANEOUS RECORD RETENTION

The needs of the individual hospital, the statute of limitations for the specific state, and possible future use of each type of record should be carefully considered before reaching a decision regarding retention periods for the individual hospital.

NURSES' BEDSIDE RECORDS

As nurses' notes are primarily a means of communication between the doctors and nurses, they have served their most important function during hospitalization of the patient. Therefore, in order to reduce the bulk and make the records less cumbersome to handle, many hospitals remove the nurses' notes when the medical record personnel assemble and check the medical record after discharge of the patient. This is done especially if the record is kept as a unit. The nurses' notes are then filed in chronological order in some place less accessible than the current files until the *statute of limitations* has expired. Then they are destroyed. By filing these records in chronological order, they can be easily found if needed; and it is a simple matter to destroy the oldest each year. However, it is wise to follow the same rules regarding nurses' notes on minors as for all other records on minors; and preserve the nurses' notes until the statute of limitations has expired after a minor has reached majority.

EMERGENCY ROOM RECORDS

These records need only be preserved for the duration of the *statute of limitations* for negligence or malpractice suits in the individual state unless needed for proof of hospital services or when an action is pending. The medical information which they contain is often of an episodic nature so they are of little value except for the protection of the hospital as a record of what was done. However, if the patient was in a serious condition, the emergency room record would become a part of the patient's medical record after admission to the hospital and thus be kept as long as the medical record.

REGISTERS: PATIENT AND DELIVERY ROOM

These registers should be kept *permanently,* because the patients' register lists all patients admitted to the hospital in chronological order. The delivery room register is a chronological listing of all infants born in the hospital. Either or both of these registers may be required by state or local law. Even if they are not, they will serve as a double check against the master patient index and will be invaluable if an adult or newborn patient's index card is lost or misfiled. If space is at a premium, or the paper on which these registers are written is deteriorating; they may be microfilmed if experience indicates such need for protection.

INDEXES

Disease and Operation Index

The period these indexes need be retained will be governed by the length of time covered by specific studies by the medical staff in each hospital. If studies are frequently made covering a 25-year period, these indexes should be kept that long. Otherwise, these indexes will have served their maximum period of usefulness usually in 10 years. Studies covering a longer period will rarely occur in hospitals not connected with medical schools. Even here, such studies will not occur frequently because of the great change in medical care even within the past decade.

Physicians' Index

These cards have generally served their purpose within a maximum period of *10 years.* In the majority of hospitals, five years would be within the margin of safety as their chief use is current. Later their chief use is in supplying information when doctors are applying to the specialty boards. This information is usually requested within a five-year period. If there is a possibility that the governing board of the hospital would want to know the amount of work which individual physicians bring to the hospital, an annual summary could be compiled and preserved rather than keeping the index after its period of general usefulness has passed.

MISCELLANEOUS

Daily and Monthly Analyses of Hospital Services

As annual reports should be compiled from the monthly reports, and should be kept permanently, the monthly reports should not be needed after a *five-year period*. The daily analysis will have served all needs usually after two years.

Birth and Death Certificates

Copies of these should be preserved *permanently* and if filed in the medical record at discharge of the patient they will automatically be preserved as long as needed.

Laboratory and X-Ray Reports

As long as the original and signed reports are in the medical records, duplicate copies need be kept *only as long as needed by the originating department.*

Narcotic Records

Normally these records do not come under the supervision of the medical record department. However, in the small hospital which would probably not have a registered pharmacist, many records are considered the responsibility of the medical record director as far as storage is concerned. Therefore, he should be aware of the fact that narcotic "records shall be kept, subject to inspection, for a period of *two years* from the date of dispensing or distributing of such drugs as opium, isonipecaine, coca leaves, opiate, and compound, salt, derivative, or preparation thereof." (U.S. Treasury Department, Bureau of Narcotics, *Regulations No. 5.* Section 2550; Section 2554. (c.) (1), (2), (4), (d); and Section 2556.)

SUMMARY

While the methods of numbering medical records and the systems of filing all have the same objective, that is, a continuous record of the patient available at all times, the centralized unit or serial-unit system automatically attains this objective because all records of a patient are filed together in one folder and in one department. If a centralized unit system is coupled with terminal digit filing in hospitals where the activity of the records is very great, efficient and improved service for the patient, doctors, and other personnel should be the result. Unless the medical record is immediately available when and where needed all the time, labor and expense in maintaining a medical record department is wasted.

Because the space required for the filing of medical records is growing rapidly, the medical record practitioner must face the problem of retention of records realistically. It is economically impractical to continue to use valuable space for records that are seldom used or needed. Therefore, periodic surveys should be made by the department head to review the types and frequency of requests made for medical records. Results of these surveys can greatly assist the administrative personnel responsible for making decisions regarding storage space, microfilming, and retention schedules.

STUDY QUESTIONS

1. Describe the following numbering systems, and list one advantage and disadvantage of each system:
   a. serial
   b. unit
2. List the four steps recommended for changing from a serial or serial-unit to a unit numbering and filing system.
3. Place the following six medical record numbers in sequence according to each filing system: 312497, 312498, 312398, 312399, 322301, 322302;
   a. straight numeric
   b. terminal digit
   c. middle digit
4. List three reasons why open-shelf filing units are preferable to file cabinets for medical record storage in the file area.
5. Depict the pattern which will appear on the terminal digit file guides in a file area requiring 2,500 total guides.
6. Define centralized and decentralized filing, and summarize the advantages of centralization for medical records.

7. Describe the three functions of a three-part requisition slip.

8. Identify those items of information or records which must be retained by a health care institution when medical records are destroyed after a period of 10 years, according to the *Statement on the Preservation of Medical Records in Health Care Institutions.*

9. List the four items one must consider when developing a plan for the destruction of inactive medical records.

10. List the minimum items needed in an automated chart location system.

REFERENCES

BLOOMROSEN, MERYL. "Successful Computer Applications in a Medical Record Department." *JAMRA,* Vol. 53, No. 3, June, 1982, pp. 34-44.

CAPOZZOLI, ELISABETH, RRA, MBA. "An Automated Approach to Medical Record Teaching." *Topics in Health Record Management,* Vol. 2, No. 2, December, 1981.

"Computers and the Medical Record Department." *Topics in Health Record Management,* Vol. 2, No. 2, December, 1981.

Counterpoint, "Social Security Number Not National Identifier." *JAMRA,* Vol. 55, No. 4, April, 1984, p. 11.

FINNEGAN, RITA, MA, RRA. "Dual Challenge: Medical Record Continuity and Availability." A Study to Determine the Practicality of the Unit Medical Records. *JAMRA,* October, 1980.

"Guide to the Retention and Preservation of Records with Destruction Schedules." 6th Hospital Ed. Chicago, Illinois: Records Controls, Inc. Hospital Financial Management Association, 1981.

MISHELEVICH, DAVID J., MD, PhD et al. "Medical Record Control and the Computer Topics in Health Record Management," Vol. 2, No. 2, December, 1981.

ROGERS, TILLIE. "Problems with a Family Numbering System." *Medical Record News.* February, 1975.

Statement Against Use of Social Security Numbers for Hospital Medical Records. American Hospital Association, 1974.

Statement on the Preservation of Patient Medical Records in Health Care Institutions. American Medical Record Association and American Hospital Association, 1974 (Under Revision).

TERRY, GEORGE R., and STALLARD, JOHN J. "Office Management and Control." 8th Ed. Homewood, Illinois: Richard D. Irwin, Inc., 1980.

"The Wonderful World of Color – Makes Records Management Easier." *Information and Records Management*. October, 1976.

WATERS, KATHLEEN A., and MURPHY, GRETCHEN FREDERICK. "Medical Records in Health Information." Aspen Systems, 1979.

chapter *11*

MICROFILMING

Microfilm or microrecords are the result of a photographic process which reduces the original document to a very small size. Microfilming, therefore, results in high density information recording. Microfilm is a recording medium that is also self-reproducible – that is, microfilm can be easily reproduced as microfilm. When combined with good file organization and indexing methods, microfilm is an excellent medium for storage and retrieval of medical records.

MICROFILM–AN HISTORICAL OVERVIEW

Historically, the use of microfilm for information storage is not new. The first microphotographs date back to the mid-nineteenth century, the early days of photography. These were made by Dagron, a French photographer, and Dancer, an English microscopist. In the Franco-Prussian War of 1870-71, hundreds of microfilmed messages were flown into the besieged city of Paris by carrier pigeon. The first commercial application of microfilm occurred during the late 1920s when it was used for the recording of cancelled checks in banks. Libraries were among the first users to use microfilm for archival purposes – that is, as a means of permanent storage. It was also found that microfilm was an excellent medium for storing rare books and manuscripts. During the earliest days of commercial use, microfilm was found to have three main advantages: (1) economy – it is the least expensive method of recording documents, (2) security – information cannot be altered and is more easily protected from accidents such as fire and flood, and (3) storage – microfilm requires a minimum of storage space.

Following World War II, technological improvements spurred the growth of microfilm equipment, materials, techniques, and microfilm systems design. It was also at this time that hospitals began microfilming records because of increased storage space requirements. Innovations in micrographic techniques have made microfilmed records easy to use and quite acceptable to the medical staff.

In 1951 federal laws were amended which allowed for the admission and acceptance of microfilmed records as primary evidence. With this firm foundation of legal acceptability and ease of usage, the application of microfilm to the health care industry for patient, departmental, and corporate records has been a common practice and has minimized expensive demands for storage space in health care facilities.

MICROPHOTOGRAPHY

Microphotography is the process of placing a document before a camera lens and photographing it. Lenses are made which can reduce the size of the image by various amounts. The actual amount of reduction is stated in terms of a reduction ratio. If the reduction ratio is 24 to 1, which is stated as 24X, the original document is reduced to an image 1/24 its original size. Reduction ratios range from 5X to more than 2,400X. As the reduction ratio number gets higher, the images get smaller; and the number of them that can be photographed on a square inch of film greatly increases. Medical records are commonly microfilmed at a reduction ratio of 24X which results in a storage savings of 95 percent.

Opposite to the reduction ratio is the magnification ratio. This ratio specifies how much the microrecord will be enlarged for each ratio number stated. For example, a one-inch square microrecord that is magnified 10 times (10X) will be 10 inches square in its enlarged form. Ideally, the magnification ratio should match the reduction ratio so that the enlarged microrecord will be the original size of the document filmed. This will make the magnified document easier to read.

The film used in the microfilm process is available in four sizes: 16 mm, 35 mm, 70 mm, and 105 mm. 16 mm film is used for recording documents up to 14 inches in width; 35 mm is used for longer documents such as blueprints and maps. 70 mm and 105 mm films are not widely used because they require highly skilled operators which make the process more expensive. Also, the larger film requires more storage space which offsets one of the primary advantages of microfilm.

MICROFILM CAMERAS

ROTARY – The rotary camera is used most frequently for microfilming, because it is the least expensive. With a rotary camera, documents move through the camera on a roller-transport system. The film moves forward with the movement of the document, each time opening the shutter and exposing one frame of film. A rotary camera can make images on 16 mm film at speeds exceeding 500 documents per minute. Approximately 2,500 images can be microfilmed on a single roll of 16 mm film. A rotary camera can be used for filming either one side of a document or the front and back of a document at the same time. The camera can operate at varying reduction ratios – usually between 24X and 45X.

PLANETARY – This type of camera is used to film x-rays and other oversized documents which require high resolution or density. Thirty-five mm film is usually used. Both the document and the film are stationary when the picture is taken. The planetary camera is more expensive than the rotary camera but produces a higher quality image.

ROTOLINE – This camera is used for continuous forms such as EEGs, computer printouts, or monitoring strips.

STEP AND REPEAT – A step and repeat camera is used to produce microfiche only. One page of the record after another is exposed directly onto film which is 4 inches wide. The film is then cut into 6-inch lengths which result in the standard 4 x 6-inch microfiche.

FACTORS IN SELECTING A MICROFORM

There are a wide variety of microforms available: roll film, microfilm jackets, microfiche, ultrafiche, aperture cards, and computer output microfilm (COM). When selecting a microform, a major consideration should be in selecting the microform to match the needs of the user. Other criteria include:

1. type of information to be stored;
2. overall cost of the system;
3. accessibility of information at any desired number of locations;
4. capability and cost of making duplicates and whether duplicates are to be on microfilm or hard copy;
5. frequency file is changed or updated;
6. need for file integrity (assurance that no file is lost or misfiled);
7. means of reading and duplication both at central and/or remote locations; and
8. compatibility with other information systems within the organization.

TYPES OF MICROFORMS

Roll Film

Roll film is the least expensive microform to prepare and results in the greatest storage density. A 100-foot roll of 16 mm film stored in file in boxes measuring 4 x 4 x 1 inches is the equivalent in content to a well-organized file drawer – up to 2,500 letter-size images. Roll film can be updated by splicing new images onto the roll of film. This procedure is not often used for medical records, however, as it destroys the security of the roll film. Also, splicing sometimes destroys the legal acceptability of the film. As a permanent record, roll film is excellent; since documents committed to roll film are "locked in" and cannot be misfiled.

In high reference files, roll film can be packaged in either cartridges or cassettes that facilitate film loading onto microfilm readers. Cartridges are self-loaded onto a microfilm reader; that is, the film does not have to be manually threaded onto the reader. After viewing, the film must be rewound back into the cartridge. Cassettes contain two small film reels – feed and take up – for the roll film. Cassettes do not require rewinding when removed from the reader as do cartridges and unpackaged roll film. Systems using cartridges and cassettes may sometimes provide terminals such as the one shown in Figure 1, when frequent access is required. Cartridges and cassettes are advantageous in that they protect the film from fingerprints, dust, and dirt.

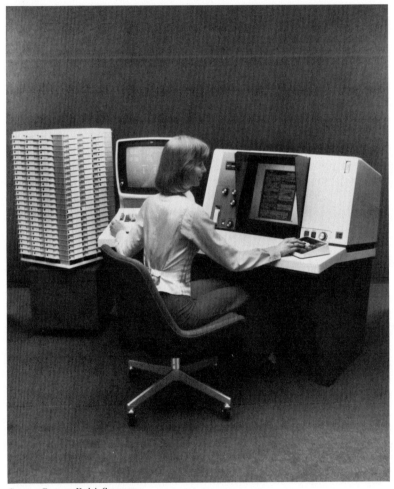

Courtesy Eastman Kodak Company

FIG. 1 – THE KODAK IMT-150 MICROIMAGE TERMINAL

Also, in files where there is a high level of reference activity, duplicate rolls of film are prepared for the reference file; and the processed camera film is stored as the master record. Duplicates can be made regardless of the type of microform chosen.

Retrieval of information from roll films is highly dependent on both file organization and film indexing. As used in most record systems, the contents are noted on the storage carton, cassette, or cartridge. Labeling the beginning and ending medical record number on each roll of film is the usual method of identification. On the roll film itself, a target sheet containing the medical record number in large characters marks the beginning of each record. Targets serve the same purpose as guides in a regular numeric or alphabetic filing system.

Other methods of indexing roll film are image count, bar or code line, and photo-optical binary code. In the image count method, marks (blips) below each image are counted electronically and used by the machine to control image retrieval in a linear sequence. In the bar or code line method, bars or lines between the frames have positional value as related to a scale along the edge of the reader or reader-printer screen. And, in the photo-optical binary code method, document numbers or index terms are recorded in optical binary code adjacent to each document. This method must be used with an electronic logic system for retrieval.

Obviously, the equipment selected for reading the microfilm must be compatible with the indexing method selected. The user will need to decide on an indexing method before selecting equipment.

Since roll film cannot be easily updated, it is not recommended for use with either the serial-unit or unit methods of numbering. The integrity of the unit record cannot be maintained with roll microfilm. The best application of roll microfilm is in situations where serial numbering is used.

Unitized Microforms

Unitized microforms result in a unit medical record. Unitization is more costly than roll film; but the additional cost is often fully justified in terms of greater file flexibility, more rapid record retrieval, and the ability to provide a copy of the unitized microform rapidly and inexpensively. In teaching and research institutions, the latter may be the most important consideration in the design of the system.

There are several types of unitized microforms: microfilm jackets, microfiche, and ultrafiche.

1. **Microfilm jackets** are composed of two panels of very thin transparent filmlike material. The two panels are joined horizontally by lines of adhesive which form channels. Microfilmed images are inserted into these channels. The images are cut from roll film and slid into the channels of the jacket either by hand or by machine. Jackets are advantageous in that they may be updated by inserting new images into the channels.

A microfilm jacket that is 4 x 6 inches in size can hold 60 images – 5 rows of images, 12 images per row. For identification, a header, which is usually the medical record number, is lettered across the top margin of the microfilm jacket. Color-coding may also be added across the entire top margin to aid in filing and retrieval of the microfilm jacket.

2. **Microfiche** is a transparent rectangle of film containing microimages. Unlike microfilm jackets where images cut from roll film are inserted into channels, the images are photographed directly onto the film. The standard size of microfiche is 6 x 4 inches. (Standard sizes are set by the National Micrographics Association.) A microfiche of this size will hold 98 images, 7 rows, 14 images per row, filmed at a reduction ratio of 24X. With greater reduction, up to 300 images may be arranged on one standard size microfiche.

As with microfilm jackets, a header containing the medical record number is lettered at the top margin for identification. Color-coding to aid in filing and retrieval may also be added. According to a survey conducted by *Modern Office Technology* in 1983, microfiche is the most common microform in use today (Figure 2).

3. **Ultrafiche** is a variation of microfiche. The major difference is that a greater reduction ratio is used with ultrafiche. The reduction ratio range is 90X to 2,400X. Because of the great reduction ratio, thousands of images may be stored on a standard 4 x 6-inch card. For example, with a reduction ratio of 210X, 8,000 images can be stored on a 4 x 6-inch ultrafiche card. The same type of heading is used with ultrafiche as with microfiche and microfilm jackets. Color-coding can also be added.

As noted earlier, the preparation of unitized microforms involves additional costs over roll film. Depending on the method
used, the finished cost per image could be double that of roll

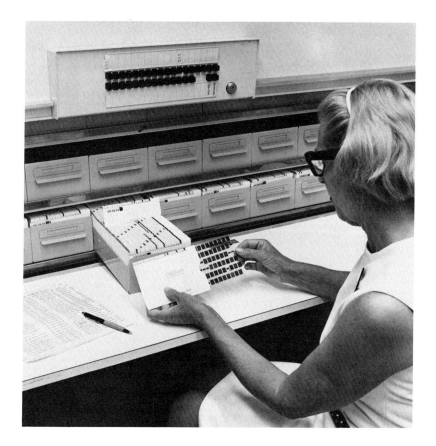

FIG. 2 – UNITIZED MASTER IN PROTECTIVE ENVELOPE FOR
AUTOMATED MICROFILM FILE

film. One must recognize, however, that this is only the cost
of converting records to microforms. In record files where there
is a high level of reference, the increased cost may be recov-
ered many times in decreased file-maintenance costs and the
ability to provide reference to a given medical record to one
or more requestors quickly without loss of control over the
master record.

Other Microforms

1. *Aperture cards* are also a type of unitized microform. Each aperture card contains an opening (aperture) cut into the card to provide a place for one to eight frames of microfilm. The frames are cut from roll film and inserted into the card. Aperture cards are not appropriate for medical record storage because they contain so few images.

Aperture cards are usually sized to be used in keypunching equipment and sorters. If aperture cards are keypunched, they can be filed and retrieved through the use of a mechanical sorter. If labeled, aperture cards can also be filed manually. In health care facilities, aperture cards are sometimes used for microfilming x-rays.

2. *Computer Output Microfilm (COM)* was developed in response to the large quantities of paper that computers generate. Such large volumes of paper require a great deal of storage space. Computer Output Microfilm greatly reduces the storage space required and speeds up the microfilming process itself.

In order to produce COM, information must first be stored in a computer. The information is stored in coded form on magnetic tape. When information is to be microfilmed, it is translated into readable form and displayed on a cathode-ray tube (CRT). A microfilm camera, called a recorder, photographs the displayed information, reducing it to microrecord size. A processor develops the film.

COM can be produced either on-line (directly connected to the computer) or off-line (not directly connected to the computer). COM is a speedy operation. A COM recorder takes a picture of the image on the screen at a rate 20 times faster than if the information were printed out by the computer. This eliminates the need to first print a paper document. This saves costs in terms of employee time, paper, and storage space.

SYSTEMS ANALYSIS AND DESIGN

Regardless of the method chosen for microfilming medical records, it should complement the existing filing system. Consideration should also be given to protection of the file in view of the sensitive nature of the records, legal requirements, and the requirements of users of the information. These should be considered during the systems analysis and design phases.

The medical record documents are first photographed on film usually 100 feet in length. The film is processed and may be left in its original roll form or converted into a unitized microform. Rolls and unitized microforms must be properly labeled and then placed in permanent storage. The procedure is illustrated in the flow process chart in Figure 3.

REASONS FOR MICROFILMING

Over the years many surveys have been conducted to determine the reasons organizations choose to microfilm records. Regardless of the type of organization, the reasons are generally the same, and they have not changed with time. These are:

1. To save both filing space and filing equipment. As much as a 98 percent savings in space and equipment can be achieved when records are microfilmed.

2. To reduce paper handling. Microrecords eliminate the need to transfer records to other places in the organization. A microfilm copy can be made from the master and sent while the original remains in the file.

3. To protect records against loss through disaster, theft, or negligence.

Other reasons for microfilming include better records management control, improved service, and reduced retrieval time. It is apparent that there are many good reasons for microfilming. The dilemma is deciding when it is appropriate to microfilm.

Cost is the major criterion to be considered when making the decision to microfilm. Factors that directly influence costs are:

1. Space savings. Converting records to microfilm can result in up to a 98 percent savings in space.

2. The length of time records are to be kept. Generally, costs and storage savings from microfilming are only realized if records are to be kept 7 to 15 years. Records that are to be kept permanently should be microfilmed unless this would make the record less convenient to use.

3. The actual cost of photographing, storing, and using microrecords. Microfilming can be expensive and time consuming because of the equipment needed for the process. Equipment needed for in-house microfilming includes

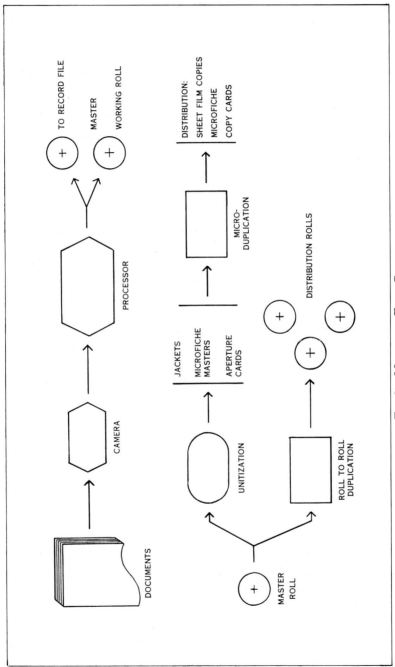

Fig. 3 – Microfilm Flow Chart

cameras to photograph the records; jacket inserters which provide enlarged viewing of film images for inspection and selection; microfilm lay-up equipment which prepares microfiche masters; and film duplication equipment which replicates the microform. In addition to the equipment needed for the microfilming process itself, any system utilizing microrecords requires readers to enlarge the microrecord for reading, reader-printers for printing hard copy records for the users, film and filing supplies, and storage equipment. Additional costs include costs for preparing records for microfilm and management costs for inspecting and indexing microrecords.

Other factors which influence the decision to microfilm include the condition or quality of the documents to be microfilmed, and accessibility of microrecords to users. Original documents that have deteriorated will result in photographs of poor quality. Carbon copies and deep shades of colored paper do not photograph well. Colors on original paper can usually be photographed but in black and white only.

From the users standpoint, viewing microrecords on readers can be difficult. In any event, readers should be widely located throughout the facility. But even with wide availability of readers, the user must still go to a fixed location to view the microfilmed record.

STEPS IN DESIGNING THE SYSTEM

There are four areas that should be studied for good microfilm system design. These are:

1. The nature of the information to be microfilmed. What are the content and value of the units of information coming into the system? Who uses the information? What is the required retention period? How and when is the information generated? How should it be added to the system?

2. The organization of the information to be microfilmed. How will users seek information? How must the information units be indexed or the collection organized to facilitate retrieval? Will in-depth indexing be required or will good file organization suffice?

3. The location of the information to be microfilmed. Where are the users of the system? Where is it desirable or necessary to have the information available? Are the users all

within the health care facility proper, or are some down the street or several miles away?

4. The size of the information units to be microfilmed. How big are the documents that will come into the system? What is the average number of pages and what is the size distribution? Are the pages all 8½ x 11 inches, or are there many other sizes to be considered? In any new system, consideration of the user is paramount. As suggested above, his needs must be determined as the basis for system design. Equally or perhaps more important, as the system is implemented, he must be oriented to its use and its benefits.

Fortunately, most of the considerations discussed throughout this text are well understood and the controls well established for medical records. Given a thorough understanding of these considerations and drawing upon the experience of medical record departments currently using microfilm, the design of a system to satisfy the requirements in a given hospital or clinic should be straightforward. In this, the medical record director can also receive invaluable help from microfilm service companies, some of which specialize in this field, and if an in-house system is indicated, from knowledgeable microfilm equipment salesmen. In addition, consultants are available to assist in system analysis, design, and implementation efforts.

PREPARATION OF RECORDS FOR FILMING

Many questions must be settled before the actual work of filming can begin. Is the medical record, as a whole, to be filmed, or are certain parts to be excluded? Some hospitals do not film the nurses' notes; others delete certain other documents. Such decisions must be made by the hospital administration with the approval of the medical staff. A distinction must also be made at this time between the medical record per se, which pertains to the care and treatment of the patient, and administrative records. The latter includes extraneous records filed in the medical record folder as a convenience. These may include, for example, continuity of care forms, bills, and items of correspondence.

If the medical records to be microfilmed are not assembled in a standard order, it may be well to do this prior to filming. The preparatory period will be longer, but time will be saved when retrieving information from film. Forms kept for the protection of the hospital at the time of patient hospitalization, such as clothing lists, may be discarded at this time. Blank sheets should be eliminated. Anything not vital to the patient's continuing care or not needed for study or legal reasons may be removed. In general, care should be exercised in preparing records. The cost of filming is low enough, that documents of any potential future value should be retained. In any event, the procedures for stripping records must be clear; and, when in doubt, clerical personnel should be instructed to consult the medical record director. In considering what should be filmed, guidance may also be found in *A Guide to Retention and Preservation of Hospital Records* published by the Hospital Financial Management Association. For a final decision, the hospital's legal counsel should be consulted.

The length of time needed for preparation varies according to the condition of the medical records to be filed. A check must always be made to ascertain that there has been no misfiling within the record, and hospital numbers must also be checked. Records filmed out of order on a roll or under wrong numbers are lost and may never come to light again.

The type of fastener used is also a factor in determining the time required for record preparation. If a fastener used on current records is difficult to remove, a change should be considered.

The time required for file preparation is generally much greater than expected. On the average, it takes two and one-half man-days to prepare the records filed in one and one-half standard letter-size file shelves. The preparation consists of:

1. Pulling all staples or removing other types of fasteners.
2. Checking all sheets in the medical records to see that they are arranged in a standard sequence.
3. Indicating two-sided records that must be copied on both sides.
4. Removing all blank sheets and miscellaneous records not being preserved by the hospital.
5. Checking all names and hospital numbers.
6. Making the target sheets that separate the records.
7. Indexing each admission; separating and indexing outpatient and emergency records if necessary.

Some hospitals prefer that record preparation be done completely by hospital personnel. However, given clearly established ground rules, reputable and experienced microfilm service companies can also perform this work satisfactorily under contract.

FILMING THE RECORD

The actual filming of records is a relatively simple process after the work of preparation is completed. While personnel can be trained to operate a camera, processor, and unitization equipment, the speed and quality with which the work is done depends upon the operator's dexterity and attitude. If space within the hospital or personnel to do the filming are not available, it may be appropriate to send the prepared medical records to a microfilm service company and have the entire job done on a contract basis; or the actual filming may take place on hospital premises with the film being processed, inspected, and unitized on a service contract.

If any part of the filming process is to be done by a microfilm service company, a formal contract should be made between the health care facility and the service company. Items to be included in the contract are: cost (usually based on a rate per 1,000 exposures); type of index system to be used on the microfilm; photography by trained technicians; processing and inspection of microfilm; retake of documents if needed; confidentiality of information; access to records being filmed, if required; transportation of records to be microfilmed and delivery of completed microfilm; and provision for destruction of original records. Original records should not be destroyed until the medical record director or his designee has spot-checked each batch of returned microfilmed records.

COMPUTER ASSISTED RETRIEVAL (CAR)

Computer assisted retrieval (CAR) is a method of locating and retrieving documents through the use of computer indexes. Computer assisted retrieval is applicable to records stored in hard copy, magnetic tape, or microfilm. The software indexing system for CAR pinpoints the location of any record in the file by file code. Computerized microfilm indexes are usually very detailed and comprehensive. On a microfilm file, a separate index for each document may be maintained; or groups of documents may be batched as one. CAR may be justified in microfilm systems where there is a high reference and retrieval rate.

MICROFILM READERS

Once medical records have been microfilmed, they must be placed on a projector, called a reader, for viewing. There are several types of readers available. The type selected will depend upon the needs of the user, the type of microform, and cost.

Basic types are:

1. **PORTABLE READERS** – Portable readers usually weigh less than 50 pounds and are designed to fit into a case similar in size to an attache case. They are often used in cars and other outside job sites. Many are battery powered. Because of their low price, many facilities use them to supplement existing microfilm equipment.

   One type of portable reader is a highly compact lap reader designed for personal use only. Lap readers are available for use with microfiche only.

2. **STATIONARY READERS** – Stationary readers may be desk top or free-standing. Stationary readers provide a wide viewing screen and a wider choice of option features than portable readers. Some readers accept a number of different microforms, while others are only suitable for one type. The number of features on any given unit will affect its cost.

3. **READER-PRINTER** – A reader-printer may be used for both viewing and producing a hard copy of a microform. Reader-printers are available for both low-volume and high-volume reproduction units to reproduce documents ranging in size from 8½ x 11 inches to 20 x 30 inches.

RECORDS MANAGEMENT AND
LEGAL CONSIDERATIONS

Sound records management is the result of an effective compromise between the desire to keep records ad infinitum and retention based upon realistic use-life and legal considerations. In general, retention is affected by the patient's age; how frequently records are used for patient care, teaching, or research purposes; and, of course, legal requirements.

Many states have laws which specify that microfilmed records are acceptable as primary evidence. In 1951 the 82nd Congress passed an amendment to Public Law 129 which provides for the admission and acceptance of microfilmed records as primary evidence. This law was reaffirmed in Section 1732 (b) in 1958. Thus, the use of microfilm as primary evidence is now legal throughout the United States regardless of whether the particular state has a law to that effect or not. In the intervening years, most state laws relating to the use of microfilm have been aligned to the federal law. Interpretation of the law, however, is the province of the legal profession; and it is well to seek counsel in the consideration of any new program. Notwithstanding the fact that the record may have been microfilmed, some records are also retained in original form for a period required in state laws which relate specifically to the retention of medical records.

In general, however, one can observe that interpretation of the law coupled with the many benefits provided by microfilm has resulted in the microfilming of medical records soon after discharge. In effect, microform records are more accessible and satisfy all reference requirements.

SUMMARY

As an information recording medium, microfilm offers a unique solution to the problems of cost-effective storage and security while at the same time making records available to qualified users.

STUDY QUESTIONS

1. Differentiate between the terms "reduction ratio" and "magnification ratio."
2. Name four types of cameras used for filming, and describe how they are used.
3. Outline the criteria to be considered when selecting a microform.
4. Describe the different types of microforms available.

5. What advantages do unitized microforms have over roll microfilm?

6. List the reasons for microfilming medical records.

7. List the steps in preparing records for filming.

8. Discuss the legality of microfilmed records as primary evidence.

REFERENCES

A Guide to the Retention and Preservation of Hospital Records. 6th Edition. Chicago, Illinois: Hospital Financial Management Association, 1981.

AVEDON, DON M. "Selecting a Service Bureau." *Journal of Micrographics.* September-October, 1976.

BROBERG, BARBARA A. "Records Evaluation for Conversion to Microfilm." *Journal of Micrographics.* September-October, 1979.

CAMPBELL, ROBERT J. "Automated Microfilm Retrieval: A Refresher Course." *Modern Office Procedures.* October, 1980.

EDLAND, LINDA B. "CAR: The Vehicle for Records Delivery." *Office Administration and Automation.* September, 1983.

Guide to Microreproduction Equipment. National Microfilm Association.

Handbook of Hospital Microfilming. Winston-Salem, North Carolina: Decodex, Inc., 1979.

JOHNSON, MINA M., and KALLAUS, NORMAN F. *Records Management,* Chapter 12. Cincinnati, Ohio: Southwestern Publishing Company, 1982.

Legality of Microfilm. Chicago, Illinois: Cohasset Associates, 1980.

NOFEL, PETER J., and FEHLNER, CHRISTINE. "Big Business Likes Its Record Small." *Modern Office Technology.* April, 1984.

PRESBY, LEONARD. "Eight-Step Study Shows Pros, Cons of Microfilming Medical Records." *Hospitals.* August 16, 1977.

"Statement on the Preservation of Patient Medical Records in Health Care Institutions." American Hospital and American Medical Record Associations.

TERRY, GEORGE R., and STALLARD, JOHN J. *Office Management and Control,* Chapter VIII. Homewood, Illinois: Richard D. Irwin, Inc., 1980.

chapter 12

NOMENCLATURE AND CLASSIFICATION SYSTEMS

Health information contained in medical records is of no value to the field of medical science if it remains stored for posterity within each health care institution. It is the comparison of health care data between individual facilities within a defined area or country, or even among countries, that is vital to the growth of medical information around the world. This sharing of information would be meaningless, however, without the use of standardized systems for the identification and classification of disease processes. Over the years, a number of standard systems have been developed for classifying and recording disease information for comparison purposes.

NOMENCLATURES AND CLASSIFICATIONS

Two terms are often heard when reference is made to the comparison of health care data – *nomenclature* and *classification*. Although often used interchangeably, the terms have different meanings when used for the comparison of disease data and should not be confused or misapplied.

An accurate study of the diseases treated in a hospital cannot be made unless a nomenclature of diseases has been carefully followed. The word "nomenclature" comes from the Latin nomen, meaning name, and clature (from calare, to call), a calling. The term thus signifies, literally, a calling of names. It is defined as a system of names used in any science or art. Thus a medical nomenclature is a recognized system of preferred terminology for naming disease processes. In the past, variations in disease terminology have made comparative studies difficult. Diseases were in many instances denoted by three or four terms; likewise, some terms were applied to a number of different diseases. For instance, Parry's disease, Graves' disease, Flajani's disease, and Basedow's disease are all known as toxic diffuse goiter. An example of two different diseases being known by one eponymic term is found in the case of Recklinghausen's disease. These are multiple neurofibromas and osteitis fibrosa cystica.

A classification system, on the other hand, emphasizes grouping of related entities to produce necessary statistical information. A medical classification system provides a method of arranging like or related disease entities in groups for the reporting of quantitative data for statistical purposes. Unlike nomenclatures, classification systems usually contain all terms – not just terms deemed proper by a nomenclature – to facilitate categorization of diagnostic or procedural data. A medical classification system standardizes the medical conditions or procedures which are to be grouped together while a medical nomenclature standardizes terminology. An effective classification system must be designed in accordance with three basic rules:

1. The set of categories should be derived from a single classification principle, such as anatomic sites, etiology, or medical specialty.
2. The set of categories should be exhaustive permitting every possible diagnostic or operative term to be placed within a category of the classification system.
3. The categories within the classification system should be mutually exclusive, so it is not possible to place a given diagnostic or treatment term within more than one category of the system.

If used properly, nomenclature and classification systems should complement each other in the recording of medical information.

NOMENCLATURES

The number of persons working in the health care field is mushrooming. This fact, coupled with an increase in the number and kinds of health care specialists, makes it vital that there is clear communication about the patient's condition. Use of standardized terminology to describe clinical progress and treatment procedures is an important means for ensuring that all persons, involved directly or indirectly in patient care, have a common understanding of the patient's disease.

Numerous attempts have been made over the years to compile accurate descriptions and identification of all the disease entities known to man. One of the earliest successful efforts was initiated in 1889 when a commission on nomenclature was appointed by the Anatomical Society (an international group), and in 1895 the report of the commission was accepted at a meeting in Basle, Switzerland. This report is now known as the Basle Nomina Anatomica (BNA); it was made necessary because of the great number of anatomical terms in use, there being at that time a total of 50,000 in the literature for about 4,500 structures. The BNA includes only names of descriptive gross anatomic structures. Revisions of this work have continued to appear, and the majority of the nomenclatures of disease have based the terminology of their anatomical classification on this valuable report by the Anatomical Society.

EARLY NOMENCLATURES IN THE UNITED STATES

Although several early nomenclatures were published in the United States including the *Bellevue Hospital Nomenclature of Diseases* in 1903, the *Classification of Diseases* adopted by Massachusetts General in 1914, *An Alphabetical Nomenclature of Diseases and Operations* by Thomas Ponton in 1927, the *Terminology of Operations of the University of Chicago* by Hilger Perry Jenkins in 1935, the *New York Hospital Classification of Nomenclature and Operations* in 1938, the *Standard Nomenclature of Diseases and Operations* was the first medical nomenclature to be accepted universally.

The *Standard Classified Nomenclature of Disease*, the forerunner of the later *Standard Nomenclature of Diseases and Operations*, originated in 1928 when the New York Academy of Medicine called a conference; the primary object of the meeting being to formulate a nomenclature that would be acceptable as a standard throughout this country. Diseases were to be arranged in a logical and orderly manner, with no overlapping, so statistics from various hospitals would be comparable. At this meeting the National Conference on Nomenclature of Disease was formed, and by fall of 1930 the basic plan providing for a dual classification was adopted. Early in 1932 a paper-covered trial edition was distributed to about 50 hospitals of various sizes and types for testing. Each disease was classified according to both anatomical location and the etiology, or cause. Code numbers, comparable to the classification number on books in a library, were adopted for convenience in filing and finding, since it was felt that a number would give a more accurate description of a disease than a name. The first official edition was published in 1933 and the second edition in 1935.

By 1937, in the belief that with the sponsorship of the American Medical Association the revisions would not be dependent on any one individual or on the necessity of securing private funds, the copyright and editing were transferred. In 1942 the third edition of the *Standard Nomenclature of Diseases* and the first edition of the *Standard Nomenclature of Operations* were published in one volume, entitled *Standard Nomenclature of Diseases and Standard Nomenclature of Operations.*

After the American Medical Association had indicated its willingness to be responsible for continuing the revision of the *Standard Nomenclature,* publication of other systems was halted in favor of the *Standard Nomenclature* in order to attain uniformity. The last (fifth) edition of *Standard Nomenclature of Diseases and Operations* was published in 1961.

NOMENCLATURES IN USE TODAY

Standard Nomenclature of Diseases and Operations (SNDO)

The *Standard Nomenclature of Diseases and Operations* was designed to be used as a medical nomenclature and to provide an authoritative list of acceptable terms for describing a patient's illness and treatment. Its numerical and logical arrangement of code numbers to describe diseases, conditions, and operations facilitated the retrieval of data for research and statistical purposes for more than thirty years in North America and some other countries throughout the world. And even though its last revision was in 1961, the terminology, while not including new terms and conditions since then, is considered to be acceptable and almost classic.

Several reasons are given for the AMA's not continuing to re-publish the SNDO which include the cost of maintaining a staff for revising and updating the materials, and the fact that its meticulous attention to detail and the necessity of adhering to coding rules made it difficult to use on a worldwide basis. A brief discussion of SNDO follows because there are several decades of medical data indexed by this system which medical record practitioners may need to access.

Dual System – The *Standard Nomenclature of Diseases and Operations* (SNDO) is also a dual system of classification. Each disease entity is described in two ways: first, according to the disease site (organ or portion of the body concerned) or topography; and second, according to the cause of the disease or etiology. Similarly, operative procedures are classified according to the site, or topography, and according to the operative technique or procedure employed on that site. The following sample entries serve to demonstrate this point:

461 – 942	Arteriosclerosis of aorta
site etiology	*etiology site*
461 – 16	Biopsy of aorta
site procedure	*procedure site*

Every disease and operative code number consists of two parts separated by a hyphen. In both the disease and the operative codes, the portion to the left of the hyphen represents the site, or topography. The etiology is shown in the digits to the right of the hyphen in a disease code, while the procedure is shown in the digits to the right of the hyphen in an operative code. Every disease code must contain a minimum of six digits, three topographical and three etiological. Operative codes range from three topographical digits and two procedural digits, to a maximum of ten digits.

To retrieve records from an SNDO index, the medical record practitioner should be familiar with the following characteristics of SNDO: decimal digits are used to add further detail to the topography or etiology portion of a code; the meanings of the decimal digits differ from category to category; open end codes and master codes require completion by referring to the classification listings in the front of SNDO; and neoplastic disease codes contain behavior letters to show pathologic behavior.

Example: 640-8091.0H – Adenocarcinoma of stomach with metastasis, differentiation not determined.

640 – Stomach
8091 – Adenocarcinoma
.0 – With metastasis
H – Differentiation not determined

Current Medical Information and Terminology (CMIT)

Current Medical Information and Terminology, published by the American Medical Association, is a system adopted to name and describe diseases for reference in clinical recording and reporting. It is an alphabetical listing of preferred disease terms with accompanying descriptions.

Each disease is described according to: additional terms, synonyms and eponyms; etiology; symptoms; signs; complications; laboratory data; x-rays; and pathology. Each entry is assigned a six-digit code applicable to computerized indexing. The first two digits of the number specify the body system affected by the disease. This is followed by a four-digit random computer number assigned to that disease term. An example of a CMIT code would be:

Alzheimer's Disease   09   4992
                Body System   Random Computer Number

CMIT contains two indexes. The numerical index is a sequential list of four-digit numbers, and the associated disease terms and the body system index is an alphabetical listing of diseases in each body system identifying the page number of the disease description. The fifth edition of CMIT was published in 1981.

Current Procedural Terminology (CPT)

Current Procedural Terminology, currently referred to as CPT-4, was first published by the American Medical Association in 1966. It is a comprehensive listing of medical terms and codes for the uniform designation of diagnostic and therapeutic procedures in surgery, medicine, and the specialties. Its purpose is to provide standard terminology and coding for consistency and comparability in reporting for third-party reimbursement.

The main body of the book consists of five sections: Medicine, Anesthesiology, Surgery, Radiology, Pathology and Laboratory with a block of five-digit numbers assigned to each section. The five main sections are further divided into anatomic, procedural, condition or descriptor subheadings. Each CPT classification number is a single five-digit procedure or service code, such as "93280 cardiac fluoroscopy."

The index is arranged alphabetically and contains six categories of entries: procedure or service, organ, condition, synonyms, eponyms, and abbreviations.

CPT is designed for physician use in reporting procedures or services rendered, the amount of time involved, and the location at which the procedures were performed. Any procedure or service in any section of the book may be used to designate the services rendered by any qualified physician. Most physicians report a significant portion of their services using codes from the Medicine section, for it provides separate five-digit designations for new and established patients, as well as the degree of service required for patient treatment (brief service, limited service, etc.). Procedures are also coded to identify place of occurrence such as office, hospital, nursing home, emergency room, etc. Additional two-digit modifier codes with a hyphen are provided to indicate that a service or procedure has been altered by some specific circumstance but not changed in its definition or code. These two-digit codes with a hyphen are placed after the five-digit procedure code to indicate circumstances such as "a service or procedure has both a professional and technical component," "a bilateral procedure was performed," or "unusual events occurred." For example, -76 placed after 90784 – 90784-76 – indicates "repeat procedure by same physician."

Each section of CPT-4 contains a number of specific code numbers designated for reporting unlisted procedures, for it is recognized that there may be services or procedures performed by physicians that are not found in CPT-4. To maintain the effectiveness of CPT, the AMA revises and publishes CPT-4 on an annual basis.

Systematized Nomenclature of Pathology (SNOP)

The *Systematized Nomenclature of Pathology* was published in 1965 by the American College of Pathologists. It provides a system for classifying and indexing pathological specimens. The JCAH standards specify that diagnoses made from surgical specimens and necropsies shall be expressed in acceptable terminology of a recognized disease nomenclature and shall be indexed for retrieval.

The SNOP coding system is the first classification system to code diseases on a multifield basis. The classification principle used by SNOP is that disease may be defined in terms of topography – part of body affected by disease; morphology – structural change in tissue; etiology – the cause of the disease or injury; and function – physiological or chemical disorders and alterations resulting from a disease or injury.

Example: Orchitis due to mumps

T	–7800	Testis NOS
M	–4000	Inflammation NOS
E	–3250	Mumps virus
F	–9414	Mumps

Code numbers for etiology or function may occasionally be used in place of a morphological code number if there is no structural change associated with the disease. An etiological or functional code number might be placed under a site-morphology code number to indicate a certain symptom.

Although the primary aim of this nomenclature is to help pathologists organize and utilize their material, it may be used by the medical record administrator in several ways: assisting the department of pathology in setting up a SNOP index, as a coding reference, or to report data to a discharge data service. SNOP has also been used successfully for the coding and indexing of health records by some medical record departments.

Systematized Nomenclature of Medicine (SNOMED)

In 1977 the American College of Pathologists published the *Systematized Nomenclature of Medicine* which represented a major expansion of SNOP. It is the most recent and most comprehensive nomenclature in the health field. SNOMED has seven axes:

Axis 1 is a hierarchical anatomic nomenclature called "Topography."

Axis 2 represents abnormal anatomy called "Morphology."

Axis 3 lists all causes and causal agents of disease, dysfunctions, and morphological alterations that occur in the human body and is called "Etiology."

Axis 4 contains the normal and abnormal functions, functional states and physiological units of the body and the major organ systems and is called "Function."

These axes comprise the nomenclature components of the system, and various combinations are necessary to obtain a disease. For this reason, the fifth axis, called "Disease," is an organized list of classes of diseases, complex disease entities, and syndromes. SNOMED can actually express all the necessary diagnostic detail to manage the patient's signs, symptoms, problems, and disease components as well as place the final diagnosis in the disease classification axis for statistical reporting utilizing the preceding five categories.

INTEGRATION OF CODABLE FINDINGS INTO A CLASSIFICATION OF DISEASE					
Nomenclature					Classification
Topography +	Morphology +	Etiology +	Function	=	Disease
Crystalline lens +	Cataract, mature +	Acquired +	Low vision	=	Disease of lens
T-XX700	M-51120	E-0024	F-X0050	=	D-X080

However, the sixth axis, called "Procedures," is used to describe the actions of the health care team. It contains a list of administrative, diagnostic, therapeutic, and preventive procedures. Axis 7, called "Occupation," has been added to permit the comparison and correlation of information in data banks on labor forces with medical information.

The structure of SNOMED allows practically all health care information recorded on patients' records to be stored for data retrieval. Because SNOMED was designed for computer storage and automatic encoding, it has not been widely used, since computers are only now becoming available for this purpose in most health care facilities. Some anatomic pathology laboratories are utilizing automatic encoding programs to assign SNOMED codes.

Specialty Nomenclatures

Some specialty groups have developed nomenclatures to improve communications, storage, and retrieval of specialty information. These nomenclatures describe the diseases and disorders associated with the specialty and provide useful information to assist coders in correctly classifying various diagnoses.

In 1973 the New York Heart Association published the seventh edition of the **Nomenclature and Criteria for Diagnoses of Diseases of the Heart and Great Vessels.** This nomenclature describes diseases of the heart and great vessels and lists criteria required for the diagnosis such as:

"Myocarditis due to rheumatic fever – a change in heart size or the appearance of ventricular failure in association with one or more of the following: evidence of infection with beta-hemolytic streptococcus of group A or one of the other major or minor criteria of rheumatic fever."

The Council for International Organizations of Medical Science and the World Health Organization issued the first edition of **Diseases of the Lower Respiratory Tract** (bronchi, lungs, and pleura) and the **International Nomenclature of Diseases** (IND) in 1979. This nomenclature identifies recommended terms and describes each disease or syndrome for which a name is recommended. It serves as a complement to ICD; and the names recommended in the IND will be used, as appropriate, in the tenth revision of the ICD. For example:

Bronchial asthma is described as: An episodic increase in airway resistance or airflow obstruction resulting in attacks of difficulty in breathing, especially on expiration. Wheezing is a typical feature. The changes in resistance are due to smooth-muscle hyperreactivity, mucosal vascular congestion, edema, and excessive mucous secretion. These bronchial wall changes are induced ("triggered") by many different factors including common environmental allergens, inhaled irritants, exercise, infections, and psychological stimuli. *Synonyms:* asthma convulsivum, essential asthma, nervous asthma, spasmodic asthma, true asthma.

Standard Nomenclature of Athletic Injuries

In 1964 the American Medical Association began the development of a standard nomenclature relating to degree and type of injury in sports, so meaningful records and statistics concerning sports injuries and their cause and prevention could be maintained. A revised nomenclature was published in 1976. For

---

Anterior Tibial Compartment Syndrome

Additional Term: Volkmann's Ischemia of Leg

ETIOLOGY
Unaccustomed repetitive activity; chronic overuse; direct trauma; localized infection.

SYMPTOMS
Severe pain made more severe by function, not disappearing with rest.

SIGNS
Loss of function of anterior tibial and toe extensor muscles with ensuing footdrop; passive stretching of involved muscles produces red, glossy, and warm skin over area; marked tenderness and hardness of fascia over involved space; occasionally accompanied by peroneal nerve injury and consequent sensory loss over dorsum of foot, lateral side of lower leg.

COMPLICATIONS
Severe disability, if unrecognized early, due to ischemic necrosis and irreparable scarring.

PATHOLOGY
Rapid swelling of muscle within anterior tibial compartment or hemorrhage into this space; edema, extravasation of red blood cells; replacement of muscles by fibrous scarring and inelastic noncontractile muscle groups.

FIG. 1 – DESCRIPTIVE INFORMATION OF TYPICAL ENTRY

each term, descriptive information is provided to assist sports medicine practitioners to differentiate one clinical entity from another. A typical entry appears in Figure 1.

Standard Nomenclature of Veterinary Diseases and Operations (SNVDO)

A standard nomenclature in veterinary medicine developed in 1964 out of the National Cancer Institute's attempt to acquire retrospective data on animal neoplasia. A second abridged edition of SNVDO was published in 1975 by the Public Health Service. It is designed to assign acceptable terminology and a unique descriptive code number to conditions common to domestic animal species in the United States and Canada. SNVDO classifies diseases according to the portion of the body affected (topography) and the cause of the disorder (etiology). A diagnostic code contains three parts:

Characters 1-4   represent the part of the body affected.
Characters 5-8   represent cause of the disease process.
Character 9   represents a particular pathologic state if it exists and is usually considered part of the etiology.

Example: Adenocarcinoma of biliary passages, differentiated, 6820-8091F

6820 – topography – biliary tract
8091 – adenocarcinoma
F   – malignant neoplasm differentiated

An operative code number contains three characters to denote the location of the site of the surgical procedure, the last character being dropped from the topography code. Two digits are used after a hyphen to represent the procedure. For example, open reduction of femur would be assigned code: 235-54 with 235 representing the femur site and 54 open reduction, generally or unspecified including fixation. The structure of SNVDO and many of its codes are based on the *Standard Nomenclature of Diseases and Operations.*

NOMENCLATURE USAGE

Regardless of the nomenclature used, disease and operative terms must be expressed with sufficient clarity and specificity for the data to be correctly identified and coded.

The nature of acceptable terminology for stating final diagnoses and operations is clear once the following basic rules are learned. Every diagnosis must contain a specific site and etiology, every operation a site and a procedure, insofar as possible. If the physician is unable to specify site or etiology because of inconclusive results from x-rays, laboratory tests, or other examinations, he must state that a particular disease is suspected or that the diagnosis is incomplete. If the physician can state only symptoms and no disease, he must record the diagnosis as deferred or unknown. The following examples illustrate some of these points.

	INCORRECT TERMINOLOGY	CORRECT TERMINOLOGY
1.	Embolism of artery (no topography)	Embolism of pulmonary artery
2.	Emphysema (no etiology)	Emphysema due to infection
3.	Arthrotomy (no topography)	Arthrotomy of knee joint
4.	Headache	Undiagnosed disease manifested by headache
5.	Plastic operation of arm with full-thickness skin graft	Plastic operation of arm with full-thickness skin graft Excision of skin of leg for graft, donor site
6.	Infarction of myocardium from arteriosclerotic coronary thrombosis	Infarction of myocardium from arteriosclerotic coronary thrombosis
	Polydipsia	Diabetes mellitus, Polydipsia

(The symptom, polydipsia, cannot be explained by the infarction; therefore, another disease must be present.)

7.	Hives	Urticaria

(The physician has used an unacceptable term. The disease index refers the coder to urticaria, the correct term for this condition.)

8.	Pott's disease	Tuberculosis of the vertebra

(An eponym is a name of a disease, organ, operation, etc., in which the name of a person is included. Certain eponyms are so commonly used that they are acceptable as a diagnosis, i.e., Laennec's cirrhosis. In most cases, eponyms are no substitute for a diagnosis stating site and etiology.)

The above examples point out some of the common errors in diagnostic and operative terminology. In many instances, the physician unknowingly makes these errors and will be willing to provide more specificity of data. The medical record practitioner may assist physicians in documenting their patients' diagnoses. Only the physician who actually treats the patient is in a position to make the diagnosis.

STATISTICAL CLASSIFICATIONS

Classification systems are used to organize health care data for easy and meaningful retrieval. Frequently, the medical record practitioner is responsible for selecting an appropriate classification system for classifying, storing, and retrieving patient health information from patient/client health records.

HISTORY OF CLASSIFICATION SYSTEMS

Attempts to group data on disease processes in a relevant manner date back many years. The early Greeks, following the pathology of Hippocrates, classified diseases into four types, known as the four humors – blood, which being from the heart, represents heat; black bile, which comes from the spleen and stomach, represents wetness; yellow bile, which is secreted by the liver, represents dryness; and phlegm, which comes from the brain and is diffused through the whole body, represents cold. These various types of diseases were, in turn, classified according to their respective systems of the body.

In the seventeenth century, Captain John Graunt, of London, began directing the attention of the world to morbidity and mortality statistics in his *London Bills of Mortality*. This was the first real attempt to study disease from a statistical point of view.

As early as 1837, William Farr, Registrar General of England and Wales, worked to achieve better classification and international uniformity in the use of statistics. The general arrangement and the principle of classifying diseases by anatomical site proposed by Farr have survived as the basis of the *International List of Causes of Death*. Thus the foundation was laid for our present-day vital statistics.

INTERNATIONAL CLASSIFICATION OF
DISEASES (ICD)

Dr. Jacques Bertillon developed the *Bertillon Classification of Causes of Death* in 1893. In 1898 the American Public Health Association recommended that the *Bertillon Classification* be adopted by registrars in Canada, Mexico, and the United States; and that the classification be revised every ten years. Revisions were completed in 1900, 1920, 1929, and 1938 entitled the *International Classification of Causes of Death*. In 1948, under the auspices of the World Health Organization, the sixth revision was published and included, for the first time, lists for the tabulation of morbidity as well as mortality. After the appearance of the sixth revision of the *International Statistical Classification* containing morbidity listings, hospitals began experiments using ICD for classifying diseases. In 1956 a pilot study was undertaken by the American Hospital Association and the American Medical Record Association, supported by a research grant from the Public Health Service. Fourteen hospitals in the United States carried out the pilot study using a modified version of the *International Statistical Classification of Diseases, Injuries and Causes of Death* with the *Standard Nomenclature of Diseases and Operations* being used as a control. The findings of the study pointed up the fact that the modified version of the International was suitable for hospital indexing purposes. Coding and posting took less time using the International; and in answering requests for certain disease entities, more pertinent records were found by using the International listing, although more nonpertinent records were also pulled.

The results of this study were promising enough to warrant the appointment of a committee to consolidate the findings of the tests into a volume which could be used as a hospital indexing tool. The completion of this task resulted in Public Health Service Publication 719, the **International Classification of Diseases, Adapted for Indexing Hospital Records by Diseases and Operations** (ICDA) in 1959 and revised in 1962. Modifications were made to provide greater detail; and, in some instances, changes were made at the three-digit category level. A classification of surgical operations was introduced to meet the classification needs of hospitals.

Eighth Revision, International Classification of Diseases (ICDA-8)

The World Health Organization took into consideration the increased specificity required for indexing hospital records in preparing the eighth revision of ICD. Although the eighth revision was constructed with hospital indexing in mind, it was recognized that the basic classification might provide inadequate detail for diagnostic indexing in some countries. In the United States, the Public Health Service asked a group of consultants to study the eighth revision for applicability for the various uses in the United States. The recommendations of this group resulted in the preparation of an adaptation that gave greater detail and specificity than provided in the World Health Organization's publication. The *Eighth Revision, International Classification of Diseases, Adapted for Use in the United States*, published in 1968, served as the basis for coding diagnostic data for official morbidity and mortality statistics in the United States and also proved to be suitable for use by hospitals in indexing hospital records by diagnoses and operations.

The International has evolved from an international listing of causes of death to a comprehensive classification of both morbidity and mortality. Over the years, international cooperation in the field of vital and health statistics has improved, which coupled with better medical education, caused an exchange of information that greatly contributed to the betterment of health standards all over the world.

Hospital Adaptation – (H-ICDA)

A variation of the ICDA-8 classification system was published in 1968 by the Commission on Professional and Hospital Activities for use with its Professional Activities Study (PAS) data recording system. The *Hospital Adaptation of ICDA* followed the basic format of ICDA-8 with certain modifications. Those hospitals using the PAS data system were required to use the H-ICDA for coding and indexing patient information. In 1973 a second edition of the H-ICDA was published for use by PAS-participating hospitals. This edition was used until the *Hospital Adaptation of ICDA* was replaced in 1979 by the *International Classification of Diseases, Ninth Revision, Clinical Modification*.

Ninth Revision of ICD (ICD-9)

Although participating countries had been working individually on updating the ninth edition, representatives came together in 1975 in Geneva, Switzerland, to make the final decision. The resulting publication, *International Classification of Diseases, Ninth Revision* became effective as the World Health Organization statistical classification in 1979. The current *International Classification of Diseases* is primarily a universal classification system for grouping illnesses. Its secondary purpose is for use in hospital disease indexing, provided it satisfactorily serves that purpose. The ICD-9 was published as three volumes, including the tabular list of diseases, alphabetic index, and a new procedure classification. Coding was expanded into greater detail by the addition of a fifth digit in specified disease categories. Dual classification numbers were introduced which combined two descriptions of disease entities into a single code number.

Clinical Modification (ICD-9-CM)

In 1977 the National Center for Health Statistics began the development of a modification of the ICD-9 for use in the United States. The *International Classification of Diseases, Ninth Revision, Clinical Modification* resulted. The term "clinical" emphasized the intent of the modification: to serve as a useful tool in the area of classification of morbidity data for reporting, compiling, and comparing health care data to assist in evaluating the appropriateness and timeliness of medical care for internal and external reviews, planning health care delivery systems, determining patterns of patient care among health care providers, analyzing payments for health service, and conducting epidemiological and clinical research.

The ICD-9-CM is published in three volumes. Volume one contains a numerical list of the disease code numbers in tabular form. An alphabetic index to the disease entries in Volume 1 is provided in Volume 2. A third volume, not present in ICDA-8, was added to ICD-9-CM to contain the classification system for surgical, diagnostic, and therapeutic procedures. Volume 3 contains a tabular list and alphabetic index for proper classification of procedures. The first two volumes of ICD-9-CM are completely compatible with ICD-9, for ICD-9-CM codes may be collapsed back to their ICD-9 counterpart. The ICD-9-CM procedure classification draws heavily on the fascicles of ICD-9, but compatability with the *ICD-9 – Classification of Procedures in Medicine* was not maintained when a different classification axis was deemed clinically more useful.

Structure of Code Numbers

The basic number of digits applied to a disease condition is three, such as 410 – acute myocardial infarction. In many instances, the code number is expanded by use of a decimal digit, .0 through .9, to amplify or permit greater detail in the classification of a disease. Some codes are further subdivided into fifth-digit subclassifications, resulting in a code number with a maximum of five digits.

Operative procedures are assigned two digits, such as 32 – excision of lung and bronchus. Here also decimal digits, .0 through .9, are assigned to describe the precise procedures, such as 32.5 – pneumonectomy, complete. An additional decimal digit is assigned for designated procedures, creating a maximum four-digit procedure number.

Other Features

In addition to the code numbers for disease and operative procedures, the ICD-9-CM contains other options designed to display valuable statistical data for those desiring this information. A supplementary classification, "Classification of Factors Influencing Health Status and Contact with Health Service" is provided to record patient visits for reasons not related to a particular disease or injury. Admission to a hospital for a voluntary sterilization only is not a disease or injury and, therefore, is coded by using the supplementary classification. These codes are commonly referred to as "V-codes," since the code number itself is always preceded by the letter "V."

The E-codes in the "Classification of External Causes of Injury and Poisoning" (E800-E998) are used in conjunction with a disease or injury code number, as they only provide supplemental information to further explain the precipitating incident.

Four additional appendices are provided in Volume 1 for reference purposes and coder information.

ICD-9-CM is required for statistical reporting purposes by the National Center for Health Statistics of the United States. For this reason, it is used extensively by hospitals and other health care facilities for indexing, storing, and retrieving health care data.

The National Center for Health Statistics (NCHS) entered into an agreement with the American Hospital Association and the American Medical Record Association in 1964 to establish an ICD clearinghouse. AHA accepted financial responsibility for maintaining the clearinghouse which answers queries on hospital coding. The agreement specified that errata and new codes would be published in the *Journal of the American Medical Record Association*. To date, three sets of errata have been issued for ICD-9-CM. To ensure accurate coding, medical record practitioners must see that published errata are entered promptly into all ICD-9-CM coding books used by medical record department coders.

The NCHS also collects input from medical record practitioners in the U.S. for use in preparing the tenth revision of ICD. The first draft of the structure of the tenth revision has been released for comment, although it is not anticipated that the use of ICD-10 will be implemented until 1993.

Educational materials to learn how to use the ICD-9-CM are available from a number of health-related agencies and organizations, including the American Medical Record Association. In addition, various modifications and adaptations of the ICD-9-CM have been developed for use by specialized health care facilities. These classification systems more clearly meet the needs of a variety of facilities and, by retaining the structure and format of the ICD-9-CM codes, are usable for reporting statistics to the National Center for Health Statistics and elsewhere.

OTHER CLASSIFICATIONS

As the delivery of health care in the United States becomes more specialized, a need emerges for specialized patient information to follow up and evaluate the effectiveness of treatment measures. The medical record practitioner must be aware of the various specialized classification systems available for the collection of statistical information. Only through the use of an appropriate coding and indexing system will the resulting collection of data be meaningful to the health care facility. Several of the more common coding systems are discussed below.

ICD-ONCOLOGY

One area requiring specific detailed information on the effectiveness and outcome of treatment is the study of tumors or neoplasms known as oncology. For adequate statistical information and follow-up of patients, a detailed classification had to be devised to record the numbers and types of tumors in the United States.

In 1968 the *Manual of Tumor Nomenclature and Coding* was published by the American Cancer Society to meet the indexing needs of those facilities involved in the treatment of neoplastic disease. Commonly referred to as MOTNAC, the *Manual of Tumor Nomenclature and Coding* combined segments of the *Systematized Nomenclature of Pathology* (SNOP) and the ICDA-8 into one detailed classification system for specialists in oncology.

In the same year, the World Health Organization requested the International Agency for Research on Cancer to begin work on the "Neoplasm" chapter for the ninth revision of the *International Classification of Diseases* (ICD-9). A recommendation was made to the World Health Organization to publish a supplemental neoplasm classification with ICD-9 for use by the field of oncology. This supplemental classification would be based on the existing *Manual of Tumor Nomenclature and Coding.* The recommendation was endorsed by the World Health Organization in 1971 and resulted in publication of the *International Classification of Diseases for Oncology* (ICD-O) in 1976. The purpose of the ICD-O is to provide a classification system for the field of oncology which contains sufficient detail to code the extensive topography, histology (morphology), and behavior of neoplasms.

The ICD-O is divided into three sections. The site or location in the body which contains the tumor is assigned a code number (four-digit code numbers which run from 140.0 to 199.9). The "Morphology-Numerical List" contains code numbers which are used to specify the type of tumor found and its behavior. The morphology terms have five-digit code numbers which run from 8000/0 to 9990/6; the first four digits indicate the specific histologic terms, and the fifth digit after the slash is a behavior code. An optional sixth digit may be added to the morphology code number which indicates differentiation of the tumor mass. Anatomical sites and morphological terms are listed in the ICD-O "Alphabetic Index" for ease in selecting the appropriate code numbers to identify the neoplasms. The code numbers for topography, morphology, and behavior also appear in ICD-9-CM.

INTERNATIONAL CLASSIFICATION OF IMPAIRMENTS, DISABILITIES, AND HANDICAPS

This manual is published by the World Health Organization to measure the consequences of disease. It contains three distinct and independent classifications, each relating to a different plane of experience consequent upon disease:

> Impairments (I code) concerned with abnormalities of body structure and appearance and with organ or system function, resulting from any cause: in principle, impairments represent disturbances at the organ level.
>
> Disabilities (D code) reflecting the consequences of impairment in terms of functional performance and activity by the individual; disabilities thus represent disturbances at the level of the person.
>
> Handicaps (H code) concerned with the disadvantages experienced by the individual as a result of impairments and disabilities; handicaps thus reflect interaction with and adaptation to the individual's surroundings.

These ideas can be linked in the following manner:

DISEASE OR DISORDER → IMPAIRMENT → DISABILITY → HANDICAP

(intrinsic situation)   (exteriorized)   (objectified)   (socialized)

The first two classifications resemble the structure of ICD in that they are hierarchical (Figure 2). The structure of the H code is radically different from all other ICD related classifications, for the items are not classified according to the attributes of individuals but according to the circumstances that can be expected to place such individuals at a disadvantage in relation to their peers when viewed from the norms of society. It is not an exhaustive classification scheme but is restricted to key social roles – orientation, physical independence, mobility, occupation, social integration, and economic self-sufficiency. Specifi-

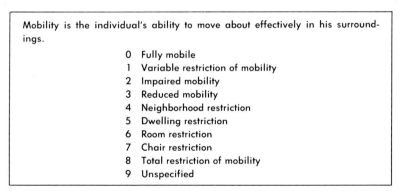

	Impairment (I codes)
37	Impairment of speech form
37.0	Impairment of speech fluency
37.1	Impairment of speech pressure
37.2	Impairment of speech patterning
	Disability (D codes)
27	Other disability in seeing and related activities
27.0	Disability in night vision
27.1	Disability in color recognition
27.2	Disability in comprehending written messages

FIG. 2 – IMPAIRMENT AND DISABILITY CODES

cation of the individual's status in regard to each dimension is required (Figure 3).

Mobility is the individual's ability to move about effectively in his surroundings.	
0	Fully mobile
1	Variable restriction of mobility
2	Impaired mobility
3	Reduced mobility
4	Neighborhood restriction
5	Dwelling restriction
6	Room restriction
7	Chair restriction
8	Total restriction of mobility
9	Unspecified

FIG. 3 – CLASSIFICATIONS OF MOBILITY

Extensive definitions are included in the classification to facilitate uniform coding. These classifications are intended to facilitate study of the consequences of disease and to provide statistics on impairments, disabilities, and handicaps.

DSM-III

Those facilities specializing in the treatment of psychiatric and mental disorders can record detailed psychiatric data by using the *Diagnostic and Statistical Manual of Mental Disorders*. First published in 1952 by the American Psychiatric Association, the *Diagnostic and Statistical Manual of Mental Disorders* (DSM-III) was an expansion of the mental disorders section of the ICD-8, both going into effect in 1968. DSM-III was published in 1980 to serve as a statistical classification and glossary of mental disorders, as well as a basis for research and administrative information. The primary purpose of DSM-III is to provide clear descriptions of diagnostic categories in order for clinicians to diagnose, communicate about, study, and treat various mental disorders. All official DSM-III codes and terms are included in ICD-9-CM although unofficial non-ICD-9-CM codes are provided in parentheses for use when greater specificity is necessary. DSM-III is not based solely on the etiology of mental disorders as this is not always known. Rather DSM-III utilizes both a descriptive and etiologic approach to the classification of mental disorders. All disorders without known etiology or pathological process are grouped together on the basis of shared clinical manifestations.

DSM-III provides specific diagnostic criteria as guides for making each diagnosis to enhance diagnostic reliability (Figure 4).

307.10 Anorexia Nervosa

Differential Diagnosis: Physical disorders with weight loss, Bulimia, Depressive disorders, Schizophrenia with bizarre eating patterns.

Diagnostic Criteria

A. Intense fear of becoming obese, which does not diminish as weight loss progresses.

B. Disturbance of body image, e.g., claiming to "feel fat" when emaciated.

C. Weight loss of at least 25 percent of original body weight or, if under 18 years of age, weight loss from original body weight plus projected weight gain expected from growth charts may be combined to make the 25 percent.

D. Refusal to maintain body weight over a minimal normal weight for age and height.

E. No known physical illness that would account for the weight loss.

FIG. 4 – DSM-III DIAGNOSTIC CRITERIA

DSM-III recommends the use of a multiaxial system (Figure 5) for evaluation to ensure that information of value in planning treatment and predicting outcome is recorded in each of five axes, the first three of which constitute an official diagnostic evaluation:

Axis I   Clinical Syndromes, Conditions Not Attributable to a Mental Disease that Are a Focus of Attention or Treatment and Additional Codes

Axis II   Personality Disorders and Specific Developmental Disorders

Axis III Physical Disorders and Conditions

Axis IV   Severity of Psychosocial Stressors

Axis V   Highest Level of Adaptive Functioning Past Year

The latter two axes are for use in special clinical or research settings.

Axis I	296.23 Major Depression, Single Episode, with Melancholia
	303.93 Alcohol Dependence, in Remission
Axis II	301.60 Dependent Personality Disorder (Provisional, R/O Borderline Personality Disorder)
Axis III	Alcoholic cirrhosis of the liver
Axis IV	Psychosocial stressors: anticipated retirement and change in residence with loss of contact with friends Severity: 4-Moderate
Axis V	Highest level of adaptive functioning past year: 3-Good

FIG. 5 – A DSM-III MULTIAXIAL EVALUATION

Some mental health facilities use DSM-III for coding and indexing. However, ICD-9-CM coding is required by most third-party payers. It is, therefore, important for each facility to evaluate its needs in establishing a coding policy. Frequently, mental health facilities will require that the diagnoses be recorded in the terminology of DSM-III but will code all diagnoses according to ICD-9-CM. There is a DSM-III-ICD-9-CM crosswalk available for those facilities who use dual coding procedures. The medical record practitioner should be thoroughly familiar with the various internal and external data requirements and needs.

CLASSIFICATION IN MENTAL RETARDATION

Since 1921 when its first manual on classification and terminology was published, the American Association of Mental Deficiency (AAMD) has been concerned about the differentiation of mental retardation from other handicapping conditions and about differences found within the population of retarded individuals. In 1983 the eighth edition was published to reflect current thinking in the field and to make it consistent with ICD-9 and DSM-III, particularly with reference to medical classification.

The AAMD system provides for making a diagnosis of mental retardation by level (same as ICD-9-CM codes), a diagnosis by etiology such as lead poisoning or Down's syndrome, and a diagnosis of concurrent problems of the individual who is diagnosed as retarded such as blindness. ICD-9-CM codes may be used for all of these diagnoses, or AAMD codes may be used for etiology because parts of the AAMD medical classification system have greater specificity with reference to etiology than are found in either ICD-9-CM or DSM-III. Examples: 14 – Postnatal hypoxia, 15 – Postnatal injury. The AAMD classification system also contains a glossary to provide some homogeneity to the professional language in the field of mental retardation. The classification is designed to facilitate communication for diagnostic, treatment, and research purposes, and to facilitate prevention efforts through identification of the cause of mental retardation.

ROENTGEN CLASSIFICATION

Other departments within the hospital may find it necessary to retain statistical information for purposes of follow-up and evaluation of patient care. The radiology department is one area which is required by the Joint Commission on Accreditation of Hospitals to retain an index of unusual and interesting radiology cases. For this purpose, the American College of Radiology has developed the *Index for Roentgen Diagnosis*, which serves as a classification system for diagnostic radiology departments.

Two sections comprise the *Index for Roentgen Diagnosis* – the listing of diagnostic code numbers and an alphabetic index. The code number describes both the anatomical site of the x-ray and the pathological process or disease. The anatomy code ranges from two to four digits before the decimal point, while the two to five decimal digits after the decimal point refer to the disease process. An optional procedural code number may be added to describe the type of radiographic examination, bringing the total possible number of digits in the code number to ten. The extent of detail to be incorporated into an individual facility's index is left to the discretion of each health care institution.

HCFA COMMON PROCEDURE CODING (HCPCS)

The federal government has tried since the late 1970s to develop a procedure labeling system which might serve all Health Care Financing Administration (HCFA) program needs for procedure information. HCFA's major use of procedure information is for the Medicare and Medicaid programs in the determination of reimbursement for professional fees. Procedure information is also used in conducting peer reviews.

HCFA's studies revealed that it would not be feasible to develop a single procedure labeling system because the purposes of *Current Procedural Terminology* (CPT-4) and ICD-9-CM are very different. The purpose of CPT-4 is to provide a listing of descriptive terms and identifying codes for reporting medical services and procedures performed by physicians. CPT-4 seeks to convey as much information as possible in a single code. ICD-9-CM is designed for the classification of morbidity and mortality information for statistical purposes and for the indexing of hospital records by disease and procedure in order to provide clinically meaningful data for research, health care planning, and quality assurance activities. ICD-9-CM may utilize several codes to completely describe a procedure.

After HCFA ruled out the development of a single procedure labeling system, the focus shifted to developing a comprehensive procedure labeling system to provide reimbursement for ancillary services such as ambulance services, prosthetic services, and the services of physicians and other independent practitioners.

HCFA's *Common Procedure Coding* (HCPCS) includes the entirety of CPT and additional codes for ancillary services. HCFA signed a limited copyright agreement with the American Medical Association to utilize CPT in HCPCS.

The objectives of HCPCS are to: establish common standards of communication among users and between providers and users; increase the compatibility of reported data; and compare physician and hospital bills and episodes of illness.

HCPCS consists of three levels:

1. CPT codes.
2. A0000-V9999 codes to designate ancillary services for which HCFA provides reimbursement, such as A4390 – Ideal bladder set; E0860 – Traction equipment, overdoor; M0722 – Physical medicine, brief inpatient hospital OMT (up to two body regions).
3. W0000-Z9999 codes for use by individual insurance carriers or state agencies for ancillary services that do not have a HCPCS code assigned to them. These codes, similar to CPT's Unlisted Procedure Codes, serve as a basis for updates to the ancillary portion of HCPCS.

HCPCS codes are utilized to obtain reimbursement under Part B of Medicare, and ICD-9-CM procedure codes are used to reimburse health care facilities for services rendered under Part A of Medicare.

NURSING DIAGNOSES

Nurses have traditionally used medical diseases as the basis of nursing treatment. However, in the early 1970s, nurses began to identify a need for a classification of nursing diagnoses. In 1976 the American Nurses Association stated that "nursing diagnosis describes actual or potential health problems which nurses are capable of treating and licensed to treat."

The physician may diagnose Parkinson's disease while the nurse diagnoses the problems that are consequences of the disease – difficulty ambulating, dependence on feeding, and poor oral secretion control.

Although no universally accepted classification of nursing diagnoses is currently available, medical record practitioners should become familiar with the references cited in this chapter.

Additionally, the American Nurses Association has requested that nursing diagnoses be included in the tenth revision of the *International Classification of Diseases.*

Nursing care is enhanced by use of standard nursing diagnoses, because each nursing diagnosis is associated with a characteristic set of nursing activities to facilitate communication between shifts and focus the development of a nursing care plan; the development of accurate staffing patterns focus quality assurance activities and permit determinations of the cost efficiency of nursing services.

CASE-MIX CLASSIFICATIONS

The purpose of a statistical compilation of disease and procedural data is primarily to furnish quantitative data on the incidence of certain diseases/procedures (morbidity) and the causes of death (mortality). Health care facilities and third-party payers in the United States, however, have other data needs; so for the last twenty years researchers have been trying to develop a useful classification system to measure the case mix (categories of patients and type) treated by a health care institution. To date, numerous approaches have been developed including diagnosis-related groups, a severity of illness index, and disease staging.

Diagnosis-Related Groups (DRGs)

Diagnosis-related groups (DRGs) represent an inpatient classification scheme to categorize patients who are medically related with respect to diagnoses and treatment, and who are statistically similar in their lengths of stay. DRGs are statistically consistent – patients in a DRG tend to consume similar amounts of hospital resources as measured by length of stay and cost. They are also medically meaningful – physician input was used to ensure that patients in a DRG have similar clinical conditions or treatment. Twenty-three major diagnostic categories (MDCs) were established to cluster patients such as:

MDC 11   Diseases and disorders of the kidney and urinary tract

12   Diseases and disorders of the male reproductive system

13   Diseases and disorders of the female reproductive system

14   Pregnancy, childbirth, and puerperium

15   Newborns and other neonates with conditions in the perinatal period

16   Diseases and disorders of the blood-forming organs and immunological disorders

The affected body system such as urinary or circulatory is the principal determinant of DRG assignment. Decision trees are utilized to display the divisions in the Major Diagnostic Categories. Patients in most MDCs are divided into two groups depending upon the presence or absence of qualifying surgery. Each procedure in ICD-9-CM was classified by physician panels as "OR" or "non-OR." After major diagnostic categories are divided into medical and surgical categories, surgical patients are further divided based on the specific surgical procedure performed, while medical patients are further divided based on the specific principal diagnosis. The medical classes in each MDC usually include a class for neoplasms and classes for symptoms and specific conditions relating to the organ system involved. Since patients can be assigned to only one DRG per episode of care, assignments are based on the Uniform Hospital Discharge Data Set definitions of principal diagnosis and principal procedure.

Principal Diagnosis – The condition established after study to be chiefly responsible for occasioning the admission of the patient to the hospital for care.

Principal Procedure – One performed for definitive treatment rather than one performed for diagnostic or exploratory purposes, or which was necessary to take care of a complication. The principal procedure is that which is most related to the principal diagnosis.

Patients with multiple procedures are assigned to the surgical DRG highest in the hierarchy within the MDC. Thus a patient having a breast biopsy and a radical mastectomy is assigned to the mastectomy DRG. Other partitions depend on the patient's age, discharge status, procedure, and/or qualifying complications/comorbidities. A complication is a secondary condition that arises during hospitalization and is thought to increase the length of stay by at least one day for approximately 75 percent of the patients. A comorbid condition is a condition that existed on admission and is thought to increase the length of stay at least one day for approximately 75 percent of the patients.

There are 467 DRGs but the case mix of many health care facilities involves primarily 25 to 30 DRGs. This grouping facilitates more analytical use of the hospital's medical record data. Many third-party payers, including the Medicare program, use DRGs to reimburse hospitals. Rates are set prospectively by DRG thus allowing the government or the insurer to fix prices in advance.

DRG assignment is usually performed by a computer with grouper software. Medical record practitioners in small facilities may assign DRGs manually utilizing the decision trees and listings of OR procedures, complications, and comorbidities. For example, "a 66-year-old female admitted with adult onset diabetes and acute abdominal colic. Workup revealed gallstones, and a cholecystectomy and common duct exploration were performed for acute cholecystitis and cholelithiasis. Patient's diabetes was out of control for most of her hospital stay." On the decision tree, this patient is tracked through total cholecystectomy and common bile duct exploration to age less than 70 and no complication/comorbidity (adult onset uncontrolled diabetes is not defined as a comorbid condition or complication) so DRG 196 is assigned (Figure 6).

Severity of Illness

The patient's stage of disease severity is not directly reflected in DRG assignment. Patients with multiple complications or comorbid conditions are assigned to the same DRG as those with one complication or comorbid condition. Health care professionals believe severity of illness must be considered to achieve equitable prospective payment and that tertiary hospitals treating proportionately more patients at the higher levels of severity may be exposed to great financial risk under a DRG prospective payment system not adjusted for severity.

Researchers at Johns Hopkins University report that an ade-

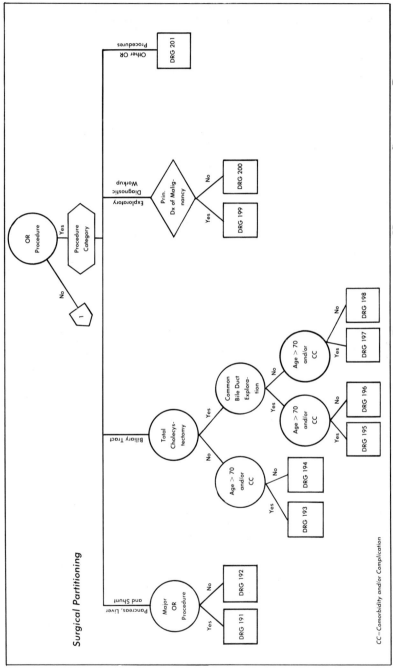

FIG. 6 — MAJOR DIAGNOSTIC CATEGORY 07: DISEASES AND DISORDERS OF THE HEPATOBILIARY SYSTEM AND PANCREAS

CC=Comorbidity and/or Complication

quate definition of inpatient severity of illness incorporates at least seven patient dimensions:

1. Stage of the principal diagnosis
2. Concurrent interacting conditions that affect the hospital course
3. Rate of response to therapy or rate of recovery and
4. Residual impairment remaining after therapy for the acute aspect of the hospitalization
5. Complications of the principal condition
6. Dependency on hospital staff
7. Extent of nonoperating room procedure

To determine the severity of illness index for each case, the patient's medical record is reviewed; and the rater scores each

TABLE 1

PATIENT SEVERITY INDEX

Characteristic		Levels			
		1	2	3	4
Stage of Principal Diagnosis		Asymptomatic	Moderate Manifestations	Major Manifestation	Catastrophic
Interactions		None	Low	Moderate	Major
Response to Therapy	Rate	Prompt	Moderate Delay	Serious Delay	No Response
	Residual	None	Minor	Moderate	Major
Complications		None or very minor	Moderate (less important than principal diagnosis)	Major (as or more important than principal diagnosis)	Catastrophic
Dependency		Low	Moderate	Major	Extreme
Procedures (Non O.R.)		Noninvasive Diagnostic	Therapeutic or Invasive Diagnostic	Nonemergency Life Sustaining	Emergency Life Sustaining
Severity rating (circle one):		1	2	3	4

Reprinted with permission of J. B. Lippincott Co., July, 1983 Issue of *Medical Care*, p. 706.

of the seven variables according to one of four levels of increasing severity. The overall severity level is then computed for the patient on a four-point scale by integrating the values of the seven variables (Table 1).

Severity of illness raters must be carefully trained in the definitions of the seven dimensions at each of four levels. Medical record practitioners, however, who have completed training programs can complete such ratings with disagreement rates comparable to those encountered for selecting principal diagnoses.

If four levels of severity of illness without a major operating room procedure and four levels with a major operating room procedure are used within the major diagnostic categories, groups are produced which are more homogenous than DRGs.

Disease Staging

Staging is another method for measuring the severity of specific well-defined diseases. In staging, diseases are divided into categories of increasing levels of severity:

Stage 1 – Conditions with no complications or problems of minimal severity.

Stage 2 – Problems limited to an organ or system, significantly increased risk of complications.

Stage 3 – Multiple site involvement, generalized systemic involvement, poor prognosis.

Stage 4 – Death.

These general stage delineations may be broken down further into subcategories to provide more specificity and to further delineate the progression of disease. Disease-staging criteria have been developed for 420 diagnoses. It is best to assign stages based on a review of the entire medical record; laboratory and pathological findings as well as vital signs and other examinations can be considered in final stage assignment.

The criteria, however, have been translated into coded criteria so they can be applied to discharge abstract data bases. Table 2 displays the coded criteria for the diagnosis *fracture of the pelvis.*

TABLE 2

DIAGNOSIS: FRACTURE OF THE PELVIS
ETIOLOGY: TRAUMA (PHYSICAL)

STAGE	COMMON DESCRIPTION OR NAME OF THE CONDITION	ICD-9-CM CODES THAT DEFINE EACH STAGE AND SUBSTAGE
1.1	Fracture of pelvis without a break in the continuity of the pelvic ring	808.20, 808.41-808.42, 808.80;
1.2	Single break in the pelvic ring	808.49;
2.1	Double breaks in the pelvic ring: 'straddle fractures'	808.43;
2.2	'Malgaigne fractures'	
2.3	Severe multiple fractures of pelvis	
2.4	Open fracture	808.30, 808.51-808.59, 808.90;
3.1	Thrombophlebitis	S1.1-S2.4 + 451.00-451.90;
3.2	Gynecological injuries or Rectal injury or Neurological injury or Urological injury	S1.1-S2.4 + 863.20-863.59, 866.00-868.19, 878.00-878.90, 879.60-879.70, 953.30, 953.50, 956.00-956.90, 958.50, 569.20-569.30;
3.3	Venous hemorrhage	S1.1-S2.4 + 459.00, 902.10-902.19, 902.31-902.39, 902.40, 902.42-50, 902.52, 902.54, 902.56-902.59, 902.82-902.90;
3.4	Arterial hemorrhage	S1.1-S2.4 + 902.00, 902.20-902.29, 902.41, 902.51, 902.53, 902.55, 902.81;
3.5	Pulmonary embolus	S1.1-S2.4 + 415.10;
3.6	Shock	S1.1-S2.4 + ZSHOCK9;
4.0	Death	S3.1-S3.6 + DEATH;

Disease staging categorizes patients so as to maximize the homogeneity within patient groups and the heterogeneity between patient groups with respect to the nature of their illnesses.

Some health care facilities are now maintaining severity of illness data, so they can determine whether physicians with patients whose bills exceed the DRG rate are indeed sicker, or whether some physicians merely utilize more services in caring for their patients. Research has demonstrated that medical rec-

ord personnel can reliably record data on the severity of a patient illness concurrently with discharge abstract coding in one
to two minutes. Software programs to facilitate assignment of
a severity index or disease stage may also be leased or purchased.

Resource Utilization Groups (RUGs)

The patient classification system called Resource Utilization
Groups is a case-mix system for long term care. This system is
still under development and is currently being studied in one
state as a reimbursement mechanism. The objective of the study
is to develop a prospective reimbursement methodology which
employs case-mix measures, allowing for adequate reimbursement of facility needs based on characteristics of the clients in
the facility.

RUGs classify patients into one of nine clusters that are relatively similar in their resource use when compared with patients in other clusters. Long term care patients are divided into
three main branches based on the variable *dress*. The first
branch, indicating those patients who dress themselves or dress
with supervision, becomes RUG group #1, the least resource-
intensive group. This group is not split further. The second
branch, indicating those who dress with support, is partitioned
into RUGs #2 and #3. RUG #2 contains patients who ambulate
by themselves or with supervision, while group #3 consists of
patients who need assistance in ambulation. The third branch,
those who are completely dependent upon others to dress, is divided into three further branches. The first branch, consisting
of those who feed themselves or are fed with supervision, is divided into final RUGs #4, #5, and #6 according to the patient's
ability to ambulate. Group #4 ambulates independently or with
supervision, group #5 ambulates with support, while group #6
ambulates only with assistance. The second branch becomes
RUG #7, those patients who need support for eating. The third
and final branch, those needing total care when fed, is partitioned into final RUGs #8 and #9 according to whether or not
fluid intake or output monitoring is performed.

Research indicates that diagnosis is not useful as a predictor
of patient resource utilization, so other measures must be found.

RUGs utilize patient characteristics which are objective and easily noted on long term care patients, but further study is necessary to determine whether RUGs can serve as the basis of a reimbursement methodology matching resources with patient needs.

CLASSIFICATION SYSTEMS FOR AMBULATORY CARE

Ambulatory care is another aspect of the health care delivery system which presents its own unique problems and needs for data retrieval. Many "occasions of service" to the ambulatory patient are not directly related to acute treatment of a specific diagnosis or condition as they are in the hospital setting. Consequently, classification systems have been designed to meet the particular needs of the ambulatory care community.

International Classification of Health Problems in Primary Care (ICHPPC)

The first edition of the *International Classification of Health Problems in Primary Care* was put together in 1975 by the Classification Committee of the World Organization of National Colleges, Academies, and Academic Associations of General Practitioners/Family Physicians (WONCA). The ICHPPC was published by the American Hospital Association. The first edition of the ICHPPC closely paralleled the ICD-8 classification system.

In 1979 the second edition of the *International Classification of Health Problems in Primary Care* (ICHPPC-2), published by the Oxford University Press, became available, following publication of the ICD-9. Both a "Tabular Classification of Health Problems" and an "Alphabetical Index" are included in ICHPPC-2. The tabular classification lists the four-digit code numbers used in ICHPPC-2, and also provides a cross-reference to corresponding code numbers in ICD-9. If a fourth digit is not necessary to fully describe the diagnosis, a three-digit code number and slash mark are assigned instead. For example, osteoporosis is assigned code number 7330, while transient cerebral ischemia is assigned 435/.

In 1983 ICHPPC-2-Defined was issued. The major new feature is that an attempt has been made to define by selection criteria the majority of terms used in the classification. For each defined rubric, one or more criteria are identified which must be fulfilled to code a problem under that diagnostic title. For example, ICHPPC code 4273 Atrial fibrillation or flutter. Inclusion in this rubric requires one of the following:

1. Demonstration of characteristic findings by electrocardiogram.

2. Totally irregular heart rate with a pulse deficit. Consider (7851) Palpitations; (7889) Tachycardia NOS.

ICHPPC-2 is designed primarily for use by health care providers who will establish the diagnosis and assign the appropriate code number. The inclusion criteria listed in ICHPPC-2-Defined are useful in training ICD-9-CM coders. The number system and content of the rubrics in the ICHPPC-2-Defined are the same as ICHPPC-2.

Reason for Visit Classification (RFV)

Another outpatient classification system which records the reasons patients seek ambulatory medical care is the *Reason for Visit Classification System*, developed by the American Medical Record Association in 1977. The *Reason for Visit Classification System* is based on a survey of patients of ambulatory care facilities conducted by the National Center for Health Statistics, entitled *National Ambulatory Medical Care Survey: Symptom Classification*. The classification is designed to collect statistical information on the symptoms, complaints, and problems which motiviated the patient to seek medical care.

The *Reason for Visit Classification System* consists of two major sections: the "Tabular List of Inclusive Terms" and the "Alphabetic Index of Terms." The tabular list is divided into seven modules: (1) Symptoms; (2) Diseases; (3) Diagnostic, screening and preventive; (4) Treatment; (5) Injuries and adverse effects; (6) Test results; and (7) Administrative.

Descriptions of signs and symptoms are included as they might be told to the physician in the patient's own words. Entries such as "runny nose," "sniffles," and "postnasal drip" are included under S400.0 Nasal congestion.

Code numbers contain three digits before the decimal point, with one decimal digit for greater detail. Fourth-digit decimal categories may be expanded at the facility's discretion to allow for greater detail and flexibility.

Reason for Encounter Classification (RFEC)

The World Health Organization recently developed the RFEC and conducted a pilot study of the new system, because there is no international classification system to identify why a person enters the health care system. RFEC is designed to classify the reasons why patients seek care at the primary level. It incorporates an expanded version of the existing *Reason for Visit Classification* and the rubrics in the diagnoses and diseases component are the same as those in the *International Classification of Health Problems in Primary Care.*

The RFEC is designed along two axes: chapter and component. Thirteen chapters have titles related to body systems, and the other three are "General," "Psychological," and "Social." Each chapter is subdivided into seven components each of which is represented by two digits in the RFEC code. The seven components are: (1) Symptoms and complaints; (2) Diagnosis and screening prevention; (3) Treatment, procedures, and medication; (4) Test results; (5) Administrative; (6) Other; and (7) Diagnoses, diseases.

The 3-character biaxial classification system has five process components, numbers 2 to 6 which have two-digit codes that are identical in all chapters. For example, the code D50 indicates the reason for the encounter is Medications, for the digestive system; A50 is Medications, general; and K50 is Medications, circulatory. RFEC has a strong nondisease orientation and is an easy classification to use.

The pilot study reveals that the RFEC can be used not only to clarify the patient's subjective statement of his or her reason for the encounter but also to interpret that reason or problem at the highest diagnostic level possible for primary care providers.

CHOOSING A CLASSIFICATION SYSTEM

The classification system chosen by a particular health care facility must be capable of supplying the information specified by federal and state regulations and accreditation requirements, as well as that desired by the facility's administration and medical staff. The type and amount of information to be collected will help determine the system or combination of systems to be used for the storage and retrieval of data. For example, an acute care facility might use the ICD-9-CM classification system to collect data on inpatients, ICHPPC for the family practice clinic, and DSM-III in the mental health clinic.

Currently, the regulations for the prospective payment system specify:

> "that all hospitals subject to the prospective payment system will be paid, for inpatient services provided, a specific amount for each discharge based on the case's classification into one of 467 diagnosis-related groups. Every hospital discharge case will fit into a DRG category and no case will apply to more than one category. The assignment is based on the principal diagnosis, secondary diagnosis (if any), procedures performed, and age, sex and discharge status of the patient. The DRGs provide coverage of the complete range of diagnoses represented in the *International Classification of Diseases 9th Revision, Clinical Modification* (ICD-9-CM) without overlay."

Acute care hospitals participating in the Medicare program, therefore, must supply ICD-9-CM codes to obtain reimbursement. However, in a health care facility where medical record personnel complete claims for the services rendered by a hospital-based group practice, CPT-4 coding would also be performed since physician reimbursement is based on CPT-4 coding. Medical record personnel may also utilize SNOP or SNOMED codes assigned by the pathologist to pathological specimens. These codes will be input into the discharge data base for retrieval purposes.

Medical record practitioners need to continually review health care literature to identify the changes being made in existing health care classification systems and to monitor the development of new systems. As alternate forms of health care delivery become more common, medical record practitioners will be required to assess the data needs of health maintenance organizations, preferred provider organizations, and skilled nursing facilities to identify classification systems appropriate for their data needs.

Data needs in the acute care setting will also require frequent reassessment, for DRGs based on ICD-9-CM codes may not continue to be the reimbursement mechanism of choice. Data, however, to describe the health care services rendered by a particular facility will continue to be necessary to plan, allocate, and evaluate the use of finite health care resources.

ENCODING SYSTEMS

An encoder has been defined in *Webster's Unabridged Dictionary* as a "cipher machine." Today's use of the word in the computer world has expanded its usage to mean the conversion of data from one type to another type. An example of this may be found in the simple act of coding a disease or condition. When done correctly and accurately, coders need to consider several variables (age, sex, complications, results, and procedures) to arrive at the proper code number.

Computer-assisted encoders are now being marketed by several vendors. These systems offer software with interactive programs to prompt the coder through a series of choices displayed on the terminal until a code is assigned for each diagnosis and procedure (Figure 7). Another vendor offers software which displays the correct pages of the ICD-9-CM index and tabular lists so the coder does not have to spend time thumbing through the code books but still is able to check all inclusion and exclusion notes to ensure assignment of the correct code.

Consistency among coders is one of the major advantages computerized coding systems offer. Encoders also promote accuracy, for the coder must go through each step of the ICD-9-CM decision process. There is no way to short-circuit the procedure by omitting a step.

Experienced coders may assign common codes more quickly working from memory and familiar code books than by working with an encoder. However, when working from memory, a coder may consistently assign an incorrect code number. Computer-assisted encoders, however, only assign codes to diagnoses input

Sex: M

Age: 74

Disposition — Choose one:

[NL]   Home — Self-Care/Home Health Service or still in hospital
  2   Left against medical advice
  3   Transferred to acute care facility
  4   Expired
  5   SNF, ICF, or other facility

Choice: NL

Principal Diagnosis
Enter Key Word: Cor

1 Cor

Which Line?

Principal Diagnosis

Cor

Cor

1. Cor Biloculare
2. Cor Bovinum or Bovis (coded as cardiac hypertrophy)
3. Cor Pulmonale
4. Cor Pulmonale with Pulmonary Hypertension
5. Cor Triatriatum or Triatrium
6. Cor Triloculare
Which Line?

Principal Diagnosis

Cor
Cor Pulmonale

Cor Pulmonale

1. Acute
2. Chronic
3. With Pulmonary Embolus
4. Unspecified

Which Line?

Principal Diagnosis

Cor
Cor Pulmonale
Acute

ICD-9-CM   Review Code
   415.0   Acute cor pulmonale

Press any key to continue

FIG. 7 – DECISION TREE – COMPUTER-ASSISTED ENCODER

by the coder. The coder must analyze the discharge information in the medical record to ensure that the physician has identified the appropriate principal diagnosis according to UHDDS definitions. Additionally, the documentation in the record must indicate that the diagnosis selected is that condition which, after study, occasioned the admission of the patient to the hospital for care.

DRG

336   Transurethral Prostatectomy (70+/cc)
       HCFA wt. 0.9974 Mean LOS 8.4 Outlier LOS (22 days)

Diagnoses

1. * 185   Malignant neoplasm of prostate
2. * 25030   Diabetes mellitus with coma, non-insulin
             dependent or unspecified (Type II)

Select alternate principal Dx or NL to continue

Procedures

602 Transurethral prostatectomy

DRG

468 *** O.R. Procedure Unrelated to Diagnosis MDC ***

       HCFA wt. 2.0818 Mean LOS 11.2 Outlier LOS 33 days

       *Note this may not be an error in coding, but
       you should carefully examine your selection of
       principal diagnosis and make sure you have
       included all surgeries.

Diagnoses:

1. * 25030 Diabetes mellitus with coma, non-insulin
           dependent or unspecified (Type II)
2.   185   Malignant neoplasm of prostate

Select alternate principal Dx or NL to continue
Procedures
* 602 Transurethral prostatectomy

FIG. 8 – ASSIGNING DIAGNOSIS CODE WITH ENCODER

Encoders can accurately assign a code to the diagnosis selected and even query the coder to ensure that the coder does not want to select a different diagnosis as the principal one (Figure 8). However, the coder makes the final decision on the identification of the principal diagnosis and other diagnoses to be reported. The encoder cannot tell which diagnoses listed by the physician affect the current stay. Yet, only those diagnoses which affect the current stay are to be reported according to the UHDDS definitions. Diagnoses that relate to an earlier episode of care which have no bearing on the current hospital stay are to be excluded.

Some vendors have developed encoders which encourage selection of the diagnosis with the highest reimbursement as the principal diagnosis. This practice is referred to as DRG creep and constitutes Medicare fraud when the medical record documentation indicates a less costly diagnosis as the principal diagnosis.

For accurate coding, either manually or with an encoder, the critical skill is searching the medical record to identify the diagnosis which fits the UHDDS definition of principal diagnosis, and all other diagnoses and procedures which affect the hospital stay.

Computer support of the coding function is expensive; for in addition to hardware and software costs, an annual license fee is assessed. After assessing the volume of coding to be completed and the proficiency and depth of a hospital's coding staff, each medical record practitioner must decide whether computer-assisted encoders can be cost effective and justified.

SUMMARY

Many disease and operation nomenclatures and classification systems have been used in the United States throughout the years. As our health care delivery system has become more specialized, so too have specialty classification systems been developed for use in recording valuable medical statistical information. Although federal and state requirements may somewhat mandate the choice of a classification system, special projects embarked upon by health care institutions often require the medical record practitioner to make individual decisions regarding an appropriate classification system for use. The medical record practitioner must constantly stay abreast of changes and innovations in published coding systems and nomenclatures. No single classification will satisfy everyone's needs. A careful appraisal of the needs of the facility and an up-to-date knowledge of coding possibilities will result in selection of an appropriate coding system by the health care institution.

STUDY QUESTIONS

1. Define nomenclature and classification system, and explain how each may be used to complement the other in recording medical information.
2. State the purpose, and describe the structure of the code numbers used in each of the following nomenclatures and classification systems:

a. CMIT	f. ICD-O
b. CPT	g. DSM-III
c. SNOP	h. ICHPPC-2
d. SNOMED	i. RFV
e. ICD-9-CM	j. RFEC

3. Define a nursing diagnosis, and identify how nursing care is enhanced by the use of standard nursing diagnoses.
4. State the purposes of case-mix classification, and describe the structure of:

   Diagnosis-Related Groups
   Severity of Illness Index
   Disease Staging
5. List some considerations which should be made when selecting an appropriate classification system for use in a health care facility.
6. Identify the strengths and weaknesses of computer-assisted encoders.

REFERENCES

American College of Radiology. *Index for Roentgen Diagnoses,* 3rd Edition. Chicago, Illinois: American College of Radiology, 1975.

BARNES, CATHLEEN A., ART. "Disease Staging: A Clinically Oriented Dimension of Case Mix." *Journal of the American Medical Record Association.* January, 1985.

CAMPBELL, CLAIRE. *Nursing Diagnosis and Intervention in Nursing Practice.* New York, New York: John Wiley and Sons, 1978.

College of American Pathologists. *Systematized Nomenclature of Medicine.* Skokie, Illinois: College of American Pathologists, 1979.

COTE, ROGER A., MD, MSc, and ROBBOY, STANLEY, MD. "Progress in Medical Information Management: Systematized Nomenclature of Medicine (SNOMED)." *Journal of the American Medical Association.* February 22/29, 1980 – Vol. 243, No. 8.

Council for International Organizations of Medical Sciences and the World Health Organization. *International Nomenclature of Diseases – Diseases of the Lower Respiratory Tract.* Geneva, Switzerland, 1979.

Current Procedural Terminology, 4th Edition. American Medical Association. Chicago, Illinois, January, 1985.

Diagnostic and Statistical Manual of Mental Disorders, 3rd Edition. American Psychiatric Association. Washington, D.C., 1980.

FINKEL, ASHER, MD, Ed. *Current Medical Information and Terminology,* 5th Edition. American Medical Association. Chicago, Illinois, 1981.

FINNEGAN, RITA, MA, RRA. *Coding for Prospective Payment.* American Medical Record Association. Chicago, Illinois, 1984.

————. *ICD-9-CM Basic Coding Handbook.* American Medical Record Association. Chicago, Illinois, September, 1980.

————. *Data Quality and DRGs.* American Medical Record Association. Chicago, Illinois, 1983.

FRIES, BRANT E., PHD, and COONEY, LEO M., JR., MD. "Resource Utilization Groups: A Patient Classification System for Long-Term Care." July, 1984.

GEBBIE, KRISTINE M., and LAVIN, MARY ANN. *Classification of Nursing Diagnoses.* St. Louis, Missouri: The C.V. Mosby Company, 1975.

GONNELLA, JOSEPH S., MD, HORNBROOK, MARK C., PHD., and LOUIS, DANIEL Z., MS. "Staging of Disease: A Case-Mix Measurement." *Journal of the American Medical Association.* February 3, 1984 – Vol. 251, No. 5.

GROSSMAN, HERBERT J., Ed. *Classification in Mental Retardation.* American Association on Mental Deficiency, 1983.

Health Care Financing Administration, U.S. Department of Health and Human Services. *Health Care Financing Administration Common Procedure Coding System, Health Care Financing Administration,* 1984.

HORN, SUSAN DADAKIS, PHD. "Measuring Severity of Illness: Comparisons Across Institutions." *American Journal of Public Health.* 1983, Vol. 73, No. 1.

International Classification of Diseases for Oncology. World Health Organization. Geneva, Switzerland, 1976.

International Classification of Health Problems in Primary Care, 3rd Edition. World Organization of National Colleges, Academies, and Academic Associations of General Practitioners/Family Physicians. Oxford University Press, 1983.

LAMBERTS, HENK, MD., MEADS, SUE, and WOOD, MAURICE, MD. "Classification of Reasons Why Persons Seeking Primary Care: Pilot Study of a New System." *Public Health Reports.* November-December, 1984, Vol. 99, No. 6.

Manual of the World Health Organization International Statistical Classification of Diseases, Injuries, and Causes of Death. World Health Organization. Geneva, Switzerland, 1977.

Nomenclature and Criteria for Diagnosis of Diseases of the Heart and Great Vessels, 7th Edition. New York Heart Association, 1973.

SIMMONS, DELANNE A. *A Classification Scheme for Client Problems in Community Health Nursing.* Department of Health and Human Services Publication No. HRA 80-16, 1980.

Standard Nomenclature of Athletic Injuries. American Medical Association. Chicago, Illinois, 1976.

Systematized Nomenclature of Pathology. College of American Pathologists. Chicago, Illinois, 1965.

THOMPSON, JAMES, MD, GREEN, DELRAY, RRA, and SAVITT, HARRY L., MPH. "Preliminary Report on Crosswalk from DSM-III to ICD-9-CM." *American Journal of Psychiatry.* February, 1983.

U.S. Department of Health, Education, and Welfare. *A Reason for Visit Classification for Ambulatory Care,* Series 2, No. 78. Hyattsville, Maryland, February, 1979.

U.S. Department of Health, Education, and Welfare. *Standard Nomenclature of Veterinary Diseases and Operations,* 2nd Edition. U.S. National Institutes of Health, 1975.

World Health Organization. *International Classification of Impairments, Disabilities, and Handicaps.* Geneva, Switzerland, 1980.

chapter 13

INDEXES AND REGISTERS

The maintenance and retrieval of health information is an important function of the medical record department. Medical record practitioners abstract, compile, analyze, store, and retrieve health information. Two tools employed to facilitate the maintenance and retrieval of this information are the index and register. According to the *American Heritage Dictionary* an index is "Anything that serves to guide, point out, or otherwise facilitate reference." A register is "A formal or official recording of items, names, or actions."

Hospitals usually maintain an admission register, a death register, a birth register, an operating room register, an emergency room register, a number index, a master patient index, a physicians' index, and disease and operative indexes. Some hospitals also maintain cancer registries.

Until the early 1970s, most indexes and registers in health care facilities were compiled by manual methods. Certain kinds of information about the patient and/or patient care were extracted from the medical record and hand-posted on ledger sheets or cards.

Indexes and registers contain much valuable information, and the types of requests and uses vary. The most familiar and traditional request for health information is by physicians for patient care management and research. Today, however, hospitals and other types of health facilities are being required to provide patient care information with great frequency by agencies that fund such care. Medicare, Medicaid, and other third-party payers want to be assured that the episode of patient care they are paying for was necessary and appropriate. Peer review organizations, accrediting agencies, and licensing bodies request health information to review the quality of the care delivered. The administration of the health care facility requests information to use as a basis for management and financial decisions.

These increasing demands for health information require the health care facility to maintain an effective and efficient information system. The use of computerized data systems with their ability to accept, store, and produce data with efficiency and ease is almost a must.

While there are many manually maintained indexes and registers still in existence, the increasing demands for information and the availability of minicomputers and microcomputers will in all probability continue to increase the computerization of these activities.

MASTER PATIENT INDEX

The master patient index identifies all patients who have ever been admitted or treated by the hospital or health care facility. The master patient index is the key to locating patient records and is one of the most important tools in the medical record department. Traditionally, the master patient index has been maintained by preparing an index card for each patient admitted or treated at a health care facility. The index cards are usually arranged alphabetically in a vertical file but can also be filed phonetically by last name. The patient index card may be prepared in the patient registration area at the time of admission or later by medical record personnel.

CONTENT OF THE PATIENT INDEX

Only information of an identifying nature necessary for prompt location of a particular medical record should be contained on the patient index card (Figure 1). This information should as a minimum include: full name, address, identifying number, birth date (month, date, and year; in cases where patients have the same name, the date of birth provides additional information for identifying and obtaining the correct health record). Additional information that might be listed on the patient index card includes: admission and discharge dates, result (discharged or died), and attending physician's name.

This identifying information may be given out in accordance with hospital policy in response to legitimate requests. The privacy necessary for maintaining confidential information should be considered before making any decision to record diagnoses and operations on patient index cards.

Smith		Richard	Alan		M	24
FAMILY NAME		FIRST NAME	MIDDLE NAME		SEX	AGE

4568 Camden Drive, Indianapolis, IN BIRTH DATE 10 18 1948

ADDRESS — MONTH DAY YEAR

ADMITTED	DISCHARGED	RESULT	PHYSICIAN	HOSP. NO.
1-12-73	1-16-73		Thomas J. Duggan	623485
7-04-76	7-05-76		Thomas J. Duggan	664273
3-11-79	3-20-79		Thomas J. Duggan	702896
11-02-80	11-05-80		Charles Johnson	720251
5-20-85	5-23-85		Charles Johnson	783651

FORM A-201 PATIENT'S INDEX CARD   PHYSICIANS' RECORD CO., BERWYN, ILLINOIS   (OVER)

Form courtesy of Physicians' Record Company

FIG. 1 – PATIENT'S INDEX CARD (3 x 5)

ARRANGEMENT OF THE MASTER PATIENT INDEX

Bound volumes or index cards may be used for the listing of patients' names. When using bound volumes, the book is divided into alphabetical sections. Names are listed under the first letter of the surname in chronological order by date of admission. This method is feasible for a very small facility, but retrieval becomes cumbersome and increasingly difficult for large facilities since a strict alphabetical sequence is not followed.

In most facilities, the patients' information is compiled on index cards and placed alphabetically in a vertical file, a separate card for each patient.

Some facilities maintain their patient index by year of admission. This practice is not recommended, because patients often forget the date of their last admission or if they were ever admitted to the facility at all. Much time is lost searching through several sections of the index for the appropriate index card. Only one index card which provides a perpetual record of the patient should be maintained per patient.

Alphabetical Filing

The following guidelines are suggested for maintenance of an alphabetical patient index:

1. Place surname first, then given name followed by middle name or initial, and file in strict alphabetical sequence.

2. Arrange cards in alphabetical order like words in a dictionary, following letter by letter to the end of the name and then by given name and initials. The telephone directory serves as a ready reference when in doubt.

3. When a given patient requires more than one card to accommodate all of his admissions, the cards will be arranged in chronological order, with the earliest date first, working from front to back in the drawer.

4. If there is more than one person with the same surname and given name, the cards are arranged alphabetically by middle initial. If no middle initial is given, the cards are arranged according to birth date, filing the oldest card first.

5. Names with prefixes of D', de, De, Des, Di, Du, La, Mc, Mac, Van, Von, etc., are filed alphabetically as D'Armand (D-A-r-m-a-n-d), De Tarnowski (D-e-T-a-r-n-o-w-s-k-i), etc.

6. Names beginning with St., as St. Peter, are filed as S-a-i-n-t.

7. Compound or hyphenated names are filed as one word; thus Craig-Stuart would be filed under C-r-a-i-g-S-t-u-a-r-t, following the name through, letter by letter.

8. Names with religious titles such as Reverend, Mother, Father, Brother, and Sister are filed under the surnames, the titles being disregarded, and then given name. Sister Mary Douglas is filed as Douglas, Mary. Religious titles should not be filed in groups such as all Sisters together, for this method is not efficient.

or as Douglas sister Mary
8a married woman · use her given name.

9. If an initial is given instead of a patient's first or middle names, the rule is "file nothing before something." Thus, M. Brown would precede M. Kay Brown and Mary Kay Brown.

10. Commercial sets of guide cards frequently have a separate division for names beginning with Mc. However, because of difficulty in distinguishing between two names with the same sound, it is permissible to combine Mac and Mc without distinction as to spelling, filing Mc as if spelled Mac. Whichever filing method is adopted, it must be adhered to throughout the file to maintain uniformity.

11. It is customary for people of Spanish descent to combine the name of the mother with the name of the father. For instance, with the name Soto Ramariz, Soto is the surname of the father, and Ramariz the maiden name of the mother. They are filed in alphabetical sequence of first, the father's name and then the mother's maiden name. Thus, the name of Maria Dolores Soto Ramariz would be filed in the S section of the file in the following order: S-o-t-o-R-a-m-a-r-i-z, Maria Dolores.

12. If a patient's name has changed since a previous admission, a cross-reference should be made to the former name. For instance, if O'Brien, Mary Catherine is admitted, a cross-reference should be made to her previous admission as McCarty, Mary Catherine. All information recorded on the original card is entered on the new card and the original card is cross-referenced to the new card.

13. When looking for a given person's name card, one must keep in mind that there may be many spellings of the same name; search must be made under every possible spelling of the name before stating there is no card for that name. For instance, there are approximately 35 ways of spelling the name Baer, 10 or more ways of spelling Burke, etc. Again, the telephone directory is an excellent reference for alternate spellings of common names.

14. For the purpose of allotting space in a file drawer, it has been determined that there are twice as many W's as A's in the majority of alphabetical files, twice as many B's as G's; and that one name in every five begins with

either M or S while names beginning with the letters Q, X, and I are proportionately few.

15. The master patient index should contain sufficient alphabetical guides for speedy reference. No more than 20 cards should be filed behind a guide. Thus, a file containing 5,000 cards would require approximately 250 alphabetical guides. Commercial companies can provide valuable assistance in determining the appropriate number of guides and divisions for the index.

16. To maintain uniformity in the master patient index when a personnel change is made, filing directions should be explicit. Wherever possible, only one person should be assigned the responsibility for filing index cards. All filing rules must be consistently adhered to if "lost" cards are to be avoided.

17. Card files should be audited regularly for misfiles, and additional training of master patient index clerks provided as necessary.

Phonetic Filing

Hospitals located in communities having large populations with foreign names may use the phonetic system for filing patient index cards. When hospitals use a phonetic method, the patient's index card is filed behind the appropriate guide for the initial letter of the surname, but according to sound rather than according to spelling. Thus, all surnames that sound alike but are spelled differently are filed together.

The English alphabet, with the exception of the vowels a, e, i, o, u and the letters w, h, and y, which are not coded, is reduced to six key letters with a corresponding three-digit numeric code as follows:

Key Letters	Code Numbers	Equivalents
b	1	p, f, v
c	2	s, k, g, j, q, x, z
d	3	t
l	4	none
m	5	n
r	6	none

Instead of indexing each name by its exact spelling, as in a straight alphabetical file, name variations are brought together

by the code number which represents the key letters. The first letter of the surname is not coded but serves as a prefix to the three-digit code number, and coding is limited to succeeding key letters or their equivalents (Figure 2).

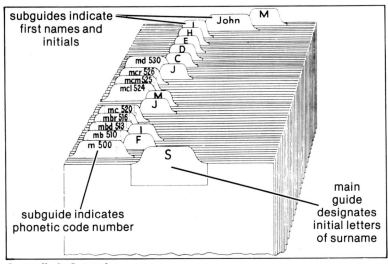

Courtesy Kardex Systems, Inc.

Fig. 2 – This phonetic arrangement of a patients' index has guides which indicate initial letters of surnames. Subguides indicate code numbers, first names, and initials.

For instance, to code the surname Martin:

M – prefix, not coded
a – vowel, not coded
r – 6 (key letter)
t – 3 (an equivalent)
i – vowel, not coded
n – 5 (an equivalent)

The name Martin is, therefore, coded 635. All variations in the spelling of the name Martin are coded 635 and will be filed together: Mardan, Marden, Mardyn, Martan, Marten, Martin, Martyn, Merten, Merton, Morden, Morten, Mortin, Morton, Murten. Thus it can be seen that names of like or similar sound will generally code the same, be grouped together in a file, and be found more quickly than if it is necessary to hunt through a completely alphabetized patient's index file.

In a file section like our illustration (Figure 2) all names beginning with the letter S will be grouped together according to their codes behind the main guide S. The letters shown on the left-hand side of the file and on the left-hand side of the following listing represent the key letters of the surname to be coded, while the number alongside represents the resulting codes for those key letters. The second-position and third-position guides are auxiliary guides for the given names and are used when there is a large group of cards with the same given name initial letters. As an example, we might find the following names in this file behind the specific guides:

mcr   526

       Singer, Anna Marie
       Sanger, Fred C.
       Singer, Ralph R.
       Senger, William T.

md   530

       Smith, Arthur E.
       Sinda, Andrew T.
       Shenit, Barbara Jean

     C

       Smith, Caroline
       Schmidt, Charles M.
       Smith, Claude R.

     D

       Smith, Dorothy Marie
       Schmidt, Dorothy P.

     E

       Smith, Earl E.
       Smith, Elmer E.
       Smythe, George T.

Duplication is avoided as names, spelled incorrectly as well as those with typographical errors, will be filed together if they sound alike.

The sponsors of this system state there are only five rules which must be observed in maintaining a phonetic file:

1. When two or more key letters or their equivalents occur together, treat them as one letter.
2. If a name contains less than three key letters, add zeros to arrive at the code number. The name "Jackson" is com-

pletely coded with the number 25, so a zero (also called a cipher) is added to assign the name a 3-digit code, J-250.

3. If two of the same key letters, or a key letter and its equivalent, are separated by h or w, code one key letter.

4. When a repeated key letter or its equivalent is separated by a, e, i, o, u, or y, the key letters or their equivalents are considered separately.

5. After coding of the surname, arrangement between the key letter guides should be alphabetical according to given name.

With a phonetic file the medical record practitioner does not have to stop and think of the various other ways the particular name for which he is searching might be spelled. The sponsors of this system claim that this method detects duplication in the files and discloses 90 percent of all transposition of letters. This system has one great disadvantage in that rules for phonetic filing must be learned; and when persons who know how to file and retrieve are not present, access to the file is limited.

MICROFILMING THE PATIENT INDEX

After a health facility has been treating patients for a number of years, it accumulates a vast number of patient index cards; and storage of these cards may become a major problem. Finding a patient's card may take a great deal of time if medical record department employees must sift through many thousands of cards. Microfilming the patient index is often considered a solution for space and retrieval problems.

The health care facility may decide to microfilm the cards of deceased patients or patients who have not been in the facility for ten years, etc., on regular roll film to reduce the size of the file. When space is a major problem, the entire file may be filmed, and a microfiche index utilized to retrieve patient index information.

To develop a microfilmed index, the entire file must be input into a computer and then output onto microfilm. This procedure also identifies duplicates and misfiles, for the computer will identify entries with different numbers but the same name and birth date. The information on each patient's card becomes a one-line entry on a microfiche containing information on 50-60 patients. When information is requested, the microfiche for the appropriate section of the alphabet is placed on a microfiche reader; and the correct entry is noted on the screen.

Multiple microfiche indexes can be provided to a hospital, so a set can be made available to the admitting department and the emergency room. Corrections and additions to the master patient index are usually maintained in a card file or on computer printout for two-week to four-week intervals until an updated set of microfiche is generated. At that point, the previous set of microfiche is destroyed. Space savings, accuracy, and rapid retrieval are advantages associated with a microfiche index. Disadvantages include cost and the necessity of maintaining a temporary file between updates of the microfiche index.

AUTOMATION OF PATIENT INDEX

The patients' index is an area which is readily adaptable to automation. In the admitting department at the time of patient registration, the patient's name is entered into the cathode-ray terminal (CRT). The computer searches its memory and displays all persons with that name and any similar sounding names, plus basic identifying information for each name (Figure 3). The admitting clerk makes the appropriate selection and re-

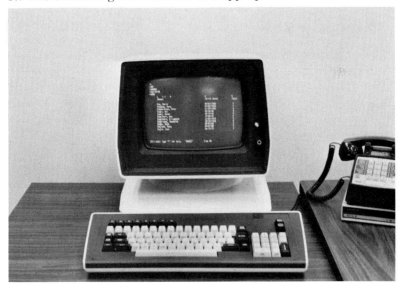

FIG. 3 – PATIENT INDEX DISPLAY – CRT

quests that all identifying data be displayed in order to make any necessary updates. If a patient is a new patient, the admitting clerk will initiate registration by calling up a registration form on the terminal and filling in the form by keyboard-data entry.

A computerized master patient index provides other departments with immediate access to the master patient index. When CRTs are located at each nursing station, discharge information is entered into the computer on the unit; and this information is disseminated to all departments that need it to perform their duties.

A computerized master patient index provides a very accurate index with fast retrieval, although it may be expensive and time consuming to computerize a very large existing index.

The American Hospital Association recommends that hospitals retain, in an index or register or on summary cards, certain basic information after the medical record has outlived the statute of limitations for that state or the time period established by the hospital for the destruction of records. Therefore, the patient index will remain in some form or other as a permanent record of all patients who have ever been admitted to the hospital.

FILING EQUIPMENT AND SUPPLIES FOR PATIENTS' INDEX CARDS

The type of equipment in which the patients' index cards will be filed depends upon the size of the cards used. Most commonly used are 3 x 5-inch cards, but this size may vary depending on the amount of information to be recorded. Facilities that file their medical records according to a serial or serial-unit number, list all admission and discharge dates and new hospital numbers for each patient on one index card.

If 3 x 5-inch cards are used, they are usually filed in vertical, eight-drawer, triple-compartment file cabinets; as these are economical both as to floor space required and cost. The number of cabinets needed will depend upon the quantity of cards to be filed and also upon the weight of the card stock. Heavier cards, of course, require more space. If average-weight stock is used, 100 cards can be filed to the inch. Thus a standard eight-drawer, triple-compartment file cabinet will hold approximately 63,000 cards with guides. When purchasing any type of filing equipment, care should be exercised to select standard styles and colors so matching cabinets can be obtained as needed. Space for at least an additional five years should be provided when equipment is purchased.

Many large hospitals with active outpatient clinics employing the unit system of numbering and filing and a centralized patients' index use impairment-size cards. These cards are usually referred to as MIB cards, which were first introduced by the insurance industry's Medical Information Bureau that kept a master file of applicants' impairments. The cards are 2¼ x 3 inches in size and require only about half the space necessary for the same number of 3 x 5 cards. With the unit system, the patient always retains the same identifying number; therefore, many hospitals feel that only minimum information is necessary on the patient's index card. Others find it is advantageous to place admission and discharge dates on these cards, in which case, both sides of the card may be used.

When impairment cards are used, a pattern must be established for the placement of information, because the cards are too small to indicate by printing where information should be recorded as is done with larger cards. Once the pattern has been established, it must be strictly followed; so everyone will know what each line means (Figure 4).

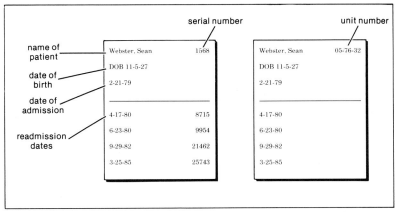

Form courtesy of Physicians' Record Company

FIG. 4 – AN IMPAIRMENT-SIZE (2¼″ x 3″) INDEX CARD SAVES TIME AND SPACE. THE CARD ON THE LEFT HAS SERIAL NUMBERING; THE CARD ON THE RIGHT HAS UNIT NUMBERING.

The impairment-size card may be filed in vertical file-drawer cabinets similar to those previously mentioned for 3 x 5 cards.

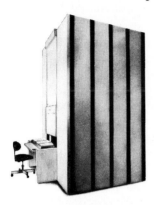

An 11-drawer, 4-compartment vertical file cabinet will hold approximately 117,000 such cards and guides. However, these cards are particularly useful if the quantity of cards is great enough, and the activity of the file is sufficient to warrant the use of mechanical or elevator files (Figure 5). This type of equipment is recommended for any file containing more than 500,000 cards if they are actively used. It saves considerable time and cuts fatigue; since the operator can sit at the file and, by the touch of a button, bring the required section of the index to a height where there is complete visibility. While hospitals using elevator files generally use MIB cards because they conserve space and time, such files can also be obtained for 3 x 5 cards.

Sylvania Commercial Electronics Corp.

Fig. 5 – Electrically Powered MPI File Designed to Conserve Space. At the Touch of a Button an Alphabetical Section is Located and Moved into Working Position.

ALPHABETICAL INDEX GUIDES

Alphabetical index guides are available from most file equipment companies for all sizes of cards. Construction is usually of heavy cardboard or plastic material. The ease with which the guides can be seen and their durability are prime considerations for purchasing index guides. A clear plastic self-indexer, which is a cover that slips over a patient's index card, is also obtainable. Being slightly larger, the top of the card with the patient's name is extended about ⅜ of an inch above the other cards, thus serving as a guide. This is particularly helpful, because these covers then serve as file guides and can be placed where they will be most useful. In addition, surnames most common to the area can be easily guided. This is an advantage as the common surnames may vary from one part of the country to another because of the settlement of different nationalities.

The performance of filing personnel may be evaluated if a self-indexer or a plain colored card is filed with each patient index card. These self-indexers or colored cards are removed as the supervisor verifies the accuracy of the filing for each patient index card. Self-indexers are also used by some facilities to identify inpatients.

THE NUMBER INDEX

The number index is important in the medical record department as the patient identification number control. It is the origin of the numbering system whether it be serial, unit, or serial-unit. It is a chronological list of the hospital numbers issued to patients and the name of the patient assigned each number. It must be remembered that a number index is a numerical listing of numbers. Therefore, if unit numbers are used, all admissions of any one patient will not be shown; while an admission register, being a chronological listing of admissions, provides a record of all admissions.

The number index may be a loose-leaf book, vertical or visible file, or a computer listing. If the hospital keeps a loose-leaf book, the sheets should be bound at the end of the year to prevent loss. If the hospital keeps a card file, a $2\frac{1}{4}$ x 3-inch card filed in a vertical file allows the greatest number of cards to be housed in a given space. If a computer is used to store the patient index, the computer can be programmed to store the number index and automatically assign a hospital number when a patient is being registered for admission. Automated assignment of identification numbers reduces the chance of skipping numbers or assigning the same number to two patients.

Because the number index is the source of hospital numbers and, therefore, used as a reference when there is doubt about the accuracy of a number, the number index should be monitored to assure its accuracy and completeness.

DISEASE AND OPERATION INDEXES

Disease and operation indexes record selected patient care information gathered by the health care facility. A disease index lists diseases and conditions according to the classification system or code numbers assigned by medical record department personnel. A listing of surgical and procedural code numbers comprises the operation index.

A physician or a medical staff committee might use the disease and operation indexes to retrieve medical records for the following purposes:

1. To review previous cases of a given disease in order to provide insight into the management of a current patient's health problems.
2. To test theories and compare data on certain diseases and/or treatments in order to conduct research and prepare scientific papers.
3. To procure data on the utilization of hospital facilities and to establish a hospital's need for new equipment, beds, staff, etc., in various departments.
4. To evaluate the quality of care in the hospital.
5. To conduct epidemiologic and infection-control studies.
6. To accumulate risk management data, such as the incidence of medical and surgical complications.

In addition to physicians' uses of the indexes, numerous requests for patient care data are received from hospital administrators and authorized personnel, planning agencies, educational programs, fiscal intermediaries, and health care agencies and organizations. Examples of other uses of these indexes include:

1. Providing patient care data required for licensing and accreditation surveys.
2. Locating a record when only the diagnosis and/or operation is known.
3. Providing data on medical practice in the hospital in order to qualify for accredited internship and residency programs.
4. Determining whether the treatment and procedures provided were necessary and appropriate for the diagnosis.
5. Providing educational material for students, grand rounds, and medical staff meetings.

Disease and operation indexes should be tailor-made to meet the needs of the institutions they serve. Consideration should be given to the need for the index, who will use it, and what information will be requested. Careful planning will result in an indexing system which will serve the medical and hospital staff well and, in addition, promote the efficiency of the indexing operation itself.

CONTENT OF THE DISEASE AND OPERATION INDEXES

Today's requests for patient information are often detailed, and provision should be made in the disease and operation indexes to respond to these requests as quickly as possible. In general, the indexes should provide sufficient detail to complete required medical and statistical reports and requests. Licensing and accrediting agencies require data for their surveys, and provision for this should be made in the index. Anticipated special requests for information may be easily incorporated into indexing procedures and promptly retrieved at the appropriate time. Data which might be routinely entered include:

1. Patient's sex.
2. Patient's age.
3. Patient's race.
4. Name of attending physician and surgeon.
5. Service on which the patient was hospitalized.
6. End results of hospitalization – this category specifies whether the patient died or was discharged. If the patient died, it may be of interest to record whether or not an autopsy was performed.
7. Date of admission and/or discharge and/or length of hospital stay. If the utilization committee actively reviews medical records, length of hospital stay may be indexed in order to evaluate utilization factors. Preoperative length of stay may also be of value in the routine evaluation of hospital utilization. There are two advantages to be realized from indexing either the date of admission or the date of discharge. First, if an indexing error is made in the recording of a patient's hospital number, it is possible to correct that error by referring to the admission and discharge list. Second, sometimes a physician requests a particular record by diagnosis and approximate admission or discharge date. Having a date indexed will result in a more rapid location of the desired entry in the index and in the pulling of fewer charts to locate the record.

8. Associated diseases and operations.

A disease and operation index may be set up either for *simple* indexing or *cross-indexing*, depending on the hospital's needs. Simple indexing means that entries for each disease and operation a patient may have had are made under their respective code numbers with no reference made to other code numbers assigned to that patient. With cross-indexing, reference is made to the code numbers for all diseases and operations a patient may have had during hospitalization for each separate entry posted in the index. If cross-indexing is done, space must be set aside for the recording of codes for associated diseases or operations. In a manual system, the time involved in entering the additional information on each card should be weighed against the need for this information. An automated indexing system often provides cross-indexing on each patient with additional designation for principal and other diagnoses.

USE OF INDEXES

The disease and operation indexes are the most expensive indexes in the department to maintain. The person who codes diagnoses and operations is usually one of the highest-paid employees in the department because of the expertise required. The person indexing must not only be a capable individual but also extremely accurate in making the entries. The more data indexed from any one record, the greater the cost to the department in terms of personnel time.

Another consideration is the expense of retrieving data from the index. A physician may request a list of all cases of cholecystitis in female patients. If the sex of patients has not been indexed, *all* of the records with a diagnosis of cholecystitis will have to be pulled. The pulling of many nonpertinent cases takes time and is, therefore, costly. Whether it would be less expensive to index more completely in the first place depends on how often the index is used.

The medical record professional must investigate how often the index is being used and for what purposes. The amount and kinds of data needed to be indexed can be determined by studying the patterns of usage. For example, if the utilization committee reviews records according to diagnoses, indexing length of stay could be worthwhile. If accreditation data are not being produced elsewhere, these needs must be considered. A distinction between principal and other diagnoses and procedures may be necessary to facilitate retrieval for patient care evaluation studies and research projects. Indexes put to a variety of uses are usually heavily used, and retrieval time should be as short as possible.

In the final analysis, the medical record practitioner must strive to attain a reasonable balance between retrieval time and indexing time, working to minimize the total hours required. An effective index requires no more time to maintain than the use of the index warrants.

AUTOMATED INDEXES

Disease, operation, and physician indexes are commonly compiled from discharge-data abstracts completed by medical record department personnel (Figure 6). These abstracts may be processed via an in-house computer or an external data service such as the Commission on Professional and Hospital Activities, the Hospital Utilization Project or McAuto. Some state hospital associations or third-party payers also process discharge data on a per discharge basis.

When data processing is considered, use of computerized capabilities within the facility should be compared to the cost of using outside data services. In-house data processing allows the medical record practitioner to design an abstracting and indexing system specific to the hospital's individual needs.

DISCHARGE DATA ABSTRACTS

Abstracting is compiling the pertinent information from the health record. The items appear on the abstract form in somewhat the same order as on the health record, so the transfer of information from the record to the abstract can be done quickly and accurately (Figure 7).

An abstract is prepared for each discharged patient, and the abstracts are batched and sent to the service agency for compilation. Any errors detected by computer edits result in the abstract being sent back to the facility. This requires more time to review the health record again, correct the error(s), and resubmit the abstract. The corrected data are then compiled to produce the disease and operation indexes and provide meaningful reports which reflect the treatment rendered in that facility.

Reports are prepared and returned to the facility on a monthly, quarterly, or semiannual basis, depending on the service agreement and the facility's needs. These reports assist the

FIG. 6 – OPERATION INDEX – AUTOMATED

Reprinted with permission of the McDonnell Douglas Health Information Systems Company

hospital in evaluating its overall performance. Commercial abstracting services also provide comparative reports on national and area-wide statistics for a small, extra cost. Access to this bank of comparative data and reports may well be worth the cost of the abstracting service to the health care facility. Approval for use of an outside service should be obtained from the medical staff and hospital administration prior to contract agreement.

An abstracting contract can provide the hospital with all the advantages of a data processing system without the expense of purchasing the necessary equipment. The medical record profes-

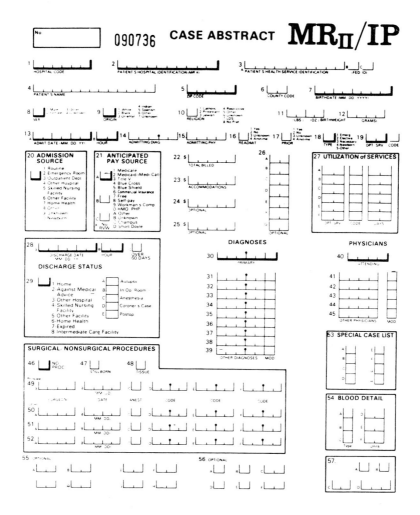

Fig. 7 – Case Abstract Form

sional must be aware, however, that use of such services lessens control over the data collected and resultant reports.

Some discharge data services and internal systems employ an on-line abstracting system utilizing CRT terminals. The screen displays the selections to complete the abstract with the proper data. Entry is accomplished by light pen or keyboard. Errors are detected at the time of entry; therefore, manhours involved in submitting corrected abstracts are eliminated. If an internal computer is being utilized, data are immediately available for research and administrative reports. The facility has the option to add or delete data items according to its needs. Data can also be quickly correlated with patient information submitted previously by other hospital departments during the patient's stay, and a total picture of the patient's stay results. For example, if administration wants to analyze the cost of treating patients with chronic obstructive pulmonary disease, financial and clinical data can be produced on one report when computer linkage exists between the medical record department and the business office.

MANUAL INDEXES

Indexing manually means that disease and operation code numbers are entered by hand or posted on each appropriate index card. Small hospitals may find it cost effective to retain manual indexes because of a low rate of requests for information. When setting up or revising a manual index file, there are three factors to be considered in designing the index card:

1. The data which will be indexed on the card.
2. The sequence of these data on the card.
3. Spacing and printing requirements.

Only those data which have been determined useful to requestors need be indexed. The placement of data on the index card is important from the standpoint of indexing efficiency. Because the hospital number is of prime importance in the retrieval operation, the column for the hospital number should be at the left-hand margin of the index card. The sequence of other data on the card should be the same as that on the summary sheet, the source sheet from which indexing is usually done. For example, if sex, race, and age appear in that order on the summary sheet, the same order should be used also on the index card. This will minimize eyestrain and speed up the indexing operation.

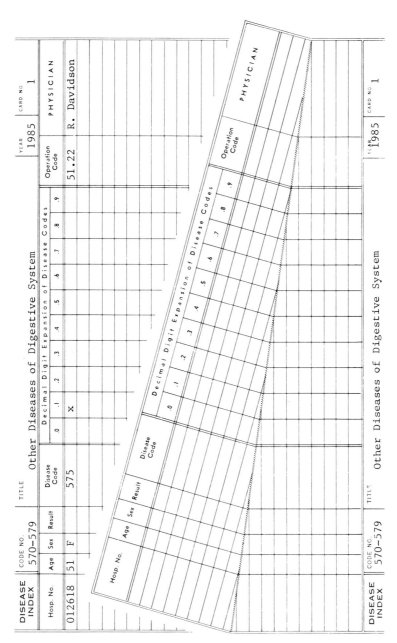

Form courtesy of Physicians' Record Company

FIG. 8 – GROUP INDEXING ON DISEASE INDEX CARD

Adequate space should be allowed so each item of data will fit easily into its appropriate column. Most entries on the cards will be handwritten; so if the columns are too small, indexing will be slow and the index card will appear cluttered. The index card should be of sufficient weight to withstand frequent handling. In establishing card size and printing arrangement, the equipment in which the cards are to be filed must be considered. For most filing arrangements, it is advisable to have the cards printed with the headings on the front and back at opposite ends. This allows cards to be turned end over end, or "tumbled," as one continues to record on the second side of the index card.

Group Indexing

In group indexing, instead of having one card for each code number in the classification system, a range of code numbers is included on each disease and operation index card. This keeps the indexes from becoming so large as to be unmanageable. This method also eliminates maintaining an index containing large numbers of cards which show only one or two entries for seldom-encountered diseases or operations. Selecting the grouping to be used will depend on the classification system used. An example of grouping with ICD-9-CM might be to prepare cards for the main headings in the classification. In sequence, then, the card headings would appear:

001-009 Intestinal Infectious Diseases
010-018 Tuberculosis
020-027 Zoonotic Bacterial Diseases
030-041 Other Bacterial Diseases

Posting to such a group card requires that a space be provided to write in the specific code on the medical record. An example of a posted disease is included in Figure 8.

Operation index cards are posted in much the same manner, with the exception that the name of the surgeon is requested.

Long term care facilities with minimal information may utilize the system for grouping illustrated in Figure 9. In this method, a large 8½ x 11 size form is used for entering all code numbers assigned in the appropriate columns across the page. A three-ring notebook is used to store these forms in chronological order by discharge date. Although it is a compact method for indexing, the retrieval of information is time consuming.

DISEASE INDEX — SKILLED NURSING FACILITY

Chart Number	Admission Date	Discharge Date	Days of Stay	Sex	Birth Date	ICD-9-CM CLASSIFICATION CODES											V	E	Doctor
						000–099	100–199	200–299	300–399	400–499	500–599	600–699	700–799	800–899	900–999				
621	7/20/85	5/6/85 T	27	F	9/30/04				374 (S)	412 (P)	582 (F)		786 (I)						J. Smith

Key to letters assigned to ICDA–8 Codes and Discharge Date:
D–Died   P–Primary diagnosis causing admission
T–Transferred to Acute   S–Secondary diseases present at time of admission
   Care Hospital   I–Diseases occurring after admission

F–Final diagnoses if different from any of the above

Form courtesy of Physicians' Record Company

FIG. 9 – DISEASE INDEX – GROUPING METHOD

The frequency of access would be the determining factor in choice of method. For an index system which is accessed infrequently, this system is adequate.

Regardless of the indexing system used, *index cards are always filed in strict numerical order*. Periodically the index should be audited to correct any misfiles. For a neater, more readable index, all captions should be made in ink or by typewriter. At the end of the calendar year, a red line should be drawn after the last entry on each card.

On the index card there is often a column for results. In order to save time, the clerk may leave this column blank if the patient was discharged alive. If the patient died but no autopsy was performed, a D should be placed in the column; an A if one was performed.

Filing Equipment for Manual Indexes

Small indexes may be conveniently filed in visible filing equipment where the titles of all cards are visible, because the edge of one card projects the width of one line beyond the edge of the previous card. The cards may be inserted in pockets which have a celluloid edge, hinged to card holders, or hung from rods. All card titles are readily visible, so errors in filing cards are minimal; and desired index cards can be located quickly.

In vertical indexes, cards stand upright in the file. It is necessary to place guides throughout the file to aid the clerk in finding a desired index card. Special tags which facilitate rapid card location may be attached to frequently used index cards.

Because vertical files require less space than visible files, they are more suitable for large indexes. However, locating individual index cards is a slower process in vertical files. Furthermore, each card on which an entry is to be posted has to be removed; a process which is not necessary with visible files.

Regardless of the type of filing equipment used, inactive index cards should be removed from the active index and stored separately to reduce bulk.

INDEXING/ABSTRACTING

To ensure timely data, it is ideal to index or abstract the medical record immediately after the chart has been assembled and coded and before it is filed into the doctors' incomplete file. However, a chart may not be clinically complete in order to code at that time, or a physician may add or change a diagnosis. To ensure that every chart is indexed or abstracted, the indexer or abstractor needs a control list, usually the daily list of discharges; and as charts are indexed or abstracted, he checks the list to show the record has been processed. Periodically these lists should be checked to see if any records have inadvertently not been indexed. Also, as the clerk indexes each code number, he should place a check mark after the code number on the admission/discharge section of the medical record. Then, after the physician has completed the record, any additions or changes in the diagnoses or procedures may be easily detected.

Of course, all indexing/abstracting may be performed after the physician has completed the record. This approach eliminates double handling of the records; however, the indexes are only as current as the physicians are in completing their records.

When a department has a temporary shortage of personnel, manual indexing may be delayed by sending all completed records to the permanent file after checking, then pulling them at a later time for indexing. The daily list of discharges is used to secure all the records requiring indexing. This method is only recommended in an emergency situation, however, as current indexes are vital to medical and statistical reports.

RETRIEVAL FROM INDEXES

When a request is made for records of a certain diagnosis, care must be taken to ensure that all records with that diagnosis are secured. Pertinent records may be found under more than one code number; therefore, medical record personnel should discuss with the requester all code numbers which might provide relevant records. The requester will then specify the exact code number or numbers. He should also be asked whether he wants only the records for a certain age group, sex, service, year, etc.

Research Files

While groups of records are being reviewed, it is advisable to keep them in a separate file where they can be readily accessible. Records removed from the permanent file for research should be signed out in the usual manner, leaving an outguide. If a record is temporarily removed from the research file, the record should be conspicuously tagged so it will be returned to the researcher.

A reasonable limit on the number of records each reviewer may hold for review, and a time limit for keeping these records are advisable. Researchers should be encouraged to complete their studies in the medical record department, if possible, in a special work area away from the work flow. Strict control over incoming and outgoing records from the research file is mandatory. A simple form, one for each study, will serve the purpose (Figure 10).

Physician's Name _____ Doe _____   Code Numbers _____ 386.0 _____

Specifications _____ Females only _____

Time Limit _____ 1 week for 20 charts _____   Years _____ 1978-1983 _____

CASE NUMBERS	RECEIVED	RETURNED	OTHER LOCATIONS
190602	4-16-84	4-19-84	
198404	4-16-84	4-19-84	
20-16-04			On microfilm
21-26-42	4-16-84		
26-49-59			Dr. Jones' incomplete file
42-94-60	4-16-84		
42-99-60	4-19-84		

FIG. 10 – RECORD REVIEW CONTROL FORM

PHYSICIANS' INDEX

TYPES

Manual/Automated

The physicians' index provides every medical staff member a record of the patients he has treated. Entries on physicians'

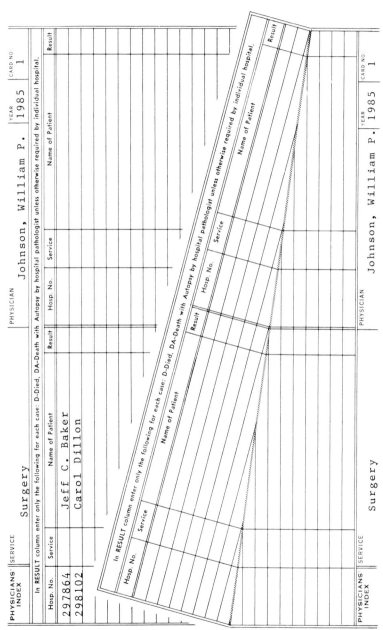

Form courtesy of Physicians' Record Company

FIG. 11 – PHYSICIANS' INDEX CARD

index cards are usually the name and hospital number of the patient but may include other data such as the hospital service and length of stay. It may also indicate those cases for which

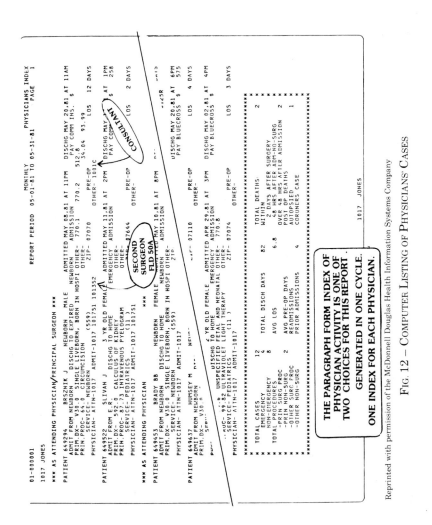

Fig. 12 – Computer Listing of Physicians' Cases

Reprinted with permission of the McDonnell Douglas Health Information Systems Company

a physician served as surgeon or consultant, the end results of hospitalization, and any other information which might be desirable. A sample of a typical index card is shown in Figure 11. If an in-house computer or a discharge data service is used for indexing diseases and operations, producing a physicians' index is a simple process. Monthly or yearly listings of physicians and their patients' names can be maintained at little extra cost (Figure 12).

USE OF THE PHYSICIANS' INDEX

Valuable use may be made of the patient data stored in the physicians' index, both by individual physicians and authorized medical staff committees.

1. The physician himself may survey his own practice. Trends in volume and types of practice are notable if service data are included in the index.
2. The credentials committee of the medical staff may use the physicians' index to identify physicians' activity profiles, distinguishing active from inactive members.
3. Data on physician use of the hospital facilities can be compiled to identify appropriate members for medical staff appointments to such committees as operating room, perinatal, morbidity, etc.
4. Hospital administration may use the index to identify needs for consultants in certain specialties and to note increases or decreases in individual physician's practices.

A physicians' index is held as a confidential record. The information contained in it is available only to the governing board and hospital administrator, to committees of the medical staff directed to review the physicians' work, and to the physician who wishes to review his own work. The index may be subpoenaed by a court. It is sometimes used in malpractice cases or for income tax investigations.

Because of the confidential nature of this index, many hospitals assign each physician a code number which appears on the card instead of the physician's name. In a computerized indexing system, a code number is essential to safeguard the confidential nature of the index. Assigned code numbers should not be reused following resignation or death of a medical staff member. It is the responsibility of the medical record professional to guard this index from unauthorized access.

Manual index cards are usually filed alphabetically by physicians' names in a visible or a vertical file or in numerical sequence according to the physician's code number. It is convenient to post to this index immediately after receipt of the discharged record.

Indexes maintained on computerized systems can provide a variety of physician profiles. Printouts can be generated on demand or displayed on a CRT screen. Because of the confidential nature of this data, access to a computerized physicians' index is available only to those authorized to have such data by hospital policy.

REGISTERS

Various registers which provide a chronological list of data are maintained in a health care facility. These registers are developed and maintained in various departments as a reference or control to basic information. Any department wishing to keep basic data to monitor their workload may maintain a register. Examples include radiology register, physical therapy register, and emergency service register. A few of the more common registers will be discussed here.

PATIENT ADMISSION AND DISCHARGE

Many states require that patient admission and discharge registers be kept within the facility. The admission register is arranged in chronological order by date and time of admission. If serial numbering is used, this register may also be used to control number assignments to patients. Each line in the admission column contains information about one patient, including the number assigned.

To avoid confusion in assigning patient numbers, the name and other information should be immediately recorded in the admission column as a patient is admitted. This practice prevents assigning the same number to two patients. The discharge register may also be arranged in chronological order by date of discharge. Information recorded in a register should be kept to the useful minimum and be sufficient to meet legal requirements. It should include only items needed for quick reference as these are most easily obtained from this source. Items which might be included in admission and discharge registers are:

Admissions	*Discharges*
Patient/Health record number	Patient/Health record number (same as assigned at admission)
Patient's name	Patient's name
Date of admission	Date of discharge or death
Physician	Physician

An analysis of survey forms and questionnaires received routinely by the facility is helpful in determining essential data for inclusion in these registers.

These registers should be kept permanently as they are a chronological list of all admissions and discharges to and from the facility. In a manual indexing system, they serve as a back-up to the master patient index if a card is misfiled. At predetermined intervals the registers may be microfilmed. In many facilities copies of daily admission and discharge lists are retained and serve as the admission/discharge register. If the health facility has the computer capacity, admission and discharge registers can be stored in computer memory and accessed through the CRT terminal or retained in the form of computer printouts.

OPERATING ROOM REGISTER

This register is kept in the operating room and should be preserved for ten years. Data included are the date of operation, patient's name and health record number, and the names of surgeons and assistants. The register provides statistical data for case-load analysis and administrative reports. After ten years these registers are no longer needed, for any information regarding an individual can be found in the medical record.

REGISTER OF BIRTHS AND DEATHS

Some states do not provide a copy of the birth, fetal death, or death certificate for the medical record. Information from birth certificates may be copied in a register of births, and information from death certificates into a register of deaths. This provides readily accessible information without referring to a medical record. In many states the law requires these registers, and the medical record director should investigate his state's requirements. If the state requires fetal death certificates and a register of births is used, fetal deaths may be entered in red ink, in chronological order with the live births; or special pages may be set aside for fetal deaths in the back of the book. Whichever method is used, the procedure should be described in the front of the register, so all will know how fetal deaths are recorded.

If a health facility has the computer capability, the computer can be programmed to provide a list of births and deaths upon command.

EMERGENCY SERVICE

A register to monitor the patients who enter the emergency service must be maintained to provide data for administrative reports and to fulfill the standards of the Joint Commission on Accreditation of Hospitals.

The JCAH specifies that a control register shall be continuously maintained and shall include at least the following information for every individual seeking care: identification, such as name, age, and sex; date, time and means of arrival; nature of the complaint; disposition; and time of departure. The names of individuals dead on arrival shall also be entered in the register.

Information from the register may aid in planning emergency service staffing and can be used to select records for evaluating the appropriateness and quality of care rendered in the emergency service.

If the facility desires detailed data, a copy of the emergency room record can be bound in chronological order and serve as the register, although this practice may create storage problems.

CANCER REGISTRY

A cancer registry is established for the collection and maintenance of comprehensive patient care data on all cancer patients. The two main objectives of a cancer registry are to provide lifetime follow-up of the cancer patient and to provide meaningful information to the physician for patient care evaluation and research.

Since 1913 the American College of Surgeons has recognized the need for improved care of cancer patients. In 1956, as part of its goal to provide cancer patients the best possible care available, the American College of Surgeons made a functioning cancer registry one of its mandatory requirements for approval of a hospital cancer program.

TYPES

Basically there are three types of cancer registries: hospital-based, central registry, and special-purpose registry. A hospital-based registry operates exclusively for cancer patients treated at a particular health care facility. A central registry can either be population-based or the main registry for a group of hospital-based registries. The central registry collects data from its designated territory, thus accumulating enough information to study trends in cancer occurrence, treatments, and results. Special purpose registries collect data on one type of cancer such as leukemias, lung cancer, breast cancer, Hodgkin's disease, etc.

Regardless of the type of registry, the collection and analysis of data on all cancer patients to improve cancer management, now and in the future, remains the basic purpose of a cancer program.

FORMAT OF THE CANCER REGISTRY

Cancer registries collect data on all inpatients and outpatients seen at a facility regardless of where the patient was originally diagnosed. A properly functioning cancer registry has four basic components to store and retrieve data in a timely manner.

Master Index File

The master index file is an alphabetical listing of all patients entered into the registry, one card per patient; these cards are never removed or destroyed, as this file is a reference to all patients listed in the registry. The information recorded on the card includes: patient's name, sex and race, birth date, hospital number, accession number, date(s) of diagnosis, age at diagnosis, diagnosis (primary site and type), and date of death. Multiple primary sites for the same patient are listed on one card.

Accession Register

The accession register is a loose leaf or bound book containing a chronological list of all cancer cases. The cases are assigned a registry or accession number by year of accession. For example, the numbering system for cases accessed in 1985 would appear 85-001, 85-002, and so forth. Additional information includes: patient's name, hospital number, diagnosis – primary site, and date of diagnosis.

The accession register is used to assess registry work load, monitor case identification, and audit the registry file for lost abstracts.

Case Files

In a manual cancer registry, it is best to file abstracts by primary site, alphabetically under year of accession. Because requests for information are usually for a specific site or cancer, this method of filing allows for timely retrieval of abstracts.

For patients with multiple primary sites, one abstract for each primary site diagnosed or treated at the facility is prepared and cross-referenced. The abstracts are updated with each readmission or annual exam.

Follow-up File

The follow-up file is the key to one of the important functions of a tumor registry: to assure that the cancer patient is seen by his physician at least annually and to record changes in the cancer and treatment.

This file identifies cases due for follow-up and is sometimes called a "tickler" file because it tickles the memory.

The file consists of two sets of guides with subdivisions for every month of the year. The first set of guides is used for filing the index cards of those patients due for follow-up in the current year. Once the patient has been successfully followed up, the card is filed behind the appropriate month for the following year. For example, after a patient is seen by his physician in August, 1985, the card will be filed behind the August, 1986, guide to remind the registrar that this patient is due for another follow-up examination at that time. This process continues for the lifetime of the patient.

A readmission constitutes a follow-up, so if a patient is due for follow-up in April, 1985, but is admitted to the facility in February, 1985, there is no need to generate a follow-up in April of 1986. Instead, the patient's card is filed behind the February guide for 1986.

Information contained on the follow-up card includes: patient name, address and phone number, medical record number and accession number, names and addresses of relatives or contacts, diagnosis, and follow-up dates. Patients having more than one primary site require only one card with each primary site and the date of diagnosis listed for cross-reference purposes.

THE TUMOR REGISTRAR

The responsibility for maintaining the cancer registry is usually assigned to the tumor registrar. This may be an RRA or an ART, or it may be someone trained on the job with supplemental workshops from the American College of Surgeons (ACS). The National Tumor Registrars Association (NTRA) certifies tumor registrars who have successfully completed the certification examination offered by NTRA.

The registrar must have a complete knowledge of the disease process and understand the methods and procedures used to diagnose cancer. The registrar must be familiar with the organization and composition of the health record and know where to find pertinent information regarding the cancer. An effective registrar must have the ability to interpret diagnostic reports and discern what is important to record on the abstract. The registrar also must possess statistical and analytical skills in order to provide meaningful reports.

CASE IDENTIFICATION

Case identification is a process to assure that all reportable cancer cases in the facility are accounted for. The medical record department is the most likely department for case identification. An employee who sees all the medical records at discharge, either the coder or employee who performs assembly and analysis, is familiarized with a list of "reportable" cases and flags these charts for the registrar. The disease index is also a source for case findings, as it is a complete list of patient discharges grouped according to diagnosis using the facility's classification system.

Another means to identify cancer cases is through the pathology, radiology, and outpatient departments, as these departments often perform tests and provide therapy to cancer patients. Procedures should be established for the registrar to routinely examine these departments' registers or to obtain copies of pertinent reports.

ABSTRACTING

The abstract is a summary of a cancer patient's hospitalization and is obtained from the medical record. The data collected on every cancer patient must meet the minimum requirements set by the American College of Surgeons for cancer program approval. Information required includes: identifying information such as age, sex, race, place of residence; the medical history of the cancer to include primary site, date of initial diagnosis, histology, etc.; procedures performed such as biopsies, x-rays and surgery, to include names, dates, and results; treatment used such as surgery, radiation, chemotherapy; and follow-up information as to subsequent treatment, and patient status.

FOLLOW-UP

One of the major functions of the cancer registry is to assure that cancer patients receive regular and continued observation and management. Once a patient is entered into the registry, follow-up is continued for the lifetime of the patient.

Each month the registrar refers to the follow-up file to determine which patients are to be followed that month and follows the sequence of events below until the status of the patient is discovered.

First, the health record is reviewed; because it will often provide information on any checkups. Next, the attending physician is sent a form letter requesting information on the health of the patient. The letter should be prepared so the physician only has to place a check next to the applicable statements. If the physician does not return the form, a second letter is routinely sent about a month later. If the physician has lost contact with the patient, the registrar must obtain consent from the attending physician to contact the patient. Because of the sensitive nature of the disease, care must be taken in the method of approach to the patient (Figure 13). No reference to

James Smith, MD
1900 West State Street
Chicago, IL 60601

THE CANCER REGISTRY IS FOLLOWING YOUR PATIENT, JANE DOE, (BIRTH DATE, 11/21/40) WITH A DIAGNOSIS OF LOBULAR CARCINOMA IN SITU OF THE BREAST, LOWER INNER QUADRANT. WE WOULD APPRECIATE ANY INFORMATION YOU MAY HAVE CONCERNING THIS PATIENT SINCE 01/84.

ALIVE	DEAD	
	DATE OF DEATH	
DATE OF CONTACT WITH PATIENT_____		
BASIS OF INFORMATION		
☐ PHYSICAL EXAMINATION TESTS	PLACE OF DEATH	
☐ OTHER (WITHOUT EXAMINATION TESTS)		
☐ HOSPITAL ADMISSION		
_____	AUTOPSY	
_____		
_____		
CONDITION OF PATIENT	☐ YES	
☐ NO EVIDENCE OF DISEASE AT THIS TIME	☐ NO	
☐ PERSISTENT TUMOR SITE(S) _____	☐ UNKNOWN	
☐ LOCAL RECURRENCE SITE(S) _____		
☐ DISTANT METASTASES SITE(S) _____		
☐ SECOND PRIMARY SITE(S) _____		
☐ UNKNOWN		
TREATMENT SINCE LAST VISIT	STATUS OF CANCER AT DEATH	
(CHECK ALL THAT ARE APPLICABLE)		
☐ RADIATION THERAPY	☐ DIED WITHOUT CANCER PRESENT	
☐ CHEMOTHERAPY	☐ UNKNOWN IF CANCER WAS PRESENT OR NOT	
☐ HORMONAL THERAPY	☐ DIED WITH CANCER PRESENT	
☐ SURGERY	(ADD ANY REMARKS YOU WOULD LIKE TO MAKE)	
☐ IMMUNOTHERAPY		
☐ NONE		
DATE TREATMENT BEGAN _____		
QUALITY OF SURVIVAL		
☐ FULLY ACTIVE		
☐ RESTRICTED ONLY FROM STRENUOUS ACTIVITY		
☐ AMBULATORY SELF CARE ONLY. UP AND ABOUT		
MORE THAN 50% OF TIME		
☐ CONFINED TO BED OR CHAIR 50% OF TIME OR MORE		
☐ COMPLETELY DISABLED		
☐ UNKNOWN		

OTHER SOURCE OF FOLLOW-UP INFORMATION

REFERRING M.D. _____

M.D. PRESENTLY FOLLOWING PATIENT (IN ADDITION TO YOU) _____

PATIENT ADDRESS _____ TELEPHONE _____

CITY _____ STATE _____ ZIP CODE _____

PLEASE RETURN TO: Diagnostic Registry
(312)942-5411

FIG. 13 – CANCER REGISTRY FOLLOW-UP LETTER

the patient's diagnosis should be made and the importance of a regular examination is to be stressed. Some registrars assist patients in making appointments with their attending physicians. In many cases, patient contact involves a great deal of time, determination, and detective work. If a patient cannot be contacted by telephone or letter, other alternatives may be to:

- send a certified letter – signed by addressee only;
- contact an employer;
- check the post office; and
- check the obituary columns in the newspaper.

A hospital cancer program must maintain a successful follow-up rate of at least 90 percent to achieve ACS approval, so one must persevere in the search for missing cancer patients.

IN-HOUSE COMPUTERIZED CANCER REGISTRY

With an on-line computerized entry and retrieval system using CRT screens with keyboards, the four main components of a cancer registry can all be maintained in computer storage. The same functions performed in a manual cancer registry apply to an automated one; they are merely a more sophisticated application of the same techniques. There are differences, though, in the time required to perform these operations and the quality of the work produced.

After a case has been identified for entry into the cancer program, the patient's name is entered via the keyboard; and the computer quickly searches its memory for that name. If the patient has previously been registered, the registrar will know that the patient's current status needs to be updated. If there are no data in the system for the patient, on command, he is automatically assigned an accession number by the computer and added to the master index file as a new cancer patient.

Because of the amount of summarizing required when abstracting a record for a cancer patient, entry directly from the medical record to the computer is a difficult task. Abstracting is first done on a form designed to correspond to the order in which the data are entered into the system. The data are coded for topography and histology using the International Classification of Diseases for Oncology (ICD-O). Staging (the measurement of the extent to which a neoplasm has progressed) is coded using the staging guide for the Surveillance, Epidemiology, and End Results (SEER) programs of the National Cancer Institute.

Computerized abstracting assures consistency in case summarizing, because the registrar is forced to search the health record to answer the queries posed by the computer.

During the entry process, the coded data appear on the screen in English so the registrar can immediately ascertain the data he entered. For the purpose of checking the validity of the data entered, the computer is programmed to only accept certain codes for each data item.

As close to discharge of the patient as possible, a case summary is printed in natural language (not coded) as specified by the American College of Surgeons. For the purpose of facilitating patient care management, copies are produced for insertion in the patient's health record, and for the attending physician; a copy is also kept in the cancer registry.

The follow-up function of a manual cancer registry is normally a time-consuming process. In the automated process, the computer generates a monthly list of patients who are due for follow-up. Letters to be sent to physicians are automatically printed from the computer much more rapidly than when prepared manually. The letters are designed for easy physician response and also to facilitate input directly into the computer (Figure 13). Letters to be sent to patients or relatives are still developed manually, since the sensitive nature of the letter requires a personal approach.

REPORT GENERATION

Manual preparation of reports is and always will be a slow and tedious process. A computerized cancer registry makes data readily available to enhance patient care management. The quality of data is very dependable and researchers enthusiastically request information.

The computer generates three kinds of reports: the case summaries, routine reports such as the accession register and master index file which are referred to daily, and nonroutine reports to respond to various requests for information. Routine reports can be printed overnight. Because every data item in computer storage can be accessed independently, reports can be generated by cancer site, histology, survival rate by cancer site, etc. Storage is arranged so every data item is a key variable and can be accessed as such.

MULTIHOSPITAL CANCER REGISTRY

A multihospital cancer registry collects cancer patient data for several participating hospitals in a geographic area. The most immediate and gratifying advantage of this arrangement is the elimination of effort duplication. Often patients initially diagnosed at one facility receive therapy and subsequent follow-up at other facilities. When this occurs, each cancer registry collects the same data and contacts the same physician for follow-up information. In a multihospital on-line system, all information for one patient is stored under one number, accessible by all facilities which treat that patient. Any facility can add data to a patient file, thereby maintaining a current registry. Only the facility which first entered data on the patient is responsible for follow-up. To maintain confidentiality, the system does not allow a facility access to a patient's file unless the patient is listed as being treated by the inquiring facility.

In a multihospital cancer registry, the data collected by each participating facility are standardized. Therefore, comparison and epidemiological studies are easy to prepare.

DATA QUALITY

Controlling the quality and quantity of coding, indexing and abstracting is the responsibility of the director of the medical record department. The JCAH standards specify that internal quality-control measures are required to assess the proficiency of personnel responsible for abstracting and coding medical record information. They further specify that verification checks for data accuracy, consistency and uniformity in recording and coding of indexes, statistical record systems, and quality assessment activities should be a regular part of the medical record abstracting process.

The importance of regular review of the coding, indexing, and abstracting functions has also been pointed out in several studies conducted by the Institute of Medicine and more recently by the Iowa study. These studies revealed serious deficiencies in data abstracted from patients' health records.

A number of problem areas were identified including incomplete documentation and errors in identifying the principal diagnosis and principal procedure. These studies indicate that the presence of multiple diagnoses reduces the reliability of the data, because an incorrect diagnosis may be sequenced as the principal diagnosis. Errors also occurred because the coder/abstractor failed to review the entire record to identify the principal diagnosis and other diagnoses which affected the current hospital stay. It is possible for two qualified coders to choose a different principal diagnosis for the same case. In some instances, a patient may be admitted with several conditions each of which would justify admission; or a patient may be admitted with multiple conditions none of which justify admission but together justify the admission.

To ensure data quality in a medical information system, specific procedures and controls must be defined within each process in the medical record data flow; for there are many opportunities for error to enter the data flow. Errors may occur when medical record data are entered in the record (documentation), when data are retrieved from the record (abstracting), when data are manipulated (coding), when data are processed manually or electronically (indexing), and when medical record data are used (interpretation). These procedures and controls may be categorized as:

1. Specifying Standards – The basis for measuring conformance to characteristics of excellence: reliability, validity, timeliness, completeness, accessibility, confidentiality, and security.
2. Quality Control – Measures performance, comparing it with standards and acting on the difference.
3. Audit – Reviewing the quality of outputs from a data system and the adequacy of quality control procedures for these systems.

For example, procedures should be developed which provide regularly for the independent development of a medical record abstract followed by comparison and reconciliation with the original abstract to evaluate the reliability of data maintained in the medical record department.

Both intrarater reliability studies which ask the question "Would the same abstractor make the same decisions or judgments twice?" and interreliability studies which ask the question "Would two different informed abstractors make the same judgments when completing an abstract?" must be performed regularly. The results obtained from such studies must be compared to the department's established standards for coding/ abstracting and corrective actions implemented as necessary.

In addition, audits should be performed to assess the accuracy and completeness of indexes and data systems outputs. Simple checks can be performed to identify sequencing errors – for example, 250.00 – uncomplicated noninsulin dependent diabetes mellitus should not appear as a principal diagnosis; for this diagnosis does not explain the reason for admission to the hospital. More sophisticated audits should also be conducted as part of the medical record department's overall quality assurance program.

SUMMARY

Indexes and registers are important sources of information commonly compiled by the medical record department staff to fulfill licensure and accreditation requirements.

The amount and type of data to be stored for each patient stay continue to rise as the demands for health information for quality assurance, reimbursement, and planning increase. To meet these demands, the director of medical records may need to develop new indexes such as case-mix indexes or registers to follow up patients with autoimmune deficiency diseases (AIDS).

In most facilities, internal or external data processing support is available to assist the staff of the medical record department to meet these increased demands for health information.

The medical record professional must keep informed about the services discharge data services can provide and also medical record applications which may be completed on personal or minicomputers in small hospitals.

Because of the important role indexes and registers play in hospital planning and reimbursement activities, data quality must be regularly assessed as part of the medical record department's quality assurance program. Additionally, procedure manuals and employee performance must be assessed regularly to ensure that timely, accurate indexes and registers are maintained in a cost-effective manner.

STUDY QUESTIONS

1. List the reasons why the master patient index is considered the most important tool in the medical record department.
2. Compare the advantages and disadvantages of using a phonetic filing system versus an alphabetical filing system.
3. State the purpose of a number index.
4. List the purposes a disease and operation index serves, and explain how to determine what data to include in the indexes.
5. Discuss the alternatives of using manual, external data service, or in-house computer systems for the abstracting and indexing function of the medical record service.
6. Describe the function of registers, and identify medical departments in which a register may be useful.
7. Describe the purposes of a cancer registry, and explain how the data collected are utilized.
8. Discuss procedures and controls which can be used in a medical record department to assure data quality, and explain how each control functions.

REFERENCES

American Heritage Dictionary of the English Language. American Heritage Publishing Co., Inc., 1973.

American Joint Committee on Cancer. *Manual for Staging of Cancer,* 2nd Ed. Philadelphia, Pennsylvania: J. B. Lippincott Co., 1983.

BRESNAHAN, MICHAEL, and COOK, JOELLEN, ART. "On-Line Medical Record Abstracting." *Medical Record News.* April, 1980.

CLIVE, ROSEMARIE E., and JAMES, BRENT, MD. "CanSur: Modern Data Management for Improved Cancer Patient Care." *American College of Surgeons,* Vol. 66, No. 9, September, 1981.

Commission on Cancer – American College of Surgeons. *Cancer Program Manual: A Supplement of the Tumor Registry,* 1981.

FINNEGAN, RITA, MA, RRA. *Data Quality and DRGs.* American Medical Record Association, 1983.

GLASS, PEGGY J., RRA. "Computer Patient Index, a Tool for Linkage of Medical Information." *Medical Record News.* April, 1975.

HOLLINSWORTH, G. "A Medical Record Department Responds to Increased Institutional Needs for Patient-Related Data." *Topics in Health Record Management: Computers and the Medical Record Department,* Vol. 2, No. 2, December, 1981.

Joint Commission on Accreditation of Hospitals. *1985 Accreditation Manual for Hospitals.* Chicago, Illinois, 1984.

MARKHAM, DANIEL et al. "A Computerized Cancer Registry Data System at a Major Teaching Hospital." *The Eighth Annual Symposium on Computer Applications in Medical Care.* November 4-7, 1984.

MURRAY, CHARLES, MD., FACP, and WALLACE, JEAN. "The Development and Use of a Computerized Cancer Data System." *Topics in Health Record Management: Computers and the Medical Record Department,* Vol. 2, No. 2, December, 1981.

PATEL, MINER K. et al. "On-Line Retrieval System at U of I Tumor Registry." *Medical Record News,* Vol. 47, June, 1976.

PRIEST, STEPHEN L. et al. "Various Experts Work to Shape Computerized Tumor Registry." *Hospitals,* Vol. 52, January 16, 1978.

U.S. Department of Health, Education, and Welfare. *Self-Instructional Manual for Tumor Registrars.* U.S. National Institutes of Health, 1975.

WATERS, KATHLEEN A., and MURPHY, GRETCHEN FREDERICK. *Medical Records in Health Information.* Aspen, 1979.

WILLIAMS, SANDRA E., and LATESSA, PHILIP. "Improving the Quality of Discharge Data." *Topics in Health Record Management.* June, 1982, pp. 41-48.

chapter 14

HEALTH CARE STATISTICS

INTRODUCTION

BASIC DATA

The medical record practitioner must realize how important the medical record department's contribution is to those who use health care data. Medical records are the prime source of data used in compiling medical care statistics. Statistics about the professional work performed in the hospital or other health care facility are compiled and provided to users for a variety of reasons. These statistics, however, mean something only when the medical record practitioner, the hospital administration, and the medical staff have a mutual understanding about the definitions of terms used, what information is tabulated, and why the data are collected. Reports to agencies and organizations outside of the hospital have meaning when everyone concerned understands the definitions and parameters of the data requested. Medical record practitioners must not only be able to define the basic data elements, but also where they originate, how they can be compiled, where they are needed, and the purposes they serve.

Statistics are facts set down as figures. To serve their purposes, such figures must be relevant, and they must be reliable if anyone is to evaluate them accurately and use them for decision making. Preparing statistics involves the collection, analysis, interpretation, and presentation of facts as numbers. In the past, medical record personnel collected and prepared the data, but the analysis and interpretation were left to medical statisticians. Today, the head of the medical record department needs a broad knowledge of statistical methods and reasoning as well as an understanding of what computers can do with raw data. He must also keep abreast of available technology for recording and retrieving data to improve professional performance facility-wide and supply more informative reports to the hospital administration, medical staff, and outside agencies.

Statistics are only as accurate as the original documents from which they are obtained. The medical record practitioner must decide whether or not the contents of medical records meet statistical needs. The kind and extent of data collected and the use made of it vary from one health care institution to another. The hospital administration and governing board use statistics to compare current operations with the past and as a guide in planning for the future. The medical staff uses statistics to appraise its own performance. Reports compiled for outside agencies and organizations on a local, state, and national level are used to list, accredit, license, and approve hospitals and other health care facilities and to disburse funds.

It is important to review the data collected every year and the methods used in collecting it. Why certain data are compiled should be questioned. What, if any, use is made of it? If medical record practitioners do not routinely question their methods and the reasons for keeping data, they may be wasting valuable time with meaningless figures and preparing reports nobody reads. Keeping up with current reporting needs will save unnecessary work and help modify collecting techniques so information kept will be accurate and useful.

UNIFORM HOSPITAL DISCHARGE DATA SET

A Uniform Hospital Discharge Data Set (UHDDS) was promulgated by the Secretary of the U.S. Department of Health, Education, and Welfare in 1974 as a minimum, common core of data on individual hospital discharges in the Medicare and Medicaid programs. In the past ten years, the UHDDS has achieved fairly widespread use as a minimum, common core of data within the Department of Health and Human Services (DHHS) in programs which require data on individual hospital discharges on a continuing basis. The data set is also used within other federal agencies and has gained acceptance and use as a standard in the nonfederal public and private sectors, such as hospital discharge abstracting services.

The UHDDS was revised in 1984 to improve the original version in the light of current needs and developments. Revisions to definitions and categories have been developed to update certain items and to improve their accuracy. The revised data set will be implemented for federal health programs on January 1, 1986.

The revised data set consists of the following items:

Number 1	Personal Identification – The unique number assigned to each patient within a hospital that distinguishes the patient and his or her hospital record from all others in that institution.
Number 2	Date of Birth – Month, day, and year of birth.
Number 3	Sex – Male or female.
Number 4a	Race – White, Black, Asian or Pacific Islander, American Indian/Eskimo/Aleut, other.
Number 4b	Ethnicity – Spanish origin/Hispanic, Non-Spanish origin/Non-Hispanic.
Number 5	Residence – Zip code, code for foreign residence.
Number 6	Hospital Identification – A unique institutional number within a data collection system.
Number 7-8	Admission and Discharge Dates – Month, day, and year of both admission and discharge.
Number 9-10	Physical Identification – Each physician must have a unique identification number within the hospital. The attending physician and the operating physician (if applicable) are to be identified.

> 9. Attending Physician – The clinician who is primarily and largely responsible for the care of the patient from the beginning of the hospital episode.
>
> 10. Operating Physician – The clinician who performed the principal procedure.

Number 11   Diagnoses – All diagnoses that affect the current hospital stay.

    a.   Principal Diagnosis is designated and defined as: the condition established after study to be chiefly responsible for occasioning the admission of the patient to the hospital for care.

    b.   Other Diagnoses are designated and defined as: all conditions that coexist at the time of admission, that develop subsequently, or that affect the treatment received and/or the length of stay. Diagnoses that relate to an earlier episode which have no bearing on the current hospital stay are to be excluded.

Number 12   Procedures and Date – All significant procedures are to be reported.

    a.   A significant procedure is one that is:

      (1) Surgical in nature, or
      (2) Carries a procedural risk, or
      (3) Carries an anesthetic risk, or
      (4) Requires specialized training.

    b.   For significant procedures, the identity (by unique number within the hospital) of the person performing the procedure and the date must be reported.

    c.   When more than one procedure is reported, the principal procedure is to be designated. In determining which of several procedures is principal, the following criteria apply:

      The principal procedure is one that was performed for diagnostic or exploratory purposes, or was necessary to take care of a complication. If there appear to be two procedures that are principal, then the one most related to the principal diagnosis should be selected as the principal procedure.

Number 13   Disposition of Patient

Discharged to home (routine discharge).

Left against medical advice.

Discharged to another short term hospital.

Discharged to a long term care institution.

Died.

Other.

Number 14   Expected Payer for Most of This Bill – Single major source that the patient expects will pay for his or her bill.

Blue Cross.

Other insurance companies.

Medicare.

Medicaid.

Workers' Compensation.

Other government payers.

Self-pay.

No charge (free, charity, special research, or teaching).

Other.

OTHER DATA SETS

There are also data sets for ambulatory and long term care patients which are discussed in Chapters 4 and 5. Although these sets are in various stages of acceptance by the National Committee on Vital and Health Statistics of the DHHS, they are recommended for use by persons who are compiling and using statistical data. Further information and explanation of terms for these data elements may be found in AMRA's publication *Glossary of Hospital Terms*.

DETERMINATION OF COLLECTION NEEDS

As has been noted, both the administration and medical staff use statistics; so they should be consulted as to their specific needs. The increased concern about health care costs has increased the demand for financial data as it relates to clinical data. Therefore, the medical record practitioner needs to consult with the administrator and financial manager on a regular basis to make certain that merged financial-clinical data will be available for regular or special request use. The latter may include, for example, cost of disease entities or costs per physician or medical staff unit.

Studies have shown that each year more than 100 outside agencies request information from hospitals on some periodic, formal basis. Data may be requested about the hospital's operation (utilization, personnel, and finances) or about patient care. Some of these agencies are: American Hospital Association (annual survey of hospitals), state hospital associations, state hospital licensure and planning agencies, Joint Commission on Accreditation of Hospitals, Blue Cross and Blue Shield, American Medical Association (residency data), Health Systems Agencies, Peer Review Organizations, Internal Revenue Service, insurance companies in the accident and health field, Social Security Administration and their intermediaries, and local and state welfare departments. It would be advisable for medical record practitioners to study the reports and instructions for completing the forms received from these agencies before setting up or revising a data collection system. A review of the following publications will identify the data needed by three of these organizations: *Guide to the Health Care Field*, American Hospital Association; *Directory of Residency Training Programs*, American Medical Association; *Accreditation Manual for Hospitals* and *Accreditation Manual for Long Term Care Facilities*, Joint Commission on Accreditation of Hospitals.

The Joint Commission on Accreditation of Hospitals uses a survey questionnaire in its hospital accreditation process. Prior to the surveyor's scheduled visit, the hospital receives two copies of the Hospital Survey Profile – a working copy and an official copy. The working copy should be completed by the appropriate individuals. From it, the responses are transcribed onto the official copy which is returned to the Joint Commission upon its completion. The returned questionnaire is used in a presurvey study and the on-site survey.

Hospitals having approved residencies receive a form from the Division of Medical Education, Department of Graduate Medical Education of the American Medical Association, for completion and return. The medical record practitioner may be requested to furnish data to the directors of the residency programs within the hospital or complete the form for them, but the director of each approved program should verify the information submitted.

State hospital associations and licensing agencies often have unique data needs to approve hospitals for licensure and health care planning requirements. A composite picture of the health care provided in a given area may be published as a result.

There are other state and national organizations which approve specific hospital programs or other health care facility programs. The medical record professional should find out from the facility's administrator what programs have received approval and whether or not plans are being made to seek further approvals. If the latter is the case, medical record personnel can have the information needed for such approval available when it is requested.

Questions the medical record practitioner must ask to determine what data to collect include: What reports are needed by the hospital administration and medical staff? What reports are required by outside agencies? And what information is requested on them? Copies of these reports should be studied and a list of the data elements must be compiled. Medical record practitioners should know why data are needed and how they are used. When a questioning attitude about statistics is developed and maintained, unneeded information is not kept from year to year. A review of statistics and reports compiled should be conducted annually.

GLOSSARY OF HOSPITAL TERMS

Because of the need for uniformity in definitions throughout the country, the *Glossary of Hospital Terms* was developed by the American Medical Record Association after much research into statistical reporting and consultation with representatives from twenty-two health-related organizations. The terms in the *Glossary*, first published in 1969, are those common to short term hospitals and their patients. A second edition was published in 1979 which broadened the original glossary of hospital terms to a glossary of health care terms. Reference is now made to terms used in health care corporations, health maintenance organizations, and many other health-related programs and facilities.

The *Glossary of Hospital Terms* should be available to those preparing statistical reports. When a definition is given on a report form, that definition should be followed; when a term is not defined, the *Glossary* should be used to identify the appropriate definition for the term to ensure uniform reporting. This way more of the statistics collected will have meaning, will be reliable, will be comparable, and will serve a useful purpose.

MEDICAL SERVICES AND MEDICAL CARE UNIT

From the *Glossary* it can be seen that the words "medical," "department," "service" (as in "clinical service," "type of service"), and "clinic" have been overused. Each has many meanings. The *Glossary* defines *medical services* as "the activities related to medical care performed by physicians, nurses, and other professional and technical personnel under the direction of a physician." It covers the services rendered by all persons who care for patients, and does not distinguish medical services from surgical services.

The word "service" as in "clinical service," has had, heretofore, at least three meanings: It could be a "division or unit of medical staff responsibility," a "group of inpatient beds," or a "group of discharged patients with related diseases or treatments." The *Glossary* suggests that the term "medical care unit" be substituted and used to describe the various types of patient care facilities in which inpatient beds are located and related services performed. The definition of *medical care unit* is given as "an assemblage of inpatient beds (or newborn bassinets) and related facilities and assigned personnel in which medical services are provided to a defined and limited class of patients according to their particular medical care needs."

Medical care units do not always correspond to organized *medical staff units*, defined as "one of the departments, divisions, or specialties into which the organized medical staff of a hospital is divided in order to fulfill medical staff responsibility." For example, a hospital may have obstetric, newborn, pediatric, intensive care, medical, and surgical care units. This same hospital may have organized *staff* units of medicine, surgery, otorhinolaryngology, obstetrics and gynecology, and pediatrics.

OTHER GLOSSARY DEFINITIONS

Other definitions which relate to the organizational structure of the hospital have been specified in the *Glossary*. A *unit* is defined as "an organizational entity of a hospital." Hospitals are organized both physically and functionally into units. An *inpatient care unit* is defined as "an assemblage of inpatient beds (or newborn bassinets) and related facilities and assigned personnel."

The terms "inpatient hospitalization," "inpatient admission," and "inpatient discharge" are used in this discussion of statistics; therefore, the definition of each, as it appears in the *Glossary*, is given here.

Inpatient Hospitalization – "a period in a person's life during which he is an inpatient in a single hospital without interruption except by possible intervening leaves of absence."

Inpatient Admission – "the formal acceptance by a hospital of a patient who is to be provided with room, board, and continuous nursing service in an area of the hospital where patients generally stay at least overnight."

Inpatient Discharge – "the termination of a period of inpatient hospitalization through the formal release of the inpatient by the hospital." The term inpatient discharge includes the end of a hospitalization by order of the physician, against advice, or by death. Unless otherwise specified, discharges include deaths.

Medical record practitioners should familiarize themselves with other definitions in the *Glossary*.

DATA COLLECTION

After it has been determined what data are needed, much of this data must be abstracted daily in some organized form from the discharged medical records of the previous day. The necessary items may be hand-posted on work sheets or entered on abstracts for input into a commercial or in-house data processing system. Manual data collection procedures utilizing work sheets with columnar headings for services, results, and optional data with hand entries for each patient by case number have been replaced in all but a few small hospitals by discharge data abstracts. In either case, a procedure should be developed for receiving all records of patients discharged from the hospital by the morning following discharge. A list of patients discharged each day will serve as a checklist for records received. This list may be arranged in order by hospital number or alphabetically by patients' surnames. The order most convenient for those checking the records of discharged patients in the department should be used. The admitting office, business office, nursing office, or medical record department may be responsible for preparing the discharge list; or computer printouts of admissions and discharges may be distributed daily from a data processing system.

DAILY DISCHARGE ANALYSIS

The compilation of data concerning patients discharged from the hospital is called a discharge service analysis or analysis of hospital service. A true discharge analysis provides data describing the professional activities of the existing organized medical staff units and/or specialty clinical education programs (teaching programs for residents) of a particular hospital.

Assigning Patients to Medical Staff Units

When data are kept according to existing organized medical staff units, a true analysis of hospital service is available. The practice of arbitrarily assigning each discharged patient by principal diagnosis (the diagnosis chiefly responsible for occasioning the admission of the patient) to a "service," "clinical service," or "disease service" at the hospital level generally does not provide a true analysis of hospital service but, instead, gives a tabulation of patients based on arbitrary groupings of clinical diagnoses.

In this practice, discharged patients are assigned not only to existing organized medical staff units but also to nonexistent medical staff units. For example, a hospital has four organized medical staff units – medicine, surgery, obstetrics, and newborn. One day 10 patients are discharged from the hospital. It is the practice in this hospital to assign discharged patients, according to principal diagnosis, to the "service" which would ordinarily render treatment to the patient. Following this procedure, three patients are assigned to medicine, three patients are assigned to surgery, two patients are assigned to psychiatry, and two patients are assigned to orthopedics. The two patients assigned to psychiatry and the two patients assigned to orthopedics are being assigned to "services" which represent medical specialties, but these medical specialties are not represented in this particular hospital's medical staff structure. The patients assigned to psychiatry and orthopedics were assigned in the discharge analysis to nonexistent medical staff units. The resulting data, therefore, do not give a true picture of the care rendered by the physicians on the existing medical staff units. Another practice carries this one step further. In addition to assigning some discharged patients to nonexistent "services" in the discharge analysis, other discharged patients may be assigned to "services" representing disease conditions, e.g., fracture, tuberculosis, and tumor. Such classification further dilutes the picture of the professional activities of the organized medical staff units. There is no consistent method of performing an analysis of hospital services, so not all discharge analyses give a true picture of the care rendered by physicians on existing organized medical staff units. As a result, very little comparable data are available between hospitals. Whenever possible, discharge analysis at the hospital level should be tabulated according to the organized medical staff units caring for patients rather than arbitrary assignments based on the principal diagnosis.

The number of medical staff units in a hospital will vary according to the size of the hospital, the number of physicians on the medical staff, the type of treatment rendered to patients, and the type of medical staff organization. The medical staff units (departments, divisions, or specialties) or specialty clinical education programs (residency training programs) into which the medical staff of a hospital is organized should be included in the bylaws, rules, and regulations of the medical staff. When preparing a discharge analysis, patients should be entered under only those units into which the medical staff is formally organized. In a facility with a structured medical staff, physicians will only treat patients within the medical staff unit of their specialty, so accurate statistics can easily be gathered about the care given by the physicians in that unit.

There are some hospitals where the medical staff is formally organized, but physicians may be granted privileges to render care in more than one medical staff unit. Evaluation of physicians' activities within each unit is more difficult. For purposes of internal evaluation in these hospitals, discharged patients should be grouped according to principal diagnosis and operation, and charged to the most appropriate medical staff unit. When a family practitioner admits a patient who receives medical treatment, the patient should be assigned to the medical unit of the medical staff; if the patient receives surgical treatment, he should be assigned to the surgical unit of the medical staff. (If a family practice medical staff unit is organized, patients cared for by family practitioners will be assigned to this unit.)

When a hospital's medical staff is not organized into units, data should be classified by the medical care provided according to the three basic units: medicine, surgery, and obstetrics. Also, for statistical purposes, a newborn unit is necessary. Infants newly born in the hospital should not be grouped in the three basic units. This is true even if the newborn infant receives care from an obstetrician rather than a pediatrician. Certain arbitrary decisions will be necessary to determine if a patient should be classified as receiving medical or surgical care. It is recommended that the determining factor be whether or not a surgical operation was performed in the operating room. The one exception to the rule is obstetrical surgery, e.g., cesarean section. If the surgical operation is related to pregnancy or delivery, the patient should be counted as obstetrical, not surgical.

Transfers Between Medical Care Units

In larger hospitals, medical care units (beds) will be restricted to the care of patients assigned to a specific medical staff unit or clinical education program. In either case, or both, the statistics for each medical staff unit or clinical education program must be preserved. The integrity of these statistics is achieved by having the medical record, census figures, and all reports indicate clearly whenever patients transfer from one medical care unit to another during their periods of hospitalization. This information can be included on the discharge analysis work sheets or computer printouts by adding two columns per medical staff unit. One column will show patients transferred off the unit; the other will indicate the days before transfer. By this means, credit is given for patient care to each medical staff unit rather than just the unit discharging the patient; and the number of days of care rendered the patient on each unit can be tabulated. The discharge analysis will show that the patient was discharged from the unit which last cared for him, but the days credited to the discharging unit will be only the days he was actually on that unit.

Division of Adults and Children

In some hospitals, a division by adults and children under each medical staff unit may be required. Pediatric patients and child patients are, however, not synonymous. To avoid confusion, the term "pediatric patients" should be used for those children cared for by the organized medical staff unit of pediatrics. If patients are divided into adult and child categories, the upper age limit used should be specified. Hospitals in the United States have no standard dividing line between children and adults. Most often, patients 13 years of age and younger are considered children; but, almost as often, patients 14 years of age and younger are considered to be children. Whenever possible upon admission, the actual age of each patient should be recorded. If grouping of ages is necessary, the purpose for which the information will be used should determine the ranges of each group. The narrowest grouping of age should be used whenever possible.

Newborn and Obstetrical Patients

The following information concerning newborn and obstetrical patients will be helpful when tabulating patients who are cared for by physicians on these medical staff units:

Newborn (alive at birth) – This category includes only infants born in the hospital. Infants who are born at home or who are born on the way to the hospital are not hospital newborn inpatients but are, instead, hospital inpatients other than newborn.

Obstetrics – Includes all patients having diseases and conditions of pregnancy, labor, and the puerperium, whether normal or pathological. Pregnancy commences with conception, and the puerperium ends six weeks after delivery. If desired, obstetrical patients may be subdivided into one of the following four categories:

Delivered in Hospital – Includes mothers for whom the pregnancy has terminated in the hospital, regardless of whether the infant is liveborn or is a fetal death.

Admitted After Delivery – Includes mothers for whom the pregnancy terminated before reaching the hospital, regardless of whether the infant is liveborn or is a fetal death. Some may classify these mothers as "Not Delivered." Patients in this category include women who have delivered outside the hospital and are brought in for the puerperium, those patients with retained placentas, postpartum hemorrhages, and other puerperal conditions immediately following delivery.

Aborted – Includes mothers for whom the pregnancy has terminated in less than the time specified by the health agency for a viable infant.

Not Delivered – Includes pregnant women admitted for a condition of pregnancy but not delivered of a liveborn or stillborn infant in the hospital. Patients so classified have conditions such as threatened abortions which have been prevented from terminating and false labors.

Other Discharge Analysis Items

If institutional infections are included in the discharge analysis, this data must first be determined by the appropriate medical staff committee or the individual given the responsibility for making this medical judgment. The same is true of anesthesia deaths and analysis of tissue removed during surgery.

MONTHLY AND ANNUAL REPORTS

Daily statistics are accumulated for monthly and annual reports to be presented to the administration and medical staff for periodic special reports. Other sources of statistics for these reports may include monthly data from therapeutic and diagnostic departments (surgery, clinical and pathology laboratory, x-ray, physical therapy, etc.) and the daily census to be explained later in this chapter. The monthly analysis report concerning professional care rendered to patients will reflect only those medical staff units of the hospital included in the daily discharge analysis even though Figure 1, a commonly

ANALYSIS OF HOSPITAL SERVICE Month of

CLASSIFICATION or SERVICE (List each patient once only)	Number of Patients	Hospital Days	CONSULTATIONS			Infections	DEATHS			AUTOPSIES	
			Total	Rendered	Recorded		Total	Post-oper.	Anesthetic	Total	Over 48 hrs.
Medicine											
Surgery											
Obstetrics											
Delivered in Hospital											
Admitted After Delivery											
Aborted											
Not Delivered											
Newborn											
Term, Born Alive											
Immature, Born Alive											
Gynecology											
Ophthalmology											
Otorhinolaryngology											
Urology											
Orthopedics											
Dermatology											
Pediatrics											
Neurology											
Neurosurgery											
Psychiatry											
Thoracic Surgery											
Total Discharges											

RECAPITULATION OF PATIENTS IN HOSPITAL		
Patients in hospital midnight last day previous month		
Patients admitted during month (exclude newborn)		
Newborn this month		
Total patients treated this month		
Patients discharged this month (exclude deaths)		
Deaths this month		
Total patients in hospital last day this month		

RESULTS (List each patient once only)	Number of Patients
Discharged Alive	
Deaths - under 48 hours	
over 48 hours	
Total Discharges and Deaths	
Late Fetal Deaths (stillbirths)	

DEATHS
(List additional deaths on a separate sheet)

FORM C-619 PHYSICIANS' RECORD CO. BERWYN, ILLINOIS • PRINTED IN U.S.A. (OVER)

Form courtesy of Physicians' Record Company

FIG. 1 – MONTHLY ANALYSIS OF HOSPITAL SERVICE (front)

used form, makes provision for additional medical staff units. Its reverse side (Figure 2) contains an example of other information which may be needed by the hospital administration or outside agencies. Each hospital should decide whether this form contains enough or too much information. If it does not meet the hospital's needs, another form should be designed. For ex-

COMPARATIVE REPORT OF PROFESSIONAL PERFORMANCE				
Month_____19_____	THIS MONTH	THIS MONTH LAST YEAR	THIS YEAR TO DATE	LAST YEAR TO DATE
TOTAL PATIENTS DISCHARGED (including deaths)				
Adults and Children				
Newborn Infants				
DAYS OF CARE TO PATIENTS DISCHARGED (including deaths)				
Adults and Children				
Newborn Infants				
AVERAGE LENGTH OF STAY (based on days of care to patients discharged, including deaths)				
Adults and Children				
Newborn Infants				
TOTAL DEATHS				
Deaths - under 48 hours				
over 48 hours				
Net Death Rate				
Maternal Death Rate				
Infant Death Rate				
Postoperative Death Rate				
Late Fetal Deaths (stillbirths)				
TOTAL AUTOPSIES (on discharged patients, exclusive of stillbirths)				
Gross Autopsy Rate				
Coroner's or Medical Examiner's Cases				
Coroner's or Medical Examiner's Cases Autopsied at Hospital				
Net Autopsy Rate			—	—
TOTAL PATIENTS ADMITTED				
Adults and Children				
Newborn Infants (born alive)				
DAILY CENSUS OF HOSPITAL PATIENTS				
Maximum on Any One Day This Month (including newborn)				
Minimum on Any One Day This Month (including newborn)				
Total Patient Days Care to Patients in Hospital				
Adults and Children				
Newborn Infants				
Average Daily Census				
Adults and Children				
Newborn Infants				
Average Percentage of Occupancy				
Adults and Children				
Newborn Infants				
OPERATIONS PERFORMED (total patients operated upon)				
Postoperative Infection Rate (on clean cases)				
Normal Tissue Removed				
Total Cesarean Sections Performed				
Cesarean Section Rate				
Total Primary Sterilizations				
Total Therapeutic Abortions				

FIG. 2 – COMPARATIVE REPORT OF PROFESSIONAL PERFORMANCE
(back of Fig. 1)

ample, diagnostic and therapeutic department reports may be included. Medical record practitioners can make a valuable contribution by suggesting inclusions in the monthly report not currently compiled (e.g., comparison of the current month's data with that of the same month of the previous year and the total to date of the current year).

The monthly report prepared by the medical record department is important to the hospital administration and governing board for future planning and control of activities. These reports serve as a valuable management tool, as do the financial and other reports the administration receives from other areas of the hospital. The chairman of the medical staff units and/or chiefs of the clinical education programs and department heads use the reports to analyze the results of their current work and compare it with past performance.

The reports give hospital administration and the governing board a greater appreciation of the work performed by medical record personnel and also provide timely data to complete reports for outside agencies.

An annual report, which is a compilation of twelve monthly reports, is easily prepared if the figures are cumulated each month just as the monthly report is cumulated daily by manual or computer methods.

If the report is to be reviewed by persons not familiar with the source of the data on the report, there should be a sufficient number of explanations or legends to identify the source and manner of arriving at the statistics presented. Any report emanating from the medical record department should, above all, be accurate, dated, and contain sufficient explanation of the information so it can be easily and correctly interpreted.

USE OF AUTOMATED SYSTEMS

In many hospitals today, a data processing system assists with the collection of all or portions of the statistical data. Regardless of whether information is processed in-house or by an outside data processing service, a large amount of valuable hospital data can be retrieved for use in tracking patient care, research and planning efforts, and reporting to federal, state, and other health-related organizations.

The daily census is often one of the first reports automated by a facility when converting from a manual to a computerized statistical reporting system. From the census information fed into the computer, a daily list of admissions, discharges, and transfers is printed and distributed to those areas of the hospital requiring this information.

Programs can be written or purchased to organize data entered in the computer to produce a discharge analysis of hospital services. Monthly, semiannual, and annual reports provide comparative data on the professional care rendered to patients in the facility. Computation of percentages and ratios required for statistical reporting can be done manually or programmed into the computer and retrieved as required.

As a word of caution, however, changeovers to computerized operations must not be underestimated as to their planning and implementation time. If a service company has a packaged program which provides all the calculations desired, in all probability it would work well easily and require only minimal planning of procedural changes within the medical record department. If, on the other hand, the desired computerization is to be introduced as a new program – whether in-house or to a service company – considerably more time and effort will be required to plan, implement, adjust, and readjust the program until it works smoothly and efficiently.

Computer applications are discussed further in Chapter 15.

COMPUTATION OF PERCENTAGES (RATIOS)

Using figures from the monthly report form, which in turn were derived from manual or computer abstracting of records of discharged patients, medical record practitioners can compute percentages to make their reports meaningful. However, a percentage based on too few items may be misleading. It should not be calculated on a base of less than 20. Some percentages, therefore, need not be calculated monthly but should be calculated annually.

A percentage is computed on the basis of the whole divided into 100 parts. A percentage is a part of the whole expressed in hundreds. Percentage is a name used when fractional parts are converted into units of 100. Any two-place decimal fraction (.54) is a part of 100, and it can be expressed as percent (per 100) by moving the decimal point two places to the right and adding the percent sign (54%). Any percentage (24%) may be expressed as a decimal fraction (.24) by moving the decimal point two places to the left and dropping the percent sign.

A fraction such as ⅛ may be written as a percentage by dividing the numerator (1) by the denominator (8), multiplying the quotient (.125) by 100 (12.5%), which involves moving the decimal point two places to the right, and adding the percent sign.

To convert a one-place decimal fraction (.2) to percent, a zero must be added when the decimal point is moved two places to the right and the percent sign is added (20%).

It is impossible to work all percentages out to whole numbers. Therefore, each hospital should establish its own policy as to the number of decimal places to be used in computing and reporting percentages. Regardless of the policy established, the division process should always be carried out to one more figure in the quotient than is desired. The quotient is then rounded to the desired number by applying the following rule: drop the last figure if it is less than the number 5; add one unit to the preceding figure if the last figure is the number 5 or greater, then drop the undesired figure.

Example: It is a hospital's policy that all percentages, or ratios, on a report are to be carried out to one decimal place. Therefore, division should be carried out to two decimal places, e.g., 19.43%, and the quotient should be rounded to one decimal place. Applying the rule given above, the last figure (the one to be dropped) in the example is 3. As this is less than 5, the percent is reported as 19.4%. If the division worked out to be 20.68%, applying the rule, the last figure (the one to be dropped) is 8. Since it is greater than 5, one unit is added to the number preceding it; and the resulting percentage in accordance with the hospital's policy is 20.7%.

The term "ratio" is frequently used instead of percentage. A ratio expresses the quantitative relation of one thing to another, such as the relation of births to deaths or of deaths to discharges. A ratio may be written as a fraction (5/2) or 5:2. A ratio thus expressed can be reduced to a decimal fraction and from a decimal fraction to a percent. A ratio can be expressed as parts of 100 (percent) and a percent can be expressed as a ratio. A ratio of 15 to 100 may be expressed as 15%, and 25% may be expressed as a ratio of 25 to 100. After a percentage has been determined, the result may be referred to as a rate.

Careful attention must be given all figures. Many mathematical errors occur because of misplaced decimal points. All figures should be double-checked to be sure they make sense and are accurate. After calculating a rate, it is important to consider its size for correct interpretation.

If a percentage of given totals is desired or if the ratio between the total of the numbers being compared is to be found, the percentage should be figured on the given totals. It is *incorrect to add percentages.*

Example:

Service	No. of Patients	No. Deaths	% Deaths
Medicine	42	2	5
Surgery	63	5	8
Obstetrics	25	0	0
Newborn	25	1	4
TOTAL	155	8	5

If the individual percentages of deaths in the above example had been added, the result would indicate the percentage of deaths was 17%. Actually, 8 deaths out of 155 cases is 5%.

Statistics are facts represented by figures which mean something only if they can be compared with comparable numbers. Also, when making a comparison, the reason for the observed difference must be explained. Meaningful comparisons can be made and differences explained only if the definitions of the items compared and counted are identical. The factors a measure is made from must be clearly stated before the data can be used to make meaningful decisions. Data compiled and compared in one health care facility cannot be compared to data compiled in another facility unless uniform definitions of the factors involved are used.

There is one bit of common-sense reasoning that will help the medical record practitioner when computing a rate. A rate should be considered as the number of times something did happen compared to the number of times something could have happened. When expressing this ratio as a percentage, the number of times a thing happened is divided by the number of times it could have happened.

In the formulas for computing various percentages which follow, the numerator is stated above a line which means "divided by." Beneath this line is the denominator.

COMMON HOSPITAL PERCENTAGES AND RATES

The percentages or rates commonly computed by the medical record practitioner are defined and exemplified below. There is no rule that says these rates must be computed each month or year. Judgment needs to be used by the medical record practitioner after consulting with the administration and medical staff, as well as careful review of agency and accreditation requests (e.g., AHA, AMA, PRO, HSA, state health departments, certification boards, accreditation agencies, and federal government agencies).

DEATH RATES (MORTALITY)

Various death rates may be computed: gross death rate, net death rate, anesthesia death rate, postoperative death rate, maternal death rate, neonatal death rate, etc. Deaths are included in discharges because, like discharges, deaths are terminations of inpatient hospitalizations. The hospital death rate is defined in the *Glossary of Hospital Terms* as "the proportion of inpatient hospitalizations that end in death, usually expressed as a percentage." Counts of deaths occurring both within 48 hours and those over 48 hours of admission (postoperative, maternal, and perinatal deaths, as well as stillbirths) are currently needed in reports to various health-related agencies.

Patients who are dead on arrival (DOA) are not included when figuring these rates. Patients who die in the emergency room where there has been no administrative decision to provide them with room, board, or continuous nursing service in an area of the hospital where patients generally stay overnight are not included when figuring this rate. When such administrative decision has been made and the patient dies when receiving lifesaving services in any unit (e.g., operating room, recovery room) of the hospital other than the emergency unit, this patient is considered a hospital inpatient and, therefore, a hospital death. Fetal deaths are not included when figuring the death rate. However, their number should be counted separately. If newborn inpatients are included in the numerator, all newborn inpatient discharges (including deaths) must be included in the denominator.

Death rates can be computed for deaths occurring both before and after 48 hours of admission and are sometimes requested in this manner by reporting agencies. However, as an indicator of hospital care, it would probably be more useful to examine all deaths that occur regardless of how soon after admission the patient dies. The medical record practitioner needs to know what accreditation and certifying agencies, as well as data collection agencies, are requesting in their forms in order to decide which of these rates will be computed regularly.

Hospital Death Rate (Gross Death Rate) – The proportion of inpatient hospitalizations that end in death, usually expressed as a percentage. The percentage is computed as follows:

$$\frac{\text{Number of deaths of inpatients in a period} \times 100}{\text{Number of discharges (including deaths) in the same period}}$$

Example: A hospital had a total of 21 deaths during May. These included inpatient deaths of all ages, those occurring under and over 48 hours, and coroner's or medical examiner's cases. A total of 650 patients were discharged (including deaths) during the month. To figure the hospital death rate according to the formula, $21 \times 100 \div 650 = 3.23\%$. Therefore, the gross percentage of deaths, or the hospital death rate, for May was 3.23%. Some hospitals would round this figure to the nearest tenth of one percent which would be 3.2%. Hospitals reporting percentages in whole numbers would report 3%.

Net Death Rate (Institutional Death Rate) – The ratio of the total number of deaths for a period occurring in the hospital 48 hours or more after admission to the total number of discharges and deaths 48 hours and over for that period. The formula for figuring the percentage is:

$$\frac{\text{Deaths (including newborn) minus those under 48 hours for a period} \times 100}{\text{Total number of discharges (including deaths and newborn) minus deaths under 48 hours for the period}}$$

Example: Taking the example given under hospital death rate, we find that of the 21 deaths during May, 6 died in under 48 hours, 15 died 48 hours or more after admission to the hospital. The total discharges including deaths were 650. Expressed in figures according to the formula, this is $(21 - 6) \times 100 \div (650 - 6) = 15 \times 100 \div 644 = 2.33\%$. The net, or institutional, death rate or percentage of deaths which occurred in this hospital in May was 2.3% or 2%.

Anesthesia Death Rate – This rate is infrequently computed; but it may be useful to a particular administration, medical staff, certifying, or accrediting body. If computed, this is the ratio of deaths caused by anesthetic agents for a period to the number of anesthetics administered for the period. Since anesthesia deaths occur infrequently, this rate may not be computed more frequently than annually. An anesthetic death is defined as a death that takes place while the patient is under anesthesia or which is caused by anesthetics or other agents used by an anesthetist or anesthesiologist in the practice of his/her profession. This determination can be made only by a physician. Even so, a cause-and-effect relationship is difficult to establish. It may be more meaningful to relate the incidence of death after using a specific anesthetic to the total use of anesthetics.

The number of anesthetics administered is obtained from the anesthesiology department or the operating room. The formula for figuring this percentage is:

$$\frac{\text{Total number of deaths caused by anesthetic agents for a period} \times 100}{\text{Total number of anesthetics administered for the period}}$$

Example: A total of 987 anesthetics was administered in July. One patient's death was attributed to the anesthetic agent which had been used in surgery. Expressed in terms of the formula, this is $1 \times 100 \div 987 = 0.10\%$. Therefore, the anesthesia death rate, rounded to the first decimal place, for this hospital for July was 0.1%.

Maternal Death Rate (Maternal Mortality Rate) – This ratio represents maternal deaths for a period to the total number of obstetrical patients discharged (including deaths). Most general hospitals do not compute this rate but, rather, carefully review every maternal death. Since maternal deaths occur infrequently and are carefully documented, the rate can be easily computed on a request basis. When computing, count only patients whose death is a result of an obstetric complication of the pregnancy, labor, or the puerperium; or from interventions, omissions, or treatment; or a chain of events resulting from any of these. This is called a *direct obstetric death. Indirect obstetric deaths* are those deaths of obstetrical patients resulting from a previously existing disease which is aggravated by the physiologic effects of pregnancy. A *nonmaternal death* is an obstetric death resulting from accidental or incidental causes and related to pregnancy or its management, e.g., gunshot wound or concurrent malignancy.

A woman who dies following an abortion is a maternal death, as is an obstetrical patient who dies before delivery of a cause due to pregnancy.

The formula for figuring the percentage of hospital maternal deaths (direct) is:

Total number of direct maternal deaths for a period × 100

―――――――――――――――――――――――――――――――――

Total number of obstetrical discharges (including deaths) for the period

Example: During August, General Hospital had 1 maternal death and discharged 164 obstetrical patients (the number discharged included the death). Expressed in terms of the formula, this is 1 × 100 ÷ 164 = 0.609%. Therefore, the hospital maternal death rate for August was 0.61% or 0.6%.

Neonatal Death Rate (Infant Mortality Rate) – This ratio reflects the deaths of infants born in the hospital (newborn inpatient deaths) to the number of infants discharged and died for a period. Fetal deaths are not included because they are not newborn inpatients. Infants born outside of the hospital and admitted should be recorded as child inpatients, not as newborn inpatients.

In the *Glossary of Hospital Terms*, a hospital newborn inpatient is defined as "a hospital patient who was born in the hospital at the beginning of his current inpatient hospitalization." For all practical purposes, the number of hospital live births is the same as the number of hospital newborn inpatients admitted in the period.

The formula for figuring the percentage of infant deaths is:

Total number of newborn deaths for a period × 100

―――――――――――――――――――――――――――――――――

Total number of newborn infant discharges (including deaths) for the period

Example: During April, the hospital had 1 newborn death and discharged 135 newborn infants including the death. In the terms of the formula, this is 1 × 100 ÷ 135 = 0.740%. Therefore, the percentage of infant deaths is 0.74% or 0.7% for the month of April.

Postoperative Death Rate – This ratio compares the deaths within ten days after surgery to the total number of patients operated upon for the period. The formula for figuring this percentage is:

$$\frac{\text{Total number of deaths within ten days postoperative}}{\text{Total number of patients operated upon for the period}}$$

Rather than compute this rate, some hospitals prefer to examine the relationship between deaths and surgical operations by *selected groups* of patients operated on, such as all cholecystectomies.

Fetal Death Rate (Stillbirth Rate) – This ratio computes the number of fetal deaths to total births in a given period. In a recent survey of hospitals regarding statistics that were maintained, this rate was computed in only about one-third of U.S. hospitals. Therefore, the facility's needs should be carefully investigated before making the decision to compute it on a regular basis. In hospital statistics, fetal deaths are classified according to the number of weeks' gestation or by fetal weight.

In accordance with the number of weeks' gestation, fetal deaths may be divided into those having completed less than 20 weeks' gestation (500 grams or less – early fetal death – abortion); and those having completed 20 or more weeks' gestation (intermediate – 20 completed weeks' gestation but less than 28 – 501 to 1,000 grams, and/or late – 28 completed weeks' gestation and over 1,001 grams – stillbirths). The percentage for the intermediate and/or late fetal deaths is requested most frequently. The formula for computing the percentage is:

$$\frac{\text{Total number of intermediate and/or late fetal deaths}}{\text{Total number of births including intermediate and late}}$$
$$\text{fetal deaths (stillbirths) for the period}$$

Example: A hospital had 256 births (infants born alive or dead who had completed 20 or more weeks' gestation or who weighed 501 grams or more) during March. Of the 256 births, 6 were born dead (infants did not show any evidence of life, such as beating of the heart, pulsation of the umbilical cord, or definite movement of voluntary muscles). According to the formula, this is $6 \times 100 \div 256 = 2.34\%$. Therefore, the hospital fetal death percentage for March was 2.3% or 2%.

Since state regulations vary with regard to reporting fetal deaths, the state requirements must be determined. A fetal death is no more an admission or inpatient than is a patient who is dead on arrival (DOA) at the hospital. The use of the term "fetal death" is encouraged rather than the terms "stillbirth" or "abortion."

Perinatal Mortality Rate – Perinatal death is a general term referring to both intermediate and late fetal deaths, and infants who die during the neonatal period (less than 28 days from birth referred to as neonatal deaths). The hospital perinatal mortality rate refers to the deaths of fetuses and newborn infants occurring in a hospital before, during, and shortly after birth.

Neonatal deaths are infant deaths occurring under 28 days of birth. This should be distinguished from infant deaths, which refer to deaths of infants under one year of age. For purposes of study, the neonatal period may be divided into three distinct segments:

Neonatal Period I – from the hour of birth through 23 hours and 59 minutes.

Neonatal Period II – from the beginning of the 24th hour of life through 6 days, 23 hours, and 59 minutes.

Neonatal Period III – from the beginning of the 7th day of life through 27 days, 23 hours, and 59 minutes.

INFECTION RATES

Infection or Morbidity Rate – Hospital bylaws should specify that there be a hospital-wide committee charged with the responsibility to investigate, control, and prevent infections.

The primary purpose of evaluating infections is to determine the cause so repetition may be avoided. Medical judgment is needed to establish the incidence of infections and the proper control measures to be taken. The medical record practitioner may be asked to pull records of patients suspected of having had a hospital infection or call to the committee's attention specific cases according to standards set forth by the committee. However, the medical record practitioner should not make the determination as to whether or not a hospital infection occurred. Only a physician can make the determination that an obstetrical infection was not chargeable to the hospital or to the obstetrical unit, because it was due to a recurrence of a previous sinusitis; or that a suppurating wound on a surgical case was chargeable to the surgery unit. The hospital committee charged with infection control should establish procedures for the surveillance and reporting of infections. The Joint Commission on Accreditation of Hospitals requires written criteria for reporting all types of infections, including respiratory, gastrointestinal, surgical wound, skin, urinary tract, septicemias, and those identified following discharge from the hospital.

There are various methods for infection control and reporting in hospitals. These may involve having each physician complete an infection report on each patient discharged. The medical record practitioner, with the approval of the medical staff and/or infection control committee, may cooperate in this endeavor by seeing that this report is completed by each physician. This can be accomplished if a rule is established by the medical staff whereby the medical record is considered incomplete until the infection report is properly completed by the physician and forwarded to the infection committee by the medical record department.

Hospital Infection Rate – If this rate is desired by the medical staff, medical record personnel should compute and report it on a regular basis. An infection rate for the entire hospital may be desired, and/or infection rates for specific medical care units where infections were reported may be requested. In computing any of these rates, remember a rate is the number of times a thing (in this case infection) happens (in the hospital as a whole or on a specific medical care unit) compared to the number of times it could have happened (discharges including deaths for the hospital as a whole or from a specific medical care unit).

Postoperative Infection Rate – This rate represents the ratio of all infections in clean surgical cases to the number of surgical operations. The postoperative infection rate may also be required on statistical reports. A recent random sampling of hospitals showed less than half using this rate on a regular basis; therefore, the medical record practitioner must make a decision based on need in a particular hospital. The medical staff can give guidance on what constitutes clean surgical cases.

The *Glossary of Hospital Terms* gives a definition of a surgical procedure and of a surgical operation. A *surgical procedure* is defined as "any single separate systematic manipulation upon or within the body which can be complete in itself, normally performed by a physician, dentist, or other licensed practitioner, either with or without instruments, to restore disunited or deficient parts, to remove diseased or injured tissues, to extract foreign matter, to assist in obstetrical delivery, or to aid in diagnosis." A *surgical operation* is defined as "one or more surgical procedures performed at one time for one patient via a common approach or for a common purpose."

A formula which may be used for computing the postoperative infection rate is:

$$\frac{\text{Number of infections in clean surgical cases for a period} \times 100}{\text{Number of surgical operations for the period}}$$

Example: During the month of May, 626 operations were performed. The infection committee reported 1 postoperative infection in a clean surgical case for the month. According to the formula, this is $1 \times 100 \div 626 = 0.159\%$. Therefore, the postoperative infection rate for May was 0.16% or 0.2%.

AUTOPSY RATES

The autopsy rate is the ratio of autopsies to deaths. Some hospitals consider only autopsies performed on inpatient deaths when computing this rate. This excludes autopsies performed by a hospital pathologist or physician of the medical staff on bodies of persons who were inpatients, but were discharged and died elsewhere. Any autopsy performed by a hospital pathologist or medical staff physician authorized to perform autopsies is valuable for education and research purposes.

In the *Glossary of Hospital Terms*, the following definition of hospital autopsy is given: "Postmortem examination performed by a hospital pathologist or a physician of the medical staff to whom the responsibility has been delegated, wherever performed, on the body of a person who has at some time been a hospital patient." This definition breaks with tradition. It brings out the following facts: (1) Most autopsies are performed in hospitals, but some hospitals do not have facilities for doing an autopsy. This definition allows *hospital* autopsies to be performed in local funeral homes or other places. (2) Autopsies performed on former patients are just as valuable for the improvement of clinical knowledge as those performed on patients who die in the hospital.

Autopsies performed on fetal deaths (stillborn infants) are not included when computing the hospital autopsy rate.

Hospital Autopsy Rate

The formula for computing the percentage is as follows:

$$\frac{\text{Total hospital autopsies} \times 100}{\text{Number of deaths of hospital patients whose bodies are available for hospital autopsy}}$$

The bodies of hospital patients included are: (1) Those of inpatients except the bodies of those removed by legal authorities such as coroners, medical examiners, anatomical boards, etc. If, however, the hospital pathologist or delegated medical staff physician acts as an agent for the coroner or medical examiner and performs an autopsy on any of these cases, the autopsy and death are included in computing the percentage. (2) Other hospital patients including ambulatory care patients, hospital home care patients, and former hospital patients who died elsewhere, but whose bodies have been made available for the performance of hospital autopsies by the hospital pathologist or delegated medical staff physician. The number of these autopsies and deaths will be included when computing the percentage.

Other than hospital inpatients who die, it is impossible to determine the number of former hospital patients who die in any given period. "Available for hospital autopsy" in the formula implies that at least the following conditions prevail: (1) the autopsy is performed by the hospital pathologist or delegated medical staff physician on the body of a patient who was treated by the hospital at some time, (2) the report of autopsy will be filed in the patient's medical record and in the hospital laboratory or pathology department, and (3) the tissue specimens will be filed in the hospital laboratory.

Net Autopsy Rate – This is the ratio during any given time period of all inpatient autopsies to all inpatient deaths minus unautopsied coroners' or medical examiners' cases. The formula for computing the net autopsy rate is:

$$\frac{\text{Total inpatient autopsies for a given period} \times 100}{\text{Total inpatient deaths minus unautopsied coroners' or medical examiners' cases}}$$

Example: During the month of August, 42 inpatient deaths occurred. Among these were four deaths that had to be reported to the medical examiner (coroner); two of these bodies were removed from the hospital, and no hospital autopsy was performed; hospital autopsies were performed on the other two cases. These were two of the 14 hospital autopsies performed following inpatient deaths during the month. The *net hospital rate* for the month was 35% computed as follows: 14 × 100 ÷ 40 = 35%. In addition to the 14 autopsies performed on inpatient deaths, hospital autopsies were performed on the following cases:

1. A child known to have congenital heart disease who died in the emergency room four hours after being brought in, and the parents authorized performance of a hospital autopsy.
2. A former inpatient who died in an extended care facility two months following discharge from the hospital, and the body was brought to the hospital for autopsy.
3. A former hospital patient who was discharged three months previously with an undetermined progressive illness who died at home, and his body was brought back to the hospital for an autopsy.
4. A patient who had been receiving radiation therapy treatment for three years died of an apparent myocardial infarction on the x-ray therapy table, and a hospital autopsy was performed on his body.
5. A hospital home care patient died in his home, and his body was brought to the hospital for an autopsy.
6. A patient who had had eight inpatient hospitalizations during the past four years died in an ambulance on her way back to the hospital. A hospital autopsy was performed on her body.

Therefore, these six deaths are added to the 40 available inpatient deaths; and the six additional hospital autopsies are counted. The *hospital autopsy rate*, which truly gives an accurate picture of the service rendered by the hospital pathologist for teaching and scientific purposes, is computed as follows: 20 × 100 ÷ 46 = 43.47%. The hospital autopsy rate (adjusted) for the month of August is 43.5% or 44%.

Deaths and autopsies performed on newborn inpatients are included when figuring the autopsy percentage, unless it is requested that they be excluded and figured separately. Also, the medical record practitioner may be requested to keep figures on autopsies performed on patients who expire 48 hours or over after admission, postoperative deaths, maternal deaths, anesthesia deaths, and coroner's or medical examiner's cases which were autopsied in the hospital.

When specific autopsy (or other) percentages are not required by an outside agency or organization, each hospital should establish criteria suitable for achieving its highest standard of patient care.

CESAREAN SECTION RATE

If this is computed, which is done regularly in about 40 percent of U.S. hospitals, it is the ratio of cesarean sections performed to actual deliveries in the period, not the number of obstetrical discharges. In the *Glossary of Hospital Terms*, delivery is defined as "the act of giving birth to either a living child or a dead fetus." For statistical purposes, when a delivery results in a multiple birth (more than one liveborn infant or fetus) it is counted as only one delivery. The formula for computing the percentage is:

$$\frac{\text{Total number of cesarean sections performed in a period} \times 100}{\text{Total number of deliveries in the period}}$$

Example: During the month of June, 224 deliveries occurred. Of this number 4 deliveries were by cesarean section. According to the formula, this is 4 × 100 ÷ 224 = 1.79%. The cesarean section rate for June was 1.8% or 2%.

LENGTH OF STAY CALCULATIONS

Length of Stay (for one inpatient) – This number reflects calendar days from admission to discharge. To compute a patient's length of stay, the date of admission is subtracted from the date of discharge when the patient is admitted and discharged in the same month. For example, Joe Jones was admitted June 27 and discharged June 30. His length of stay was 3 days. If he was admitted and discharged the same day, his length of stay was one day because a partial day's stay is never reported as a fraction of a day. If he was admitted June 27 and discharged July 3, his length of stay was 6 days.

Total Length of Stay (for all inpatients) – Also known as discharge days, total inpatient days of stay is the sum of the days' stay of any group of inpatients discharged during a specific period of time. This total has been termed "discharge days" or "days of care rendered to patients discharged or died." Total discharge days are necessary to compute the average length of stay. The total inpatient service or census days (days' of care rendered to patients in the institution) are *not* to be used when computing this average.

Average Length of Stay (Average Stay) – This figure reflects the average hospitalization stay of inpatients discharged during the period under consideration. The average length of stay for newborn inpatients is reported separately.

The formula for computing the average length of stay is:

$$\frac{\text{Total length of stay (discharge days)}}{\text{Total discharges}}$$

Example: A hospital discharged 1,251 patients (including deaths; excluding newborns) during April. Their combined length of stay was 6,792 days. According to the formula, divide 6,792 by 1,251 which equals 5.4. The average length of stay of the patients discharged from this hospital during April, therefore, could be rounded off at 5 days.

INPATIENT CENSUS AND RATES COMPUTED FROM IT

TERMS AND DEFINITIONS

Whether or not the medical record practitioner is responsible for compiling the census of the hospital, he should be familiar with the principles involved. The best starting point is to define the terms used. The terms below and their definitions are given in the *Glossary of Hospital Terms.*

Inpatient Census – the number of inpatients present at any one time.

Daily Inpatient Census – the number of inpatients present at the census-taking time each day, plus any inpatients who were both admitted and discharged after the census-taking time the previous day.

Inpatient Service Day (inpatient day, census day, bed occupancy day) – a unit of measure denoting the services received by one inpatient in one 24-hour period.

Total Inpatient Service Days – the sum of all inpatient service days for each of the days in the period under consideration.

Average Daily Inpatient Census (average daily census, average census, average daily number of inpatients) – average number of inpatients present each day for a given period of time.

The census may be compiled by the admitting/registration department, nursing service, business office, or medical record department; and it may be collected manually or by computer. When it is done manually, nursing service personnel usually compile the census for each floor or each inpatient care unit of the hospital (Figure 3) at a specified census-taking time, usually midnight. It may be taken at any convenient time, but it must be taken at the same hour each day. A census report from each nursing unit is sent to the department responsible for combining them into a complete master census. If the census is done by computer, the necessary data (admissions, discharges, and transfers) are entered into the computer as they occur.

The newborn infant census is reported separately. The newborn nursery census is the number of newborn inpatients occupying hospital newborn bassinets. *Hospital newborn bassinets* include bassinets, incubators, and isolettes in a newborn nursery and/or a newborn intensive care unit.

CALCULATION OF CENSUS AND PATIENT SERVICE DAY

Inpatient Census – Calculated as follows: The patients remaining in the hospital at the census-taking time for a specific day, plus the admissions for the next day, minus the discharges (including deaths) for that day, equal the patients remaining at the next census-taking time. This figure is the inpatient census for the day.

Inpatient Service Day – This measures the services received by one inpatient in one 24-hour period. The "24-hour period" is the time between the census-taking hours on two successive days. When the census-taking time is midnight, the 24-hour period will be 12:01 A.M. through 12:00 P.M., which is the same as the calendar day. The day of admission is counted as an inpatient day, but the day of discharge is not. One inpatient day must be counted for each inpatient admitted and discharged the same day – between two successive census-taking hours. If this is not done, credit for the medical services rendered to these patients will be lost. The days a patient does not use his bed because he is on a leave of absence are excluded. An absence of

DAILY FLOOR CENSUS

For the 24 Hours Ended Midnight

FLOOR ______ SECTION ______ DATE ______ 19__

ADMITTED (Record Total on LINE 2 of Summary)

HOSP. NO.	ROOM NO.	NAME	TIME

DISCHARGED (Record Total on LINE 5 of Summary)

HOSP. NO.	ROOM NO.	NAME	TIME

RECEIVED by Transfer from Other Floor (Record Total on LINE 3 of Summary)

DISCHARGED by Transfer to Other Floor (Record Total on LINE 6 of Summary)

DIED (Record Total on LINE 7 of Summary)

STILLBIRTHS (Not to be Recorded on Summary)

TRANSFERRED (Not to be Recorded on Summary)

FROM	TO		

SUMMARY FOR DAY

LINE NO.		NO. OF ADULTS & CHILDREN	NUMBER OF NEWBORN
1	Remaining Last Report		
2	Admitted		
3	Received by Transfer from Other Floor		
4	TOTAL (Sum of lines 1, 2, & 3)		
5	Discharged		
6	Discharged by Transfer to Other Floor		
7	Died		
8	TOTAL OF DISCHARGES and DEATHS (Sum of lines 5, 6, & 7)		
9	Remaining 12:00 Midnight (Line 4 Minus Line 8)		

Record the number of patients remaining at 12:00 Midnight (Line 9 of Summary of this report) on Line 1 of Summary of next day's report before sending this form to bookkeeping department.

SIGNED ______

FORM P-644

PHYSICIANS' RECORD CO., BERWYN, ILLINOIS - PRINTED IN U.S.A.

Form courtesy of Physicians' Record Company

FIG. 3 – DAILY FLOOR CENSUS

less than one day is not considered a leave of absence in compiling statistics. The unit of one inpatient service day should never be reported as a fraction of one day.

Computing the Census for Adults and Children

Example: The census-taking time is midnight. The number of adult and child patients remaining at midnight on April 29 is 455. On April 30, 21 adult and child patients are admitted, 18 patients are discharged (including deaths). Therefore, the midnight inpatient census of adults and children on April 30 is 458 (455 + 21 − 18). On April 30, 3 adult and child patients are admitted and discharged. These three patients do not show on the midnight census because they are added when they are admitted and subtracted when they are discharged, both of which occurred between census-taking times. Each, however, received one inpatient service day (one patient day's care). To account for the services rendered these patients, 3 inpatient service days must be added to 458, the midnight census of adults and children for April 30. The total inpatient service days for adults and child patients on April 30 is, therefore, 461.

In this example, the inpatient census was compiled for adults and children only. The newborn infant census must also be figured. If 80 newborn inpatients remained at midnight on April 29 and 9 newborn infants are admitted and 4 discharged on April 30, the midnight newborn census on April 30 is 85. No newborn inpatients were both admitted and discharged (including deaths) April 30. Therefore, the newborn inpatient service days and the inpatient census are both 85.

If the hospital administration or medical staff desires to study the inpatient census and/or inpatient service days on any specific medical care unit, e.g., newborn intensive care unit, the census for that unit can be separated for purposes of the study or for any valid reason just as the newborns are separated from adults.

Computing Census for All Patients

Another illustration of the inpatient census and inpatient service days for April 30 follows. This example includes all of the inpatient care units of the hospital including the newborn nursery. It is again assumed that the census-taking time is midnight.

	Number of patients in the hospital at midnight April 29	535
Plus	Number of patients admitted April 30	+ 30
		565

Minus	Patients discharged (including deaths) April 30	−22

	Patients in hospital at 12 P.M., (Midnight) April 30 (Inpatient census)	543
Plus	Patients both admitted and discharged (including deaths) on April 30	+ 3

	Inpatient service days April 30	546

Computing Intensive Care Unit Census and Service Days

The medical record practitioner must have an understanding of how the census can be used to study separate medical care units. Let us take, for example, an intensive care unit (ICU) which contains 10 beds. The census shows transfers on and off the unit as subdivisions of patients admitted to and discharged from the unit. An intrahospitalization transfer is defined in the *Glossary of Hospital Terms* as "a change in medical care unit, medical staff unit, or responsible physician, of an inpatient during hospitalization." The transfers are added to the information kept routinely. Much more information, e.g., sex, age group, may also be added to the analysis of patients in the intensive care unit if this is desired; but there should be a definite purpose for collecting this additional data to justify the time spent making the tabulation.

	Patients remaining midnight April 29	8
Plus	Patients admitted April 30	+1
Plus	Patients transferred to unit from another unit in hospital (intrahospital transfer)	+1
Minus	Patients discharged	−0
Minus	Patients died	−2
Minus	Patients transferred off unit to another unit in hospital	−1

	MIDNIGHT INPATIENT CENSUS APRIL 30	7
Plus	Patients both admitted and discharged on April 30 (These patients have already been counted as admission and discharges or deaths. However, since their patient census days have been cancelled out by adding them as admissions and subtracting them as discharges, they must be added again in order to determine the total inpatient service days on this unit.)	+1

	ICU INPATIENT SERVICE DAYS FOR APRIL 30	8

Average Daily Inpatient Census (Average Daily Census) records the average number of inpatients present each day for a given period of time. To arrive at the average number of inpatients in the hospital, the total inpatient service days for the period must first be determined. This figure is taken from the census forms. Every inpatient receives one inpatient service day (patient-day's care) each day he is hospitalized. A hospital renders as many inpatient service days on any one day as there are patients remaining in the hospital at midnight that day plus one inpatient service day for each patient both admitted and discharged the same day. The formula to obtain the average daily inpatient census for a hospital is:

$$\frac{\text{Total inpatient service days for a period}}{\text{Total number of days in the period}}$$

The *average daily newborn inpatient census* (average daily census) for newborn inpatients is generally reported separately. When it is, the following formula is used to determine the average daily inpatient census excluding newborn:

$$\frac{\text{Total inpatient service days for a period (excluding newborn)}}{\text{Total number of days in the period}}$$

Example: A hospital rendered 3,650 inpatient service days to adults and children during April (the sum of adults and children inpatient service days for each day of April). April has 30 days. According to the formula, this $3,650 \div 30 = 121.7$. Therefore, the average daily inpatient census during April was 122 adult and child patients.

The formula for determining the *average daily newborn inpatient census* is:

$$\frac{\text{Total newborn inpatient service days for a period}}{\text{Total number of days in the period}}$$

The formula for determining the average daily inpatient census for a specific medical care unit would be:

$$\frac{\text{Total inpatient service days for the medical care unit}}{\text{Total number of days in the period}}$$

Inpatient Bed Occupancy Rate (Percent of Occupancy) is the proportion of inpatient beds occupied. It is defined as the ratio of inpatient service days to inpatient bed-count days in a period under consideration. It is generally expressed as a percent. The following terms and definitions taken from the *Glossary of Hospital Terms* will be helpful in this discussion:

> *Inpatient Bed Count* (bed complement) – the number of available hospital inpatient beds, both occupied and vacant, on a given day.
>
> *Newborn Bassinet Count* – the number of available hospital newborn bassinets, both occupied and vacant, on a given day.
>
> *Inpatient Bed-Count Day* – a unit of measure denoting the presence of one inpatient bed, either occupied or vacant, set up and staffed for use in one 24-hour period. This is easily adapted to describe a newborn bassinet-count day. The "24-hour period" is the period between the census-taking hours on two successive days.

The inpatient beds and newborn bassinets counted are only those which are set up, staffed, and ready for patients. Beds in examining, therapy, labor, and recovery rooms, which are usually used by patients who have other beds, are not included in the count. Beds set up for temporary use (cots, beds in hall, beds on sun porch, etc.) are not included in the inpatient bed count.

The inpatient bed occupancy ratio can be computed at any specified point in time or for any specified day. To compute the percentage for a specified day, the inpatient service days for that day are multiplied by 100 and divided by the inpatient bed count for that day. To obtain the inpatient bed occupancy ratio as a daily average in a longer period, the formula is:

$$\frac{\text{Total inpatient service days for a period} \times 100}{\text{Total inpatient bed count days} \times \text{number of days in the period}}$$

Example: A hospital has an inpatient bed count (bed complement) of 150 (excluding the newborn bassinet count of 15). During April, the hospital rendered 3,650 inpatient service days to adults and children. April has 30 days. According to the formula, this is (3,650 × 100) ÷ (150 × 30) or 365,000 ÷ 4,500 = 81.11%. Therefore, the inpatient bed occupancy ratio for April was 81.1% or 81%.

It is generally accepted practice to exclude newborn inpatients when figuring the average daily inpatient census (average daily census), the average length of stay, and the inpatient bed occupancy rate (percentage of occupancy). When this procedure is followed, the newborn infant census, newborn average length of stay, and newborn inpatient bed occupancy ratio are computed separately to obtain a complete picture of the work of the hospital. The hospital administration and the medical staff should set a definite policy regarding the procedure to be followed in such computations.

All of the rates based on the census and inpatient service days are being computed in many hospitals today by computers programmed to use the formulas in this section.

MEASURES OF CENTRAL TENDENCY

When performing statistical analysis, an important step in some instances is to determine the one score value from a group of related figures that best characterizes the entire group. This value is called the *measure of central tendency*. There are three measures of central tendency: the mean, median, and mode. The medical record practitioner should know how these differ from one another and be familiar with their computation.

MEAN

The mean is the arithmetic average and this chapter has already dealt with such mean values as the average length of stay and the average daily inpatient census. To obtain the mean, one sums all the available scores and divides this sum by the number of scores involved.

MEDIAN

The median is defined as the midpoint (center) of the distribution of scores. It is the point above and below which 50% of the scores lie. This measure is used to avoid one extreme value presenting a misleading picture. For example, if one patient in a group stays considerably longer than the others, a median length of stay would be better than the mean.

MODE

The mode is defined as the most recurring or most frequent score in a set of scores. The mode is not used in routine medical record statistical computation.

Example: Suppose the following distribution of lengths of stay exists: 5, 1, 2, 3, 4, 5, 3, 1, 2, 1, 5, 1, 18, 8, 1. The total of these stays is 60. Dividing 60 by the number of patients, 15, we have an average length of stay, or mean, of 4 days.

Rearranging these numbers in descending order in one column and their frequency of occurrence in another column, one can readily visualize the median and mode.

STAY	FREQUENCY OF OCCURRENCE
18	1
8	1
5	3
4	1
3	2 – midpoint here so median is 3
2	2
1	5 – the most frequently recurring stay so mode is 1

Because most of the patients were short stay, a median of three is more reflective of the hospital length of stay than is the mean of four.

If the medical record practitioner has a need for a knowledge of more general statistical methods such as distribution curve and standard deviation, this information is available in any standard statistics text.

PRESENTATION OF DATA

Statistical data should be presented in a manner which catches the reader's eye and entices interest. Presentation of data extends from simple tables to elaborate graphs.

In presenting data in any form, it is important to be very conscious of the users of the reports, their degree of sophistication in reading and interpreting data, and whether or not their interest needs to be stimulated by graphs or other pictorial presentations.

TABLES

Presenting data in the form of tables of figures needs little explanation here; as we all know how to construct columns of figures, being certain to correctly identify the entire table with a title. (It may be necessary for clarity to label each column if the title does not clearly identify them.) However, there are some rules governing frequency distribution tables in which there are ranges rather than simple numbers to enter in each column.

Frequency Distribution Tables

Grouping data into a number of classes with the corresponding number in each class constitutes a frequency distribution table. See Table 1. The following are some basic rules for choosing the classes into which the data are to be grouped and the range of each.

TABLE 1

AGE DISTRIBUTION FOR INPATIENTS EXCLUDING NEWBORN

DECEMBER, 1984

Under 16	98
16 – 34	34
35 – 49	107
50 – 64	238
65 and over	393
	870

1. Do not use fewer than six or more than fifteen classes as a general rule. This choice depends mostly on the number of observations to be grouped.
2. Choose classes which cover the smallest and largest values and do not produce gaps between classes.
3. Make certain each item can go into only one class. Avoid successive classes which overlap or have one or more values in common.

Correct	*Incorrect*
Under 10	0 - 10
10 - 19	10 - 20
20 - 29	20 - 30
30 and Over	Over 30

4. Whenever feasible, classes should cover equal ranges of values. It is generally good to make these ranges (inter-

vals) multiples of 5, 10, 100 or others which facilitate tallying. This rule does not always apply to the open classes at the beginning and end.

GRAPHS

Data presented graphically usually have more appeal than tables of numerical listings. The graph helps the reader to obtain a quick overall grasp of the material presented. It should be simple in content and self-explanatory (correctly labeled). All graphs should be titled. When color is used, a key is necessary; and when more than one variable is shown, each should be differentiated by means of a key(s).

Construction of a Graph

The graph proceeds from left to right (horizontal axis) and from bottom to top (vertical axis). Along the horizontal axis, classes, ranges, midpoints, categories, etc., are drawn at equal increments. The frequency divisions are placed along the vertical scale. The vertical scale should always start with zero. A misleading impression can be created by failing to show the total range of possibilities when one starts at a figure other than zero.

If the zero line is omitted because the frequency spread is at the upper levels, the user should be alerted to this by the use of a device usually referred to as a "lightning mark."

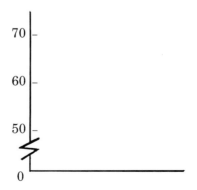

Sometimes a "tear line" is used for the same purpose.

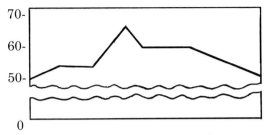

If there is one extreme value which cannot be accommodated on the vertical axis, it must be indicated within the graph rectangle.

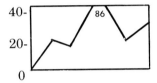

Different impressions are given by stretching or contracting the vertical and horizontal axes, easily accomplished by increasing or decreasing the number of subdivisions along either line. A general rule is that the vertical axis should be subdivided so the height of the maximum point is approximately equal to three-quarters of the length of the horizontal axis. See Figure 4.

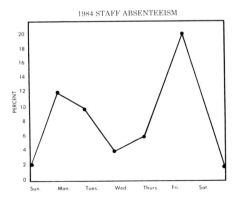

Fig. 4 – Line Graph

Class intervals (groups) can also be represented on a line graph by connecting the midpoint of each interval.

Histograms

Histograms are constructed by representing class intervals (frequency groups) on the horizontal axis, the class frequencies on the vertical axis, and drawing rectangles whose bases equal the class interval and whose heights are determined by the respective class frequencies. Be certain that the horizontal axis is identified and the entire graph has a title. It may be necessary to identify the vertical axis as well (e.g., percentages). See Figure 5.

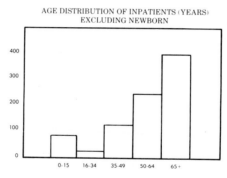

FIG. 5 – HISTOGRAM

Bar Graphs

Bar graphs are similar to histograms in construction, but there is no continuous horizontal scale (bars are spread out with space between). See Figure 6. The horizontal values may or may

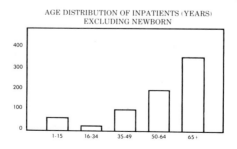

FIG. 6 – BAR GRAPH

not represent groups as they do in a histogram. Bar graphs may be vertical or horizontal. A good rule to use in determining the direction is that if the "legend" describing each bar can be written under it when drawn vertically, the vertical graph should be used. The interval markings on the vertical axis may be omitted in favor of inserting the highest score at the top of each bar. See Figure 7. Bar graphs may also be used for comparative purposes. See Figure 8. Note the inclusion of the key to interpret shading.

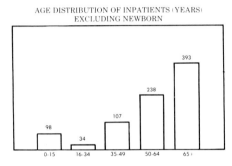

FIG. 7 – BAR GRAPH WITH FREQUENCY SPECIFIED

A few rules for drawing histograms and bar graphs follow:

1. Establish between 5-15 classes (horizontal axis).
2. Form classes of equal width, if possible, to prevent distortion.
3. Draw bars the same width and distribute them evenly.
4. Always form nonoverlapping classes.

Pictorial Presentation

Just as the visual appeal of histograms and bar graphs exceeds that of tables, even more interest may be aroused by pictorial presentations. The ways in which data can be displayed pictorially are unlimited and depend on the imagination and artistic talent of the person preparing the presentation. A form sometimes seen is called the pictogram in which symbols are used (usually drawings representing people, male and female symbols or matchstick drawings) with each symbol representing a *specified* number. By far the most common pictorial presentation is the pie graph.

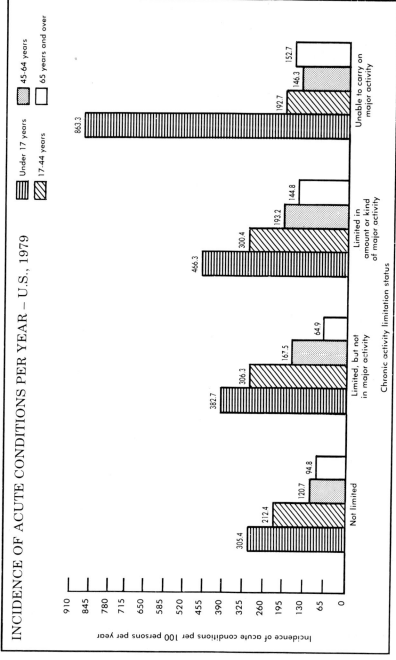

Fig. 8 – Bar Graph with Legend

Pie Graph

A pie graph is a circle divided into pie-shaped wedges which are proportional in size to the frequencies of the categories. A

PERCENTAGE OF DEFICIENCIES RELATED TO DIAGNOSIS-SPECIFIC CRITERIA FOR CEREBROVASCULAR ACCIDENT JANUARY – JUNE 1985

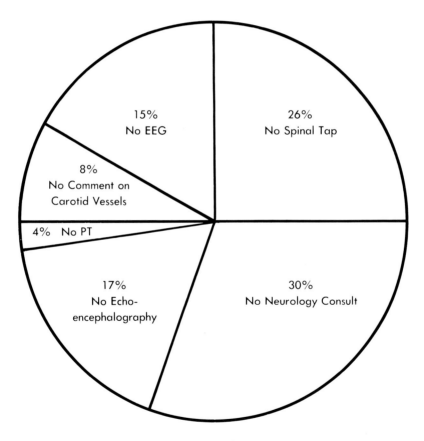

15%
No EEG

26%
No Spinal Tap

8%
No Comment on
Carotid Vessels

4% No PT

17%
No Echo-
encephalography

30%
No Neurology Consult

FIG. 9 – PIE GRAPH

pie graph always represents percentages so one must always convert the distribution into a percentage distribution. (Divide each frequency by the total number of items grouped and multiply by 100.) Divide the 360° circumference according to the percentage of each category. See Figure 9. Pie graphs have added visual appeal when sections are colored or shaded, or a piece of the pie is "cut out" to draw attention to a particular category.

Medical record practitioners would be wise to take careful note of the manner in which graphs are presented by advertisers for later application in their own departmental reports. Most ads are clever and tell their stories efficiently.

The computer frequently condenses data into readable and usable form (including graphs). However, the computer must be told what mix and match is needed and in what format data are to be presented. The medical record practitioner has an important role in designing computer outputs.

CASE-MIX MANAGEMENT

The categories of patients (type and volume) treated by a hospital represent the complexity of the hospital's case load and are called "case mix." Under the Medicare prospective payment system, hospitals are paid for services rendered Medicare patients according to fixed prices. Other payers such as Medicaid and Blue Cross also reimburse hospitals according to a DRG fixed-price system in many states.

A standard blended rate is determined for each hospital from the hospital's base-year costs, updating factor, wage index, and the regional rate. This rate is then multiplied by the published weight for each DRG to determine the fixed price a hospital will receive for a specific case. For example, a patient discharged with the principal diagnosis of anteroseptal wall myocardial infarction and other diagnoses of congestive heart failure, cardiac arrhythmia, hypokalemia, and arteriosclerotic heart disease is classified into DRG 121. If the hospital's blended rate is $3,500 and the weight of DRG 121 is 1.8454, the hospital's fixed rate for DRG 121 is $6,459. The published weights are issued annually by the federal government for the government's fiscal year October 1 to September 30.

When payment is tied directly to DRGs, a hospital must be able to identify the type and volume of patients it treats by DRGs. Therefore, one of the first reports management needs to review is the hospital's discharges by DRG. The following graph (Figure 10) shows a total of 4,800 discharges for the period January to December, 1984. Approximately 37 percent (1,771) of the discharges were included in the first ten DRGs listed. The rapid decline shown in the graph clearly indicates the hospital's dependence on a relatively few DRGs.

Case-mix management reports can vary from the most elementary to the most sophisticated depending on the data elements collected to produce the reports. Basic data reported might include the following:

1. DRG
2. Number of patients per DRG (in summary or detailed)
3. Weight value
4. National mean LOS per DRG
5. Actual or average LOS
6. Reimbursement per DRG
7. Actual or average charges/costs
8. Variance between mean LOS and actual or average LOS
9. Variance between reimbursement and actual or average charges/costs

TOTAL DISCHARGES BY DRG
January–December 1984
4,800 Total Discharges

DRG		Number	% Dsch.
391	★★★	416	8.7
373	★★★	398	8.3
430	★★★★★★★★★★★★★★★★★★★★★★★★★★★★★★★★★★★★★	285	5.9
243	★★★★★★★★★★★★★★★★★★★★★★★	141	2.9
371	★★★★★★★★★★★★★★★★★★★	130	2.7
390	★★★★★★★★★★★★★★★★	93	1.9
60	★★★★★★★★★★★★★	84	1.8
389	★★★★★★★★★	76	1.5
55	★★★★★★★★★	74	1.5
355	★★★★★★★★★	74	1.5
225	★★★★★★★★★	73	1.5

FIG. 10 – DISCHARGES BY DRG

Other elements could include level of care, discharge status, inlier/outlier designation, special care days, financial category, clinical service per DRG, utilization profile per pay source, and ancillary charges. The latter will play a major role in determining overutilization or underutilization as well as productivity indicators. Some facilities have shown an interest in displaying the average daily cost per DRG, diagnosis codes, and DRG ranking. Many other variables may also be used by hospitals tailoring reports to their needs.

These data elements can be flexed into a variety of case-mix reports. The use of so-called "canned" reports serves a definite purpose, generating very simple base information which can be compared to other facilities.

At a minimum, case-mix management reports should display total cases per DRG and total cases per physician within each DRG, either in detail or summary form. Sorting can then occur using any of the elements listed.

Case-mix reports are utilized by hospital management, physicians, and governing boards to identify the high cost/low reimbursement factors in provision of patient care. Careful study of the reports will determine areas of care which are cost effective versus those which may require modification to achieve a financial balance in the facility.

Cost reports can provide a breakdown of cost by DRG and attending physician and, in addition, be most helpful in establishing cost standards by DRG monitoring of ancillary service utilization by physician or department (Table 2). Comparisons among physician groups with similar case loads may prove useful, although the limitations of the data must be recognized.

For production of reports which are more complex and tailored to a specific facility for internal use, availability of reportwriter software is recommended. This software enables a hospital to "massage" data into unique reports on a one-time or demand basis. Figure 11 is an example of such data which may be prepared for medical staff analysis.

Case-mix data on physician performance should be used with extreme caution unless acuity or severity indexes are computed. A physician with above-average charges per DRG may actually treat patients with more comorbid conditions. When case-mix reports are analyzed, many questions may be identified which may be answered only by individual medical record review. The medical record practitioner must ensure that the administrator and the medical staff utilize case-mix data appropriately.

TABLE 2

DRG CHARGE/COST ANALYSIS BY PHYSICIAN

DRG	PHYSICIAN	TOT. PTS.	AVG. LOS	TOTAL CHARGE	AVG. CHARGE	AVG. COSTS
012	DEGENERATIVE DISORDER, MEDICAL					
	01063	2	10.2	$4,100.00	$2,050.00	$1,845.00
	30013	2	9.0	3,800.00	1,900.00	1,691.00
	01037	1	8.0	1,679.00	1,679.00	1,511.00
	TOTAL:	5	9.2	$9,579.00	$1,915.80	$1,713.92
015	SPECIFIC CEREBROVASCULAR DISORDER, WITH PRINCIPAL DIAGNOSIS OF TRANSIENT ISCHEMIC ATTACK, MEDICAL					
	01098	8	8.1	$15,205.00	$1,900.62	$1,710.56
	01103	6	7.0	9,534.00	1,589.00	1,422.15
	01151	5	7.2	7,745.00	1,549.00	1,401.84
	01064	1	7.0	1,306.00	1,306.00	1,306.00
	TOTAL:	20	7.2	$33,790.00	$1,689.50	$1,460.13

HOSPITAL OUTPATIENT STATISTICS

With the current concern about the increased cost of health care, more hospitals are turning to outpatient diagnosis and treatment as a means of holding down costs. When a hospital offers ambulatory care services, statistics in terms of persons, tests, and treatments must be carefully tabulated and reported for good management decision-making and control. Outpatient statistics need to be gathered consistently, using standard definitions to permit uniform reporting and comparison among similar facilities. See Chapter 4 for further discussion of terms utilized to collect data on ambulatory patients.

OTHER AMBULATORY CARE

OTHER HOSPITAL-BASED AMBULATORY CARE

Other hospital-based ambulatory care in a long or short term care facility might include partial hospitalization (day care and night care) and care units such as adult day care. Hospitals may also sponsor special programs such as a home health care pro-

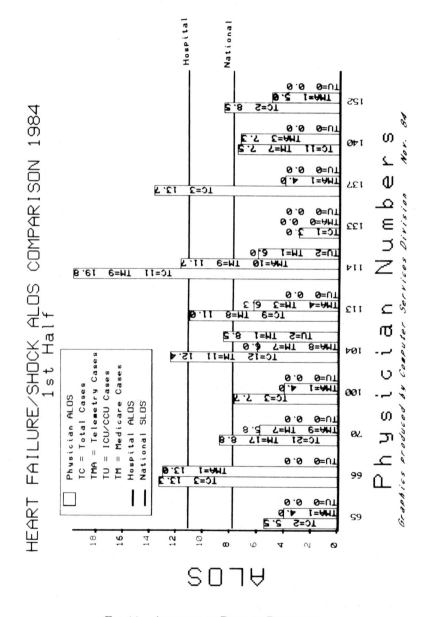

FIG. 11 – ANALYSIS OF DATA BY DIAGNOSIS

gram. While the concept of care in a hospital-based ambulatory setting is decidedly different from the usual hospital care, statistics kept are not that different. It is still necessary to have a count of patients by day, month, and year; to know the classification of medical service rendered; to compute the length of stay in the program; and to calculate mortality rates. Encounters, visits, and occasions of service will take the place of census and inpatient service days.

FREE-STANDING AMBULATORY CARE FACILITIES

The ambulatory care provided in free-standing facilities ranges from solo physician practice to group practice, outpatient surgery centers, emergency care centers, and neighborhood health centers. Some free-standing ambulatory care facilities (e.g., outpatient surgery centers) are treating patients, necessitating the compiling of the same type of statistics as hospital-based outpatient care centers. Many free-standing ambulatory facilities emphasize preventive rather than curative care, in which case statistics related to diagnosis are often meaningless. Preventive care can go on for the life of the patient which negates length-of-stay statistics. Using the hospital-based outpatient breakdown of visits, encounters, and occasions of service, one can produce meaningful data for management decision-making and control.

An important means by which free-standing ambulatory facilities can produce data for comparative purposes is through the use of the Uniform Ambulatory Medical Care Data Set (UAMCDS). The history and contents of UAMCDS can be found in the *Glossary of Hospital Terms* as well as Chapter 4 of this text.

LONG TERM CARE

Just as in short term hospitals, long term care facilities compile data needed by administration, medical staff, accreditation bodies, state health departments, federal and state government agencies, and others. Individual facility needs must be accommodated, but standard statistical compilations and computations should be used to permit uniform reporting and comparison among similar facilities.

Definitions for statistical terminology used in long term facilities are the same as for short term hospitals and are found in the *Glossary of Hospital Terms*. These are *inpatient discharge, daily inpatient census, inpatient service days,* and *length of stay*. Refer to the definitions given earlier in this chapter or to the *Glossary*.

It is important for the long term care facility to divide all its statistical compilations into categories for patients over and under 65 years of age for both reporting and managerial purposes. Additional age breakdowns may also be helpful.

It is also important to separate statistics for the different levels of care provided (e.g., skilled nursing, intermediate care, and board and care) and to carefully track transfers from one level of care to another. Separating statistics by level of care means patients must be discharged and readmitted on transfer to another level in order to obtain separate totals for each level. Levels may be further subdivided in statistical counts by type of payment (e.g., Medicare, medical assistance, and private).

Leaves of absence are included as one continuous stay in computing length of stay but are excluded, or separately tabulated, when computing bed occupancy, counting inpatient service days, or preparing the patient census.

The medical record practitioner needs to be alert to continuing changes in government and agency requests for statistical information needed from long term care facilities.

QUALITY CONTROL OF DATA COLLECTION SYSTEMS

Inputting patient information into a computer for processing and storage does not diminish the medical record department's responsibility for the accuracy and reliability of collected data. It is safe to assume that the computer can perform simple mathematical functions accurately. Quality control of input data, however, remains the responsibility of the medical record practitioner. Evaluation of the percentage of clerical error is an important consideration. Manual work sheets or computer abstracts should be randomly checked for errors. Other audit checks can be done by the computer, e.g., checking for male obstetric patients or deliveries in women over 50 years of age.

Because items are released to many recipients, it is vital that data be reliable and accurately reflect the care rendered by the facility for a given period. Periodically, the format of the data collection sheets should be evaluated to determine if the most efficient method of collection is being used. Routine quality control studies in both manual and computerized systems can ensure that the necessary collection of statistical information is done in an effective and cost-efficient manner.

Criteria may be developed to determine if each item presently collected is necessary and justified by routine use. As agency and federal reporting requirements change, data elements can be altered or deleted to satisfy revised standards. It may also be discovered that several reports carry the same items if a cross-study is done with several other departments, such as the business office, admitting department, or the hospital administration. Duplication of effort may be avoided if one consolidated report satisfies everyone's needs.

VITAL STATISTICS

Vital statistics refer to crucial events in life such as birth, marriage, death, and divorce. Birth, death, and fetal death certificates provide valuable information to private individuals, public health and welfare officials, lawyers, research persons, and social workers. A birth certificate is needed to establish citizenship or parentage, to obtain a passport, to show that a child is old enough to enter school, to register as a voter, to get a driver's license, or to obtain Social Security benefits. Statistics taken from birth certificates help in evaluating population changes and growth, evaluating birthrate trends, maternal and child health, and socioeconomic factors. Death certificates help in the settlement of life insurance claims and estates by showing proof of death. Statistics derived from death certificates help in evaluating underlying causes of death, multiple causes of death, and the frequency of certain conditions occurring together. All of this information is vital for basic research, epidemiological studies, and planning public health programs. It is, therefore, absolutely necessary that the data on these certificates be complete and accurate.

THE VITAL STATISTICS REGISTRATION SYSTEM OF THE UNITED STATES

The National Center for Health Statistics, Public Health Service, of the U.S. Department of Health and Human Services prepares standard certificates of birth, fetal death, and death. These serve as models for use by the states. The purpose of the models is to develop uniform national statistics. The certificates used by most states conform to the standard ones. Some states modify the forms because of particular needs or because of special provisions in the state's vital statistics laws. Currently the National Center for Health Statistics, in consultation with certain national and state health officers, is evaluating and revising the standard certificates. This reevaluation assures that the data collected from the certificates are useful for certain legal, medical, registration, and research needs.

When a certificate is filed, the local registrar or vital statistics office keeps a record on file and forwards the original to the state registrar. The state registrar sends a copy to the National Center for Health Statistics. The National Center prepares special statistical reports from these certificates for the United States as a whole and in comparable form for each state. The National Center also sends certain information to the World Health Organization.

The trend is to place final responsibility for vital records in the medical record department. One reason is that medical record personnel are aware of the importance of accuracy and promptness in completing forms. Another reason is that information on these certificates may be needed later and will be readily available if there is a copy in the medical record. Also, the National Center for Health Statistics recommends the use of any recognized system of disease nomenclature in certifying causes of death; and medical record personnel are most familiar with the terminology used in these publications.

DEFINITIONS FOR REPORTING OF REPRODUCTIVE HEALTH STATISTICS

Committees of the World Health Organization formulated definitions of "fetal deaths" (stillbirths, abortions) and "premature infants." This was done so reports concerning these events would be uniformly comparable throughout the United States or the world. The terms were officially adopted by the Third World Health Assembly in June, 1950. Since that time, the terms "stillbirth," "abortion," and "premature infant" have not been used in international tables. "Stillbirth" and "abortion" were replaced by "fetal death." "Premature infant" was replaced by "immature birth." Until all states amend their laws and/or health regulations to conform to the use of "fetal death" and "immature infant," hospital personnel must be familiar with all terms and know to what they refer and must use those terms adopted by agencies to which the hospital reports. The following definitions are recommended for reporting of reproductive health statistics in the United States:

Fetal Death – death prior to the complete expulsion or extraction from the mother of a product of human conception, fetus and placenta, irrespective of the duration of pregnancy; the death is indicated by the fact that, after such expulsion or extraction, the fetus does not breathe or show any other evidence of life, such as beating of the heart, pulsation of the umbilical cord, or definite movement of voluntary muscles. Heartbeats are to be distinguished from transient cardiac contractions; respirations are to be distinguished from fleeting respiratory efforts or gasps. This definition excludes induced termination of pregnancy.

Induced Termination of Pregnancy – the purposeful interruption of intrauterine pregnancy with the intention other than to produce a liveborn infant, and which does not result in a live birth. This definition excludes management of prolonged retention of products of conception following fetal death.

Live Birth – the complete expulsion or extraction from the mother of a product of human conception, irrespective of the duration of pregnancy, which, after such expulsion or extraction, breathes or shows any other evidence of life, such as beating of the heart, pulsation of the umbilical cord, or definite movement of voluntary muscles whether or not the umbilical cord has been cut or the placenta is attached. Heartbeats are to be distinguished from transient cardiac contractions; respirations are to be distinguished from fleeting respiratory efforts or gasps.

Live births may be classified as:

Low Birthweight Neonate – any neonate, regardless of gestational age, whose weight at birth is less than 2,500 grams.

Preterm Neonates – any neonate whose birth occurs before the end of the last day of the 38th week (266th day), following onset of the last menstrual period.

Term Neonate – any neonate whose birth occurs from the beginning of the first day (267th day) of the 39th week, through the end of the last day of the 42nd week (294th day), following onset of the last menstrual period.

Postterm Neonate – any neonate whose birth occurs from the beginning of the first day (295th day) of the 43rd week following onset of the last menstrual period.

COMPLETION OF CERTIFICATES

The civil laws of every state provide for the registration of births, deaths, and fetal deaths. In some states the hospital administrator is responsible for issuing birth certificates for those born in the hospital or enroute. The required information is gathered and filed with the local or state registrar. In other states, the attending physician is responsible. Although completion of birth, death, or fetal death certificates may be done by another department, the medical record practitioner should be familiar with state laws and regulations on the registration of these certificates, and should take the responsibility for prompt and accurate reporting – if reporting is the hospital's responsibility in that state. The forms, contents of the certificates used in the state, and the system for reporting these vital events should be clearly understood. To assure accurate and complete information in the medical record, a copy of the birth, death, or fetal death certificate should be included in the record. (This will be impossible in those states in which the hospital is not responsible for reporting.) This copy may be a carbon, snap-out form, stub, or multiple-copy form, depending on the type of certificates used.

SUMMARY

The information presented in this chapter covers the basic data needed by the governing board, administration, medical staff, and outside agencies. The medical record department may receive requests for nonroutine data, but such requests can be filled if data are kept in sufficient detail. Tabulations for special studies should be maintained only as needed. All statistical compilations and reports should be reviewed on an annual basis to determine their use so those not needed may be discontinued. The decision to discontinue is made only after consultation with the administration and medical staff, and review of external requests.

STUDY QUESTIONS

1. Describe how a medical record practitioner can determine the amount and type of data to be collected in a hospital data collection system.
2. Define the following terms and give the formulas for computing each:
   a. Hospital Death Rate
   b. Postoperative Death Rate
   c. Postoperative Infection Rate
   d. Neonatal Death Rate
   e. Hospital Fetal Death Rate
   f. Hospital Autopsy Rate
   g. Net Autopsy Rate
   h. Average Length of Stay
   i. Inpatient Service Day
   j. Average Daily Inpatient Census
   k. Inpatient Bed Occupancy Ratio
3. Define the following outpatient terms:
   a. Visit
   b. Encounter
   c. Episode of Care
   d. Occasion of Service
   e. Outpatient Service Day
4. Discuss who makes the decision to start compiling data for new statistical reports, and who decides to discontinue any report. Describe the precautions this decision-maker must take in this process.
5. Describe how a histogram, line graph, and bar graph are constructed and labeled.

REFERENCES

Accreditation Manual for Hospitals. Joint Commission on Accreditation of Hospitals. Chicago, Illinois, 1985.

Accreditation Manual for Long Term Care Facilities. Joint Commission on Accreditation of Hospitals. Chicago, Illinois, 1980.

American Medical Record Association. *Management for Prospective Pricing.* Workshop Materials. Chicago, Illinois, 1984.

ARMORE, SIDNEY J. *Elementary Statistics and Decision Making.* Columbus, Ohio: Charles E. Merrill Publishing Co., 1973.

AVERY, MAURINE, and IMDIEKE, BONNIE. *Medical Records in Ambulatory Care.* Rockville, Maryland: Aspen Systems Corporation, 1984.

Directory of Residency Training Programs. American Medical Association. Chicago, Illinois, 1980.

ELZEY, FREEMAN F. *A Programmed Introduction of Statistics,* 2nd Ed. Belmont, California: Brooks/Cole Publishing Co., 1971.

FINNEGAN, RITA. *Data Quality and DRGs.* American Medical Record Association. Chicago, Illinois, 1983.

FREUND, JOHN E. *Statistics.* Englewood Cliffs, New Jersey: Prentice Hall, 1970.

Glossary of Hospital Terms. American Medical Record Association. Chicago, Illinois, 1979.

Guide to the Health Care Fields. American Hospital Association. Chicago, Illinois. Published Yearly.

Handbook on the Reporting of Induced Termination of Pregnancy. PHS Publication No. 79-117, U.S. Department of Health, Education and Welfare, Public Health Service, Washington, D.C., 1979.

Hospital Handbook on Birth Registration and Fetal Death Reporting. PHS Publication No. 78-1107, U.S. Department of Health, Education and Welfare, Public Health Service, Washington, D.C., 1978.

Hospital Survey Profile. Joint Commission on Accreditation of Hospitals. Chicago, Illinois, 1984.

HUP DRG Technical Guide to Diagnostically Related Group Assignments. Hospital Utilization Project. Pittsburgh, Pennsylvania, 1984.

IOWNIE, N. M., and STARRY, A. R. *Descriptive and Inferential Statistics.* New York, New York: Harper and Row, 1977.

"Legislative Currents." *Journal of the American Medical Record Association.* American Medical Record Association. May, 1985, pp. 17-19.

Long-Term Health Care Minimum Data Set. Dept. HHS. Public Health Service, August, 1980.

Physicians' Handbook on Medical Certification: Death, Birth, Fetal Death. PHS Publication No. 78-1108, U.S. Department of Health, Education and Welfare, Public Health Service, Washington, D.C., 1978.

PIERCE, PATRICIA J. *Commonly Computed Rates and Percentages for Hospital Inpatients.* American Medical Record Association. Chicago, Illinois, 1978.

RUNYON, RICHARD P. *Winning With Statistics: A Painless First Look at Numbers, Ratios, Percentages, Means and Inference.* Reading, Massachusetts: Addison-Wesley Publishing Co., 1977.

State Definitions of Live Births, Fetal Deaths, and Gestation Periods at Which Fetal Deaths are Registered. PHS Publication No. 81-1114, U.S. Department of Health, Education and Welfare, Public Health Service, Washington, D.C., 1966.

chapter *15*

COMPUTER APPLICATIONS FOR
MEDICAL RECORDS

INTRODUCTION

Approximately twenty years ago, Dr. John Kemeny of Dartmouth College said, "Knowing how to use a computer will be as important as reading and writing." Today, the validity of Dr. Kemeny's prediction is apparent. The medical record professional now deals with both computerized and manual patient records. As costs of computer hardware decrease and as medical professionals become more aware of the increased productivity and patient care benefits of computerization, the medical record is expected to become a paperless computerized record. This is truly the Information Age. Medical record practitioners, as health information professionals, must become skilled in the areas that this technology requires. The purpose of this chapter is to introduce the reader to an overview of computer applications in health facilities with particular emphasis on medical records. Basic information on computers and what they can and cannot do is included. Readers who wish to pursue these topics in more depth are referred to the supplemental reading list at the end of this chapter.

THE HEALTH FACILITY AS A SYSTEM

An understanding of systems theory is basic to the comprehension of computer usage. A system is an integrated group of related activities or segments that work together toward a common goal or purpose. A health facility can be described as

– 506 –

a system whose goal is to provide patient care. Within the health facility are many subsystems, all working together to provide patient care. As the patient moves through the system, the care is provided by the interaction of the subsystems. These include:

- Administration
- Patient Data Base Acquisition
- Nursing
- Patient Support Services
- Diagnostic Support
- Laboratory
- Pharmacy
- Radiology
- Patient Monitoring
- Medical Records
- Medical Library

RECORD LINKAGE

Record linkage refers to "the process of connecting records on the same individual that have been generated at different times and in different places." The term "record linkage" was first introduced by H. L. Dunn in 1946 when he wrote: "Each person in the world creates a book of life. This book starts with birth and ends with death. Its pages are made up of the records of the principal events in life. Record linkage is the name given to the process of assembling the pages of this book into a volume." E. D. Acheson, a British researcher, and H. B. Newcombe, a British geneticist, have been particularly active in studying linkage possibilities, although many countries have been interested in using the concept for epidemiological and sociological research. Acheson's definition of linkage is probably the most inclusive: "a system of linked health records [that] brings together selected data of biological interest for a whole population commencing with conception and ending with death, in a series of personal cumulative files, the files organized so they can be assembled in family groups."

The computer has made record linkage more of a reality. Each hospital subsystem produces patient-related information used by care providers working within the subsystem as well as by care providers in other subsystems.

The health record acts as a communication link among the care providers and staff personnel working in these subsystems. Each patient contact provides data (input) which are processed by the care providers in the system and entered into the health record or other patient-related files such as those found in the business office.

For example, a patient is taken to radiology and given a chest x-ray. The x-ray is processed and interpreted by the radiologist, and the report is entered into the health record. Here the report is available for care providers from other subsystems to be used to institute appropriate care for the patient.

CHARACTERISTICS OF SYSTEMS

Systems have certain characteristics that affect their goal attainment. First, a health facility, as a system, must be viewed holistically as a single unit. Second, its effective functioning is the result of the interdependent actions of its subsystems. However, one must also consider the subsystems as discrete, functional units. Third, the interaction of the subsystems has a synergy that enables the subsystems to accomplish goals, in this case patient care, that would not be possible for the subsystems acting alone. Fourth, the systems exist in a hierarchical relationship to each other where the systems form layers that report to the layer above it. An example from the medical record perspective can be seen by considering the discharge abstracting function. Medical record departments perform abstracting on all discharged health records. In states with state data banks, such as Washington, the Uniform Bill #82 data set is transmitted to the state data bank maintained by the state health agency. In this example the information moves up the hierarchy from medical record departments to an official hospital data document to a state data bank, the third level of the structure. Last, control is provided for the system by input from outside forces such as changes in government regulations, marketing requirements, and the types of patients (case mix) that use the facility.

If the hospital is viewed as a system consisting of interrelated subsystems, it can be seen that the health record forms the communication link between the subsystems. It logically follows that the application of either manual or computerized methods of information handling has a significant impact on the operation of the system, both holistically and within its discrete units. Health information computer applications have been developed for both linking the subsystems together for information flow and within the subsystems for specific internal functions. An example commonly seen in health facilities is a computerized Registration-Admission, Discharge, and Transfer (R-ADT) System that affects the hospital across many subsystems. In contrast, an application such as word processing for provider dictation processing is a specific internal function usually of the medical record department.

In summary, a system is an integrated group of related subsystems whose activities are directed toward the achievement of common goals. Systems must be viewed both holistically and as discrete, differentiated subsystems. The synergy of these subsystems working together results in goal attainment. The interrelatedness of the system and subsystems is hierarchical, which provides controls on the system and its parts. The impact of computerized information systems must be considered from both a system-wide and subsystem perspective. As computer technology has become more widespread, automation of previously manual information handling functions has impacted both the subsystem where the computerized system is implemented and the facility as a whole.

COMPUTER FUNDAMENTALS

It is necessary to understand what a computer can and cannot do before examining computer applications in health care. A computer is an electronic tool for information handling. A computer will accept alphabetic and/or numeric data (words and/or numbers) as input (data entered into the computer). It will then process these data as specified by its programmed instructions. Upon request, the computer will store data and/or display the processed information in formats specified by the program so the user of the computer can view them. A computer will only do what the program tells it to do. If the programmed instructions contain errors, the computer will continue to repeat the errors until the program is changed. If the user enters invalid data that the program cannot detect as invalid, the computer will process it as valid. A common expression among computer users is "garbage in, garbage out," or GIGO.

The basic data processing cycle is shown in Figure 1. Data is input into the computer system. It is processed and either stored or output in some media for the user to utilize.

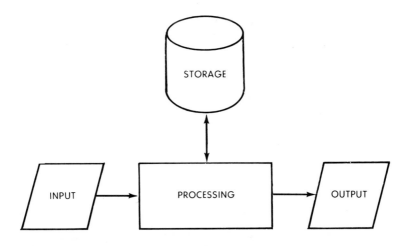

FIG. 1 – THE DATA PROCESSING CYCLE

A computer can only perform five operations. These are:

- Input: entering data into the processing unit from input device.
- Arithmetic: performing addition, subtraction, division, and multiplication.
- Logic: comparing data to identify which of two values is greater than, less than, or equal to the other. Here letters are treated as numbers by the computer.
- Output: producing processed information.
- Storage: saving the formatted data on a variety of storage devices.

These five basic processes enable computers to perform calculations, store records, sort records on any selected data element, and search for specific stored items. Computers are useful tools for data manipulation in these areas:

- Performing repeated and/or complex calculations.
- High volume data processing, such as monthly statistics, that is often repeated.
- Sorting, selecting, summarizing data for report generation, such as daily census.
- Interactive processing as the transaction is occurring, such as admitting a patient to the facility.
- Retrieving information quickly from stored files, such as a master patient index.
- Adding, updating, deleting data from files such as a discharge abstract, without retyping an entire document.
- Communicating information, such as an electronic mail which sends messages from one computer terminal to another as is found in many R-ADT systems.

COMPUTER COMPONENTS

There are two aspects to be considered when describing computer systems. The equipment or the hardware that inputs, processes, stores, and/or outputs the information, and the instructions or software that directs the hardware performance. Software is also referred to as a computer program.

Hardware Systems

The basic unit of a computer is the central processing unit (CPU), which performs the data manipulation. The CPU also has an area reserved for limited storage called primary storage or memory. The area that performs the processing is called the arithmetic and logic unit (ALU). Data input into the system goes first to the memory unit, where it waits until it is called by a third section, the control unit. The control unit acts as a "traffic cop" directing data to and from the arithmetic and logic unit as directed by the program. The reader may wish to refer to standard computer textbooks for additional information on the operation of the central processing unit.

A variety of devices can be attached to the processing unit. These are called peripheral devices. They include (1) input devices which accept data and transmit them to the CPU, (2) output devices which accept information from the central processing unit and display it in a variety of ways, and (3) secondary (or auxiliary) storage devices which hold data until the user requests output or further processing of these stored items. There is an important difference between memory and secondary storage, as these latter devices are called. Data input into memory disappears when the computer user turns off (logs off) the system. Secondary storage is designed to store information indefinitely. Files, such as the master patient index, can be stored in secondary storage and called into memory when a user such as a medical record practitioner enters (logs onto) the master patient index program. The user can ask the program to find the medical record number by entering the name of a patient who has been in the facility previously. The program will direct the central processing unit to search the file for this information and to display it, usually on a video screen, so the user can read the results of the search. The user will then log off. Data moved into the memory will disappear but the permanent copy of the file will still exist in secondary storage (Figure 2).

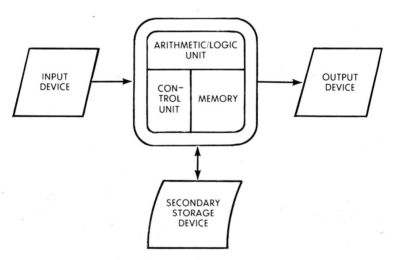

Fig. 2 – Basic Computer Configuration Showing Data Processing Cycle and Sections of the Processing Unit

Among the many devices used for data processing, by far the most common is a computer terminal. A terminal is an input/output device which may have any combination of video display screen, keyboard, light pen, printer, and even microphone.

The most common form of terminal is one with a video display or cathode-ray tube (CRT) screen for displaying what is being input as well as output, and a keyboard for data entry. These are commonly referred to as video display terminals (VDTs).

Terminals may also have a light pen attachment. The light pen is a pen-like device used to enter data in one of several ways. Some light pens read bar codes or special characters, such as may be imprinted on health record covers. The light pen is moved across the codes or characters, interpreting the pattern as data. Light pens may also be used to enter data by directing the light onto a selection from a menu displayed on a video display screen.

Some terminals are comprised of keyboards and printers, instead of video display screens. These terminals provide a hard copy of whatever data is being entered and also of information being output.

Printers, of course, may also be output devices without being terminals (i.e., they are not also capable of accepting input). Printers are often found at nursing stations where face sheets, labels, and other outputs are directed from other parts of the hospital.

Other output devices exist. Many of these also serve as storage devices. For instance, information may be output onto such storage devices as magnetic tape, magnetic disk, or computer output microfilm (COM).

Storage devices found in health facilities consist of equipment housing reels of magnetic tape, cassette tapes such as those used in tape recorders, hard magnetic disks arranged either as single disks or disk packs, and floppy disks. The media can be stored apart from the storage device in libraries, to be reattached when access is requested. Some of the media can also be shipped through the mail to other users.

Storage Capacity Requirements

All computer storage is measured in kilobytes. An in-depth discussion of memory is beyond the scope of this chapter. However, it is important to understand the concept, so data entry can be accomplished without running out of storage space. A byte is equal to one character. A kilobyte is 1,000 bytes or 1,024 bytes without rounding. Therefore, 1 kilobyte can store 1,000 characters. Medical record storage requirements can be estimated as follows:

1 Page	=	1,000 Characters
1 Average Medical Record	=	100 Pages
1 Average Medical Record	=	100,000 Characters
1 Single-Sided Floppy Disk	=	250,000 Characters
1 Double-Sided, Double- Density Floppy Disk	=	1,000,000 Characters or 1,000 Pages or 10 Medical Records

Classification by Size

Computer hardware is often classified by size. There are three general categories of computer sizes found in health facilities: (1) large scale computers, (2) minicomputers, and (3) microcomputers. Large scale computers are the most powerful. These computers have very large memories and can have many peripheral devices attached to them. They are used by large organizations to perform volumes of work, manipulate large numbers, and complete tasks which have large memory requirements.

The second category is the minicomputer. This smaller-sized computer is becoming common in hospitals. It usually has a more limited memory size and number of peripherals which it can accommodate.

The final category of computer is the microcomputer. This small computer system uses a microprocessor chip to perform operations. A microprocessor is a silicon chip with thousands of microcircuits which perform the data processing. Personal computers such as the IBM-PC are included in this group. Many medical record departments now have a microcomputer supplied by their discharge data abstracting service. All three sizes of computers process information using the five basic operations previously described. The major differences among systems relate to the size of the memory, speed of operations, and number of users who can use the system at the same time.

The terms "mainframe" and "personal" are also associated with computers to denote the location of the user with respect to the computer. A mainframe computer refers to the primary and usually large scale or minicomputer in a facility to which numerous people have access. Personal computers are used by one person at any given time. Personal computers may be grouped together into networks, but each one can operate independently.

In summary, computer hardware consists of a central processing unit and peripheral equipment. Peripherals include devices that act only as input or output units or serve both needs. The devices most commonly used by medical record professionals are VDTs and printers. The third type of peripheral device is secondary storage equipment. Minicomputers use tape drives or hard disks. Microcomputers use floppy disks and small hard disks.

Computer Software

The series of instructions that direct the computer to perform various operations is called a program or software. Programs are written by computer programmers in special languages that computers can understand. There are two basic types of programs: applications and operating systems. Most medical applications programs are written in high-level languages that resemble English. Four commonly encountered languages are (1) BASIC (Beginners All-Purpose Symbolic Instruction Code), a simple, interactive language that is found on most microcomputers as well as mini and mainframe computers; (2) RPG (Report Program Generator), for producing reports; (3) COBOL (Common Business-Oriented Language), which was designed for business applications; and (4) MUMPS (Massachusetts General Hospital Utility Multiprogramming System), an interactive language developed specifically for medical applications.

Software and the Role of the Medical Record Professional

The medical record professional's role is that of a user of applications software. Applications software refers to programs written to perform specific medical record functions such as master patient index accessing or discharge abstracting. Therefore, a knowledge of computer programming is not required for the medical record professional.

Operating System Software

Operating system programs are those used by computers to direct their internal functions. This software acts as a "traffic cop" by handling input and output operations, supervising the execution of program and memory access. Figure 3 shows a typ-

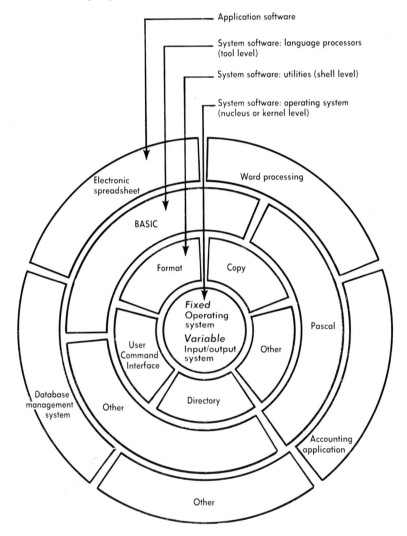

FIG. 3 – ONE VERSION OF THE SOFTWARE HIERARCHY

Reprinted with permission from Dologite, D. G. *Using Small Business Computers,* Prentice Hall, Inc., Englewood Cliffs, N.J., 1984.

ical software hierarchy which consists of the operating system program, the applications software, and other intermediary systems utility programs such as copy, formatting, libraries, and languages. The outer layer of the hierarchy consists of the applications programs found in a Hospital Information System (HIS). Operating systems greatly simplify the running of applications programs by conducting routine matters of machine access and switching, leaving the applications program free to attend solely to the application.

Currently available operating systems found on microcomputers include PC-DOS, CP/M-86, and Apple DOS. Bell Laboratories have developed the UNIX operating system which runs on both micro- and minicomputers. UNIX has a library of over 200 utility programs and unique file handling capabilities that are not available on other systems. Experts predict that UNIX will become an industry standard.

In summary, the instructions which control computer operation are coded in programs, also called software. Programs are written in a variety of high-level languages such as BASIC, COBOL, and MUMPS. There are two classes of software: (1) systems software, and (2) applications software. Systems programs operate the computer system through acting as a "traffic cop" to data and processing within the system. Applications programs perform specific tasks or functions such as accounting and word processing, as well as building data bases of stored information.

COMPUTER SYSTEMS FOUND IN HEALTH FACILITIES

Two general types of computer systems are found in health facilities today: (1) stand-alone systems, and (2) interdepartmental systems. Stand-alone systems are located within a single department, usually operating independently of other computer systems within the facility. Running encoded data on a microcomputer housed within the medical record department is an example of this type, as is a word processing system for medical record dictation located in the medical record department. Interdepartmental systems use terminals placed in various locations throughout the facility. These terminals are connected to one or more centrally located mainframe computers usually housed in the data processing department. The operation of these centrally located computers is controlled by data processing personnel. The terminals may be "dumb" terminals that can input or output data, or they may be "smart" terminals which have some processing capability as well as input and output operations. Interdepartmental computer systems may link two or more departments, such as medical records and the business office; or they may form communication linkages across the entire facility.

Health facility computer systems have a variety of names with slight differences in meaning, such as Hospital Information System (HIS), Medical Information System (MIS), or Management Information System (MIS). This chapter will refer to HIS when discussing these interdepartmental systems.

HISs have been developed to handle the large volumes of data that must be manipulated for patient care. Ball defines an HIS as "a communication network linking terminals and output devices in key patient care or service areas to a central processing unit which coordinates all essential patient care activities. Thus, the HIS provides a communications system between departments (e.g., dietary, nursing units, pharmacy, laboratory, etc.); a central information system for receipt, sorting, transmission, storage, and retrieval of information; and a high-speed data processing system for fast and economic processing of data to provide information in its most useful form." These systems exist today in various stages of completion from single applications to the entire system described above.

There are two types of HISs found today. Class A consists of a single application area which meets the needs of a specific department, such as the clinical laboratory system that generates laboratory reports. Class B refers to HISs that integrate subsystems through communication links. An example of this class is the R-ADT system previously described which switches information to several departments as the patient moves through the facility. This system is described more fully in the section on applications. Class B also includes comprehensive systems such as PHAMIS (Public Health Automated Medical Information System), and TECHNICON which hold medical record orders, laboratory results, radiology reports, pharmacy information, and other parts of the medical record on-line for provider access until the patient is discharged.

HIS CONFIGURATIONS

Computer systems found in health facilities generally fall into four basic categories:

- Large systems with one CPU
- Networks with a large CPU
- Minicomputer networks
- Microcomputer VAN and LAN networks (future trend)

Large Systems with One CPU

These systems rely on one large CPU which may be centrally located in the facility or at a remote location (see Figure 4). Ter-

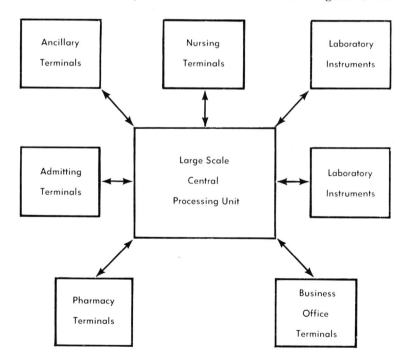

FIG. 4 – LARGE MONOLITHIC SYSTEM WITH
ONE CENTRAL PROCESSING UNIT

minals and printers are either hardwired directly to the CPU or access the CPU through a modem and telephone lines. A modem is a device which converts the digital computer signals to analog signals and transmits them over telephone lines. A modem located at the CPU site converts the signals back to digital configuration so they can be processed by the CPU. In this way, service bureaus, such as Shared Medical Systems, provide computer applications for facilities located at any location accessible by telephone. An advantage of a system of this type, whether the CPU is located in-house or at another location, is that one central data base can be established which can be used by all the terminals interactively. The major problems related to this configuration are the excessive cost of a large computer and the impact of downtime. When the computer is down (not functioning), the entire system is disabled unless a backup system is maintained.

Networks with a Mainframe and Two Minicomputers

This configuration provides a central data base and also allows additional modules to be added as needed by adding other smaller computers to the system (Figure 5). Here, subsystems such as pharmacy and laboratory have their own CPUs. These smaller CPUs are hardwired by coaxial cable to the mainframe CPU. The small CPUs communicate only with the central CPU and not with each other. All communications with terminals throughout the facility, other than within the laboratory or pharmacy systems, must go through the central CPU.

Minicomputer Networks

Minicomputer networks have a variety of configurations. A network is composed of two or more computers linked to each other and attached to several types of output and input devices. Many combinations may be used, but the preferred network design is usually a (1) star network, or (2) ring network.

Star Networks

A star network consists of a central host minicomputer and terminals and/or personal computers connected together to form a star. The star network may consist of dedicated subsystems such as the admitting, laboratory, and pharmacy systems shown in Figure 6, or as the distributed star shown in Figure 7. In each case as in the mainframe network shown above, the central host computer provides the linkage to all the subsystems located on the arms of the star. In this configuration, if the central CPU goes down, the subsystems with their own dedicated processors can continue to operate but communication throughout the entire system is not possible.

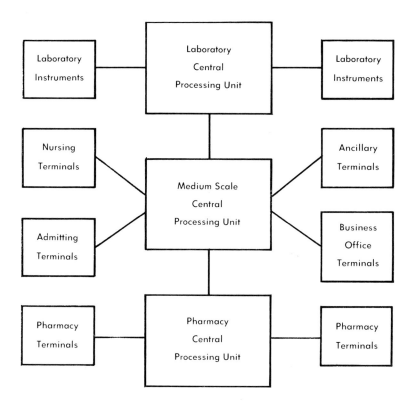

FIG. 5 – NETWORK USING MEDIUM-SIZE HOST

Reprinted with permission of Schmitz, Homer H. *Hospital Information Systems*, Aspen Systems Corporation, Germantown, 1979.

Ring Networks

A ring network uses a series of computers which communicate with each other directly without passing through a central

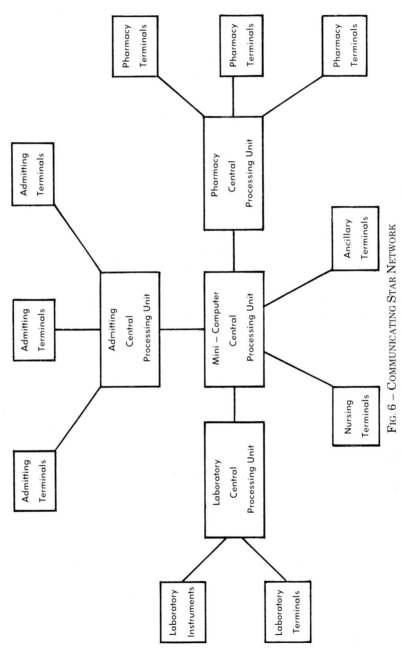

FIG. 6 – COMMUNICATING STAR NETWORK

Reprinted with permission of Schmitz, Homer H. *Hospital Information Systems,* Aspen Systems Corporation, Germantown, 1979.

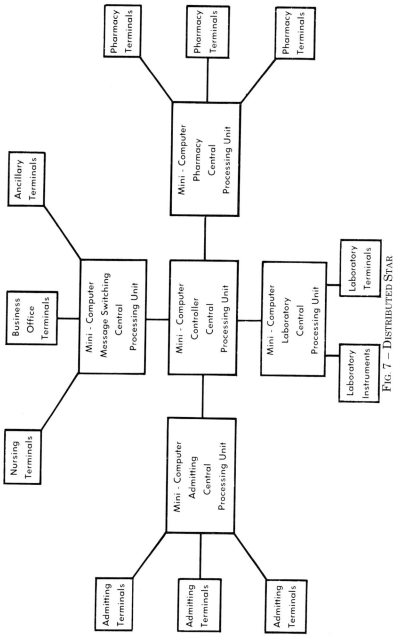

FIG. 7 – DISTRIBUTED STAR

Reprinted with permission of Schmitz, Homer H. *Hospital Information Systems,* Aspen Systems Corporation, Germantown, 1979.

host CPU. Each computer can perform all the functions of the network. If one CPU goes down, the others take over its functions until it comes back up (starts to operate again). In this system there is no interruption of service, an important consideration in the health care environment.

Small Computer Networks (VAN and LAN)

A major network type that advances in technology have recently made possible is the linkage of small computers such as personal computers (PCs), in Value Added (VAN), or Local Area (LAN) networks. A VAN utilizes a modem which connects the PCs over telephone lines. This enables the user to access large collections of information stored in data bases previously only available to libraries. There are over 1,000 health care related data bases available to PC users with modems. The listing given below describes some of these resources:

- AMA/NET: files on drugs, diseases, CPT codes, bibliographic resources.
- MED MAIL: electronic medical mail service.
- PHYCOM: physician communication service.
- BRS-MEDICAL (MIRS): stored full text of current medical books and journals in internal medicine.
- COMPUSERVE: several health data bases as well as electronic mail services. Also provides other services of interest to the general public such as stock market reports.
- DIALOG: on-line medical information from Excerpta Medica as well as other health and business related data bases including MEDLINE.
- THE SOURCE: some health related data bases as well as mail, business, news and leisure information such as airline schedules.
- ARIMIS: arthritis data base.
- ONCOCIN: cancer data base.
- PUFF: provides pulmonary function interpretation.
- CADUCEUS: uses artificial intelligence and stored information to assist providers to diagnose patient conditions.

Local Area Networks (LAN)

Local Area Networks (LAN) link personal or small computers within a limited geographic area such as a single building or a university campus. LANs were developed to allow the growing numbers of PCs and small computers found in organizations to communicate with each other through electronic mail and text transmission, share hardware resources such as letter quality printers, and to share information. The computers are connected to each other through coaxial cables in a single line, a star formation, or a ring formation. LANs are expected to be established in increasing numbers in the health care environment and have important implications for medical record professionals. With a LAN it may no longer be necessary to maintain a centralized unit record until discharge to an even greater extent than is now seen with larger HIS systems. Medical record professionals must become assertive partners in the development of these systems through interaction with data processing departments and other health professionals.

In-House Versus Shared Systems

HISs can utilize in-house computers or large host computers at remote locations which they share with other health facilities. Historically, HISs were first developed by vendors who offered increasingly sophisticated medical application software packages housed on these large computers. Facilities used terminals and modems to call the host computer to perform the functions desired. Despite the remote location of the CPU, the user experienced no appreciable time delays while interacting with the system. As costs of hardware have decreased significantly, it has become cost effective for facilities to purchase or lease their own in-house hardware. An exploding proliferation of medical application software has made it possible for facilities to purchase "off the shelf," or turnkey, software packages. These packages run on in-house computers for most of the information-related operations of hospitals, as well as many of the functions of ambulatory and long term care facilities. Future projections indicate decreased utilization of shared systems on large host computers except where a central computer system or network is owned by a large chain of health facilities or by groups of small facilities which have banded together to share the costs involved in computerization.

MEDICAL RECORD COMPUTER APPLICATIONS

The functional operations of the medical record department lend themselves well to computerization. Some of these operations are listed below:

- Maintaining the master patient index.
- Registration-Admission Discharge and Transfer (R-ADT).
- Utilization screening.
- Record completion monitoring.
- Analysis and abstracting of discharged patient records.
- Coding of diagnoses and procedures.
- Diagnosis related group assignment.
- Record access control.
- Research, case-mix analysis.
- Word processing of medical dictation and reports.

All of the functions mentioned above, as well as others not listed, have computer applications. Much of the software is available from vendors to run on computers that vary in size from PCs to mainframes. Many computer applications have been discussed in earlier chapters, including master patient index, census and statistical report generation, discharge abstracting, coding, and DRG assignments; but this chapter will describe some of the other applications found in medical record departments. Since log-on procedures vary depending on the computer manufacturer, the reader who wishes more specific information on how to use these systems is referred to departmental procedures and computer systems manuals provided by computer vendors where these systems are in operation. This chapter is intended to serve as an introduction to types of computer applications and not as a resource for actual system operations. Table 1 contains a representative listing of typical vendor system applications.

Applications that impact medical record departments exist on: (1) computers housed within the medical record department such as the discharge abstracting system previously mentioned, or (2) mainframe computers located in the data processing department which are connected by communication links to other sections of the health facility. By 1990 LANs are expected to be common in health facilities and will house applications as well.

TABLE 1
MAJOR VENDOR SYSTEMS DEVELOPMENTS

Department/Application	Number of Vendors	
	Now Offer	Plan to Offer
Nursing		
Order set entry	5	1
Charting	3	2
Patient care level tracking	3	2
Staffing requirements	5	2
Nursing notes*	5	0
Care plan*	1	6
Medication schedules*	6	2
Medication monitoring*	3	2
Pharmacy		
Patient medical profile*	7	1
Drug precaution/interaction	2	4
Unit dose care replenishment	5	2
Pharmacy inventory	3	4
Lab		
Specimen collection lists	6	1
Specimen collection labels	8	0
Results reporting*	7	0
Cumulative results*	6	1
Interface to lab computer	6	1
Radiology		
Scheduling	4	2
Report normals only*	3	3
Report all results*	2	5
Radiology index	4	2
Medical Records*		
Medical record index*	5	2
Medical record abstract*	5	2
Chart location delinquency tracking*	3	3
Emergency Room/Outpatient		
Registration*	8	0
Order entry*	8	0
Demand billing	7	0
Patient scheduling	6	2
Miscellaneous		
Preadmitting*	8	0
Computer-assigned patient ID*	8	0
Time-clocking	5	0
Surgery scheduling	2	3
Diet list preparation	7	1
Utilization review*	7	0
Cash receipts entry	6	0
Doctors' registry*	6	1

*Patient record impact.
**Some report Stats only.

Reprinted with permission from Waters, Kathleen A. and Murphy, Gretchen F. *Systems Analysis and Computer Applications.* Aspen Systems Corp., Rockville, 1983.

Most health facilities first introduced computer applications into the business office to expedite billing and financial reporting. Today even small rural facilities usually use outside computer financial services if they do not have in-house systems.

REGISTRATION-ADMISSION, DISCHARGE, AND TRANSFER SYSTEM

Many facilities have computerized the Registration-Admission, Discharge, and Transfer (R-ADT) process. The R-ADT is one of the most effective systems to implement computerization in a health facility since it integrates and provides information useful to many hospital departments. The key to this process is the establishment of a central data base of patient information available to authorized users throughout the facility through VDTs or printers.

A typical R-ADT system is shown in Figure 8. When a patient is admitted, the admissions clerk enters patient data on the VDT located in admissions. A computerized master patient index allows the clerk to assign a new medical record number or to identify a number assigned to the patient during a previous admission. The clerk also assigns the patient to a room by accessing the computerized available bed listings for the service to which the patient is to be assigned. Patients can be preregistered so all the input operations except bed assignment are performed before the patient arrives in admissions. Once the admission process is completed, the clerk transmits the data to the CPU, where the program directs the system to automatically notify the patient unit that the patient is arriving. It may also print out the medical record face sheet on the unit printer at this time. In addition, all other departments impacted by the patient's arrival are notified. These include housekeeping for notice of an occupied bed to maintain, laboratory to order diagnostic tests, dietary to begin meal services, medical records to pull previous records to send to the patient care unit, and the business office to begin the patient account.

During the patient stay, all room changes and patient transfers, such as to surgery, intensive care, radiology, and recovery, are entered into the system at VDTs or printers located throughout the facility. As procedures are performed,

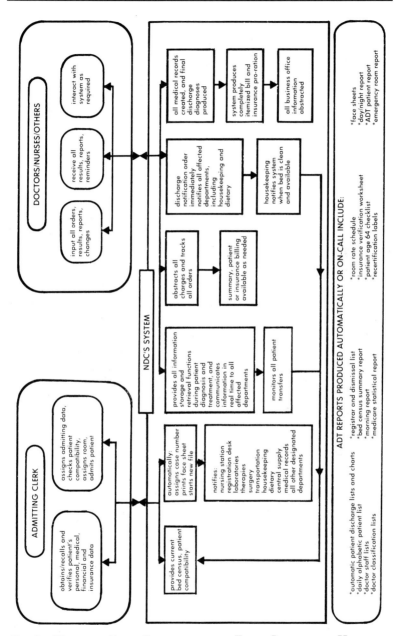

FIG. 8 – NATIONAL DATA COMMUNICATIONS FULLY INTEGRATED HOSPITAL
INFORMATION SYSTEM – ADMISSIONS/DISCHARGES/TRANSFERS SUBSYSTEM

Reprinted with permission of Charles J. Austin, *Information Systems for Hospital Administration.*
Health Administration Press, 1979.

the business office is notified so the patient bill remains current. When the patient is discharged, the nursing station personnel log (enter) the patient's discharge. This entry automatically notifies housekeeping to prepare the bed for the next patient, dietary to stop meal service, admissions that the bed is available, the business office to begin finalization of the patient bill if this has not already been completed, and medical records to obtain the patient record for discharge analysis and abstracting.

This system also generates a number of reports either automatically or on demand. These include discharge listings, daily census, morning reports, and utilization review logs. R-ADT systems are also sometimes linked to outpatient departments so clinics can be notified the patient will be coming. Some outpatient departments have separate ADT systems to follow the patient as he moves through the clinics.

UTILIZATION REVIEW SCREENING

Utilization review screening systems can be developed as part of larger R-ADT systems or can be independent systems. These systems can generate listings of review dates, days certified, review labels, and other pertinent data. They can also provide the utilization review coordinator with a patient data base when needed.

CHART COMPLETION SYSTEMS

Chart completion systems (CCS) provide the medical record department with an efficient tool for tracking physician chart completion compliance. The medical record professional can log onto the system using a VDT and call up physician data on the screen. Deficiencies can be entered and stored in computer memory. The program will then generate a number of reports upon demand by the user. A physician can request a listing of his deficient charts. Chart deficiency summary reports can also be generated which list the number of deficient charts for each physician, grouped according to service such as medicine or surgery.

CHART LOCATION AND TRACKING SYSTEMS

Many types of chart location and tracking systems are found in health facilities. PHAMIS contains a chart tracking module that not only shows where the chart is presently located, but also gives a history of where it has been by displaying clinic names and the dates when the patient chart was sent to these locations.

GENERAL PERSONAL COMPUTER BUSINESS SOFTWARE APPLICATIONS

The personal microcomputer such as the IBM-PC has software that can be utilized by medical record professionals. Some practitioners are presently using these programs to prepare budgets, maintain department files, and prepare reports with graphics applications. Future use is expected to increase as medical record professionals become more sophisticated computer users.

The electronic spreadsheet is one type which converts the video screen into a columnar matrix of cells many rows long and columns wide. These programs produce as many as 254 rows and 63 columns. The user can move the display across the matrix to view all the cells or use only a few cells. These spreadsheets operate by giving each cell of the matrix a title and type of value. Columns can be labeled with formulas which will automatically total other rows or columns or perform other desired calculations. When a change is made in one cell of the spreadsheet, the contents of all other related cells are instantly changed to reflect the new information. This enables a medical record department director preparing a budget to determine what would happen if a variety of different allocations of financial resources were applied to the budget without recalculating or redoing entire sections of the document. Some of the most popular spreadsheet programs are Visicalc and Multiplan, the latter being easiest to use.

Word processing software is also available for microcomputers. These programs allow personal computers to operate in similar fashion to the dedicated word processors that are described in the chapter on word processing. Two of the most popular software packages at the present time are Wordstar and Microsoft Word.

Another business software of use to medical record professionals is a Data Base Management System (DBMS). DBMSs store information in files on floppy disks. Users access the files by any type of data element, sort lists and search for desired items of information. These systems also generate reports that are designed by the user without the use of a programming language. The reader can readily see that these systems perform tasks similar to those described for larger facility-wide data bases. The advantage of these DBMSs is that they are controlled by the user of the software and can be used for any purpose that meets the needs of the medical record department. The family of software including FILE and REPORT are two simple examples that can be used together to produce reports. D-Base II is a more complex and powerful software DBMS. Small DBMSs are appropriate for specific department internal files such as maintaining lists and research data.

These software types have also been combined together into single programs that are called integrated software. These packages combine spreadsheets, DBMS, word processing, and graphics capability in one unit. The user can move easily from one mode to another without changing programs. This allows the user to use a spreadsheet by drawing data from a file prepared with a DBMS, and then produce graphs from these data. This information can then be included in a report written with the word processing section. Two popular examples of this type of integrated software are Lotus 123 and Symphony.

In summary, microcomputer usage will become more widespread as LANs are established in health facilities and as providers utilize VAN capability. Increasing computer literacy requirements for successful job functioning are expected to continue for the foreseeable future. The personal computer is a useful tool that can provide many applications to expedite medical record department functions.

FUTURE TRENDS

The rapid technological expansion of computerization in health care is expected to continue, limited only by the availability of funding. Automation of information handling is expected to bring opportunities for increased productivity and quality of patient care. Medical record professionals, as users of these systems, can expect to play an active role in the development and selection of application software for functions that impact their departments. Medical record professionals must, therefore, develop the knowledge, skills, and interests which allow them to participate effectively in this process.

Computers are only tools for data handling. The information that is produced by these systems is only as valid as the data entered into the system. Medical record professionals must be concerned with the quality of data used. They must also continue to protect the confidentiality and privacy of patient data that are so readily available at VDTs and printers throughout health care facilities. As the medical record becomes more fragmented and dispersed throughout these systems, safeguards must be provided to control access, accuracy, and retention throughout the HIS. An in-depth discussion of these issues is beyond the scope of this chapter, but privacy and data quality are surely two of the most significant challenges facing the medical record profession in the Information Age.

SUMMARY

This chapter is intended to serve as an introduction to computer use in health care facilities as it impacts medical record departments. Basic information on computer systems has been described including an explanation of the data processing cycle. Computer system configurations common to health facilities are defined. Applications that impact medical record departments have been illustrated. Future trends toward LAN and VAN are identified, concluding with projections of future knowledge, skills, and roles for medical record professionals.

GLOSSARY

Applications Software – Software that enables the computer to perform a function.

Bar Code – Series of lines that represents data such as MRA by a pattern of vertical lines of various widths that can be read by a light pen.

BASIC (Beginner's All-Purpose Symbolic Instruction Code) – Programming language available on most types of computers.

Coaxial Cable – Communication line consisting of a multitude of wires within a cable housing used to connect a computer system and its parts.

CPU – Central Processing Unit which performs actual processing.

CRT (Cathode-Ray Tube) – Input/output TV screenlike unit; sometimes called video terminal.

Data Bank – Large collection of information which allows information to be stored and accessed.

Data Bank Management System – Software packages called file manager systems that allow users to establish files and access them easily.

Electronic Mail (Electronic Text Transfer) – Communicates with other users through computer network.

Encode – To convert into code.

File – Collection of records.

Floppy Disk – Small oxide-coated disk used on a personal computer to store data; sometimes also called a diskette.

Hard Disk – Large oxide-coated metal disks sealed in dust-free containers used to store data.

HIS – Hospital Information System.

Input Operation – Operation that enters data into a computer system.

Integrated Software – Software packages that combine functions such as a word processor, spreadsheets, graphics, and file managers in a single package.

Local Area Network – Connected group of computers that form a communications network within a local area. (LAN).

Memory – Part of a computer system that stores data. Can be part of CPU (primary memory) or secondary storage such as hard disk or tape.

Minicomputer – Middle-size computer commonly found in HC facilities.

MIS – Management Information System.

Modem – Device that changes digital data produced by a computer to an analog signal that can be transmitted over telephone lines. It will change all analog to digital data for receipt by computer at the end of transmission.

Network – Any system of two or more computers.

On-Line – A device directly connected to a computer for interactive processing.

Operating System – Program that controls routine actions of a computer system.

Output Devices – Devices that make information generated by computer available for user.

Personal Computers – Small computers also called minicomputers.

Program – Series of instructions called software that direct a computer to perform operations.

System – Network of related procedures that performs a particular function.

Value Added Network – Data communication network that can be accessed by subscribers to the service by computer via a modem and telephone connection. (VAN).

Video Terminal – Analogous with CRT.

STUDY QUESTIONS

1. Describe a computer system.

2. Identify the five operations a computer can perform, and explain each.

3. Define a system, and identify five subsystems found in health care facilities.

4. Differentiate between input and output devices and storage. Describe two types of each device.

5. Identify and explain the difference between the three general sizes of computer systems.

6. Define software, hardware, and explain the relationship between the two concepts.

7. Define HIS, and explain the differences between type A and B systems. Describe/identify five types of medical record department applications.

8. Describe the two major types of computer figures found in health care facilities.

9. Define LAN topology. What three topologies are used with local area networks?

10.   Identify and describe one type of HIS application that impacts the entire health facility.

11.   Identify and describe three types of microcomputer business software useful in a medical record department. Define integrated software.

12.   Identify two future trends in health care computing.

REFERENCES

ACHESON, E. D. *Medical Record Linkage.* New York, New York: Oxford University Press, 1967.

AUSTIN, CHARLES J. *Information Systems for Hospital Administration.* Ann Arbor, Michigan: Health Administration Press, 1979.

BALL, MARION J. and HANNAH, KATHRYN J. *Using Computers in Nursing.* Reston: Reston Publishing Company, Inc., 1984.

BURCH, JOHN G., STRATER, FELIX R., and GRUDNITSKI, GARY. *Information Systems: Theory and Practice.* 3rd Ed. New York, New York: John Wiley & Sons, 1979.

CHRISTENSEN, WILLIAM W., and STEARNS, EUGENE I. *Microcomputers in Health Care Management.* Rockville, Maryland: Aspen Systems Corporation, 1984.

COLLEN, MORRIS F. *Hospital Computer Systems.* New York, New York: John Wiley & Sons, 1974.

COVEY, H. DOMINIC, and MCALISTER, NEIL H. *Computers in the Practice of Medicine.* Vol. 1 & 2. Reading, Massachusetts: Addison-Wesley Publishing Company, 1980.

DAYHOFF, RUTH E., Ed. *Proceedings of the Seventh Annual Symposium on Computer Applications in Medical Care.* Los Angeles, California: The Computer Society Press. IEEE Computer Society, 1983.

DOLOGITE, D. G. *Using Small Business Computers.* Englewood Cliffs, New Jersey: Prentice-Hall, Inc., 1984.

HODGE, MELVILLE. *Medical Information Systems.* Germantown, Pennsylvania: Aspen Systems Corporation, 1977.

Hospital Computer Systems Planning: Preparation of Request for Proposal. Chicago, Illinois: American Hospital Association, 1980.

JENKIN, MICHAEL A., Ed. *A Manual of Computers in Medical Practice.* Edina: Society for Computer Medicine, 1977.

KROEBER, DONALD W., and WATSON, HUGH J. *Computer-Based Information Systems: A Management Approach.* New York, New York: Macmillan Publishing Company, 1984.

LINDBERG, DONALD A. B. *The Growth of Medical Information Systems in the United States.* Lexington, Massachusetts: Lexington Books, 1979.

Proceedings of the Sixth International Congress on Medical Records, 1972.

Proceedings of the Seventh International Congress on Medical Records, 1976.

SCHMITZ, HOMER H. *Hospital Information Systems.* Germantown, Pennsylvania: Aspen Systems Corporation, 1979.

SHELLY, GARY B., and CASHMAN, THOMAS J. *Computer Fundamentals for an Information Age.* Brea, California: Anaheim Publishing Company, Inc., 1984.

SYNNOTT, WILLIAM R., and GRUBER, WILLIAM. *Information Resource Management Opportunities and Strategies for the 1980's.* New York, New York: John Wiley & Sons, 1981.

WATERS, KATHLEEN A., and MURPHY, GRETCHEN F. *Systems Analysis and Computer Applications in Health Information Management.* Rockville, Maryland: Aspen Systems Corporation, 1983.

chapter 16

WORD PROCESSING MANAGEMENT
IN TRANSCRIPTION AND
MEDICAL RECORD SERVICES

INTRODUCTION

The development of sophisticated equipment for word processing has greatly increased the hospital's ability to handle the increase of patient care data being received in and generated by the medical record department. Standard repetitive letters which are typed by a secretary; the final report of a patient care study; error-free medical transcriptions; procedure manuals; tumor registry correspondence; proposal development; all of these functions, and many more can benefit from automated word processing assistance.

In the simplest context, word processing is the use of electronic equipment to type, change, print, and permanently store information. Some say it is another generation of a typewriter. Others categorize it as a low-level computer. Many feel it is the first level of the totally automatic office, while those not as optimistic predict it is only a temporary phase in office automation. In reality, word processing is all of these things. It is a system made up of people, equipment, and procedures which has evolved to produce more efficient and economical business correspondence. Word processing has existed ever since the first spoken word was written down. From the chisel and stone records of ancient times, various revolutions in the processing of thoughts have occurred – development of paper; recording devices such as chalk, pencils, fountain pens, erasable pens; the printing press; offset printing; the phonograph; the typewriter;

dictation equipment; magnetic media; the television screen; the microchip. Emphasis on productivity in the completion of routine tasks has revolutionized the office of today.

THE EVOLUTION OF THE WORD PROCESSOR

Around the turn of the twentieth century, the mechanical typewriter eliminated the need to hand copy paperwork. It was a major revolution which brought people and equipment together to produce information and speed the process of business communication. In the 1930s automated typewriters were introduced with a device (punched rolls of paper similar to those used in player pianos) which allowed the storage and playback of individual letters or whole paragraphs. Magnetic cards and tape replaced the paper rolls in the 1960s, and a revolutionary typing element, which stayed stationary rather than moving across the carriage, made faster typing speeds possible.

In 1964 the Magnetic Tape Selectric Typewriter (MT/ST)* allowed original copy to be typed directly onto magnetic tape. Errors could be corrected by backspacing and typing over existing material. Once a final draft was entered on the tape, typewritten copy was produced by pushing a button. The correction process was very time consuming, sometimes taking more time than it would take to retype the material. These problems were solved by the development of the Mag Card Selectric Typewriter (MC/ST)* which utilized magnetic cards with a one card/one page format and won operator acceptance where the MT/ST had failed. With the Mag Card, the typist could visualize the work in progress. The Mag Tape Cassette followed in the early 1970s, and a new industry was born.

The computer evolution paralleled that of word processing; and when the video screen for the computer was added, the modern word processor was born. The typist could visualize the page before it was produced, make whatever changes were necessary, and print out the work instantly.

A word processor is a piece of equipment which captures and stores information on some type of magnetic medium. It uses the standard QWERTY Keyboard (referring to the first six letters in the second row of the standard typewriter). It differs

*Products of International Business Machines.

from a typewriter, however, because it can also store and reproduce information with a few simple commands.

COMPONENTS OF WORD PROCESSING SYSTEMS

The same components are contained in all word processing
systems. What makes each system unique, functional, and flexible is the way in which the components are put together. Each
system contains a screen, keyboard, computer, storage or memory, and a printer (see Figure 1). This comprises the hardware
of the system. The program instructions for the computer component are found in the many types of software prepared for the
system. While a standard mainframe computer processes data
representing numbers, a word processor is a computer limited
to processing data representing letters. For most standard applications, mathematical calculations are beyond the capabilities
of a word processor.

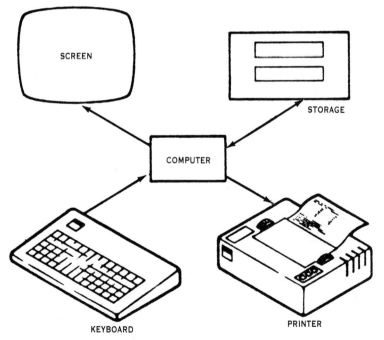

Reprinted with permission from Arthur Naiman, "Word Processing Buyer's Guide." BYTE. Copyright by McGraw-Hill.

FIG. 1 – BASIC COMPONENTS OF A WORD PROCESSOR.

Each component of the word processing system can be augmented to meet the individual needs of the user. Keyboards can be attached to the screen or can be free-standing. The memory can be stored on removable or permanent media. Printers run from very basic to sophisticated letter quality. The computer can come in many different sizes. The word processing system may be independent, or it can be an option available within a data processing system.

THE KEYBOARD

The word processing keyboard looks like and has the touch of the IBM Selectric Keyboard. In addition to the standard typewriter keys, the keyboard has a number of function keys which instruct the computer or the screen to do things which cannot be done on a typewriter. Each manufacturer has its own design of function keys, and the equipment manuals provide clear and graphic instructions to the operator on their use.

The keyboard may be attached to the screen (in which case it is known as a video display terminal or VDT), or it can be separate and movable, attached by a cable. Newer word processing equipment is being designed almost exclusively with detached keyboards, because they are more versatile and ergonomically preferred.

THE SCREEN

The screen of a word processor resembles a computer terminal screen. It is a cathode-ray tube (CRT) which produces the image of the key pressed. Screens can display a full page or a partial page and are more often designed with green or blue letters on a black/gray background to ease the eyestrain reported by users.

THE COMPUTER

The "brain" of the word processor is a computer and it has the same potential as any computer except that it is usually limited in its capacity for instructions, its mathematical programmability, and its storage capacity. In the computer are microchips, circuit boards, and central processing unit (CPU) boards in numbers and combinations necessary to service the capacity of the equipment. The computer is basically a magnetic field and is affected by all the things which bother dedicated computers – power surges, dust, heat, cigarette smoke, magnets, and static electricity. The capacity of the computer is dependent upon the equipment's ability to be expanded as far as hardware is concerned and the availability of the compatible software programs.

THE MEMORY

The storage or memory of the word processor is also flexible and usually expandable, although many models on the market are at their limit when they are sold. There are four common devices for storing material electronically: magnetic cards, magnetic tape, floppy disks, and hard or fixed disks. Magnetic cards are not as popular as they once were, and the phasing out of magnetic card equipment in offices will continue to reduce their use.

The larger the word processing systems the more likely that rigid disks will be utilized for storage. Floppies are versatile and portable, and both 5½" and 8" disks are used in word processors.

Because of a lack of standardization in the computer industry, material stored on disks cannot usually be processed by equipment from different manufacturers; so disks of the same size are often not interchangeable. The storage capacity of a word processor is measured in the same manner as a dedicated computer, in *bytes*, with each byte representing one typed character, typed space, line return, etc. The actual storage is specified in kilobytes (or thousands of characters).

The industry estimates that a business word averages 5 characters with an additional character allowed for the space between the words. Therefore, measuring the storage capacity of word processing equipment should be done using a 6-character word. The capacity should be evaluated based upon the type of material which will be stored. Table 1 summarizes guidelines for evaluating word processing capacities.

It is very important that the storage needs of the word processor are clear, because storage capacities are generally marketed at their most generous amount. However, up to 20 percent of the storage capacity is taken up by software and text organization purposes leaving only 80 percent for working purposes.

TABLE 1

EVALUATING WORD PROCESSING CAPACITIES

Byte – One character
Kilobyte (K-bytes) – One thousand twenty-four (1,024) characters
Megabyte (MB) – One thousand K-bytes or 1,048,576 bytes
32K, 48K, 64K – Common storage sizes for word processing disks

To Estimate Word Processing Capacity Needs:

"Word" equals 6 bytes: 6 characters (5-letter word plus space)

250 words (1,500 bytes) equals one page or about 1½K usually one typed page of double-spaced pica text with one-inch margins all around

Disk Capacity

5¼" disk – 50 pages (allowance for storage included)
8" disk – 600 pages (typically holds 250K)

Fixed Memory

90 Kilobytes = 15,000 words or 60 pages
1 Megabyte = 166,000 words or 664 pages
10 K-bytes should be allowed for text organization

THE PRINTER

The printer is the most important component of the word processor, because the users will judge the appearance of the finished product. Printers are often more expensive than any or all of the other components. They may require more service calls and create operator frustration.

There are various styles of printers: Impact, Dot Matrix, Jet Ink, Daisy Wheel, Thimble, and Laser printers (which do not usually have applications in medical record departments). Peripheral equipment such as sheet feeders, form tractors, acoustic covers, and envelope feeders can be added to printers depending upon the needs of the user.

The speed of the printer is important, because text production of more than a few pages will take an inordinate amount of time unless the printer operates at least 10-40 characters per second (CPS). Bidirectional printing (the printing mechanism goes from left to right, drops down and returns from right to left) is actually controlled by the computer component but is a time saver, because it reduces the traveling distance of the carriage by half over the standard typewriter style. The sophistication of the software instructions available for the printer should be weighed against the real needs of the user, because such instructions take up valuable bytes which reduce the text storage capabilities of the equipment.

WORD PROCESSING SYSTEMS

The word processing components discussed above can be arranged in stand alone, shared, or dedicated computer systems.

Stand Alone – The word processing system and the equipment are one and the same thing. The machine is self-contained and operates independently. Many stand alones are designed to be networked into bigger systems, but only one person at a time can use a stand-alone system.

Shared Resource – A clustered or shared logic system includes a variety of ways to use the components, and several persons can use the equipment simultaneously. The computer (and often the printer) are shared by several keyboards. The advantages of a shared resource system include efficient media storage and advanced software capabilities; one disadvantage is that when the system is down, all users are idle.

Dedicated Computers – Word processing software is available for most computer systems and microcomputers. The dedicated word processing equipment is easier to use and more versatile than word processing software on a mainframe; but for some applications, it may not provide enough text-editing capabilities to satisfy the needs of the user.

EVALUATING WORD PROCESSING SYSTEMS

The first step in addressing whether word processing capabilities are desirable in a medical record department is to determine where word processing can be used. Volumes of text management, text editing report writing, and updating functions lend themselves to automation. It is possible that the institution may already have made decisions about word processing equipment over which the department head has little or no control. But in most large independent offices such as medical record departments, proposals for the design of the system and its configuration are the responsibility of the manager of the area. When potential applications are considered, a feasibility study and definition of requirements should precede any equipment evaluation.

THE FEASIBILITY STUDY

Starting with the hypothesis that a word processing system would be cost effective for the facility, a feasibility study may then be undertaken. Its purpose is to make clear what word processing needs will be and how they can best be addressed. The selection of a specific system should be objective and reliable; that is, given the same set of factors, a second evaluator would follow the same steps. Because personal preference and judgment play a role in the feasibility process, another evaluator may not conclude the study with the same choice; and, therefore, the study report must identify those areas where subjective elements are present. A study cannot be done without these subjective elements, and they should not be glossed over or overlooked.

The study should include the following:

1. Discussion of the organizational structure involved (by section, department, division, or overall, whichever is appropriate to the study).

   If, for example, the hospital has committed itself to centralized information processing, acknowledgement of this policy is important. If no policy exists, that should also be mentioned.

2. Present work flow patterns and production volumes.

3. Strengths and weaknesses of the present paperwork production systems.

4. Applications to be addressed and how they will be affected (including clear projections of time and cost savings, convenience factors, and short and long term benefits).

The study should answer these three questions:

– What are the actual needs of the department?

– Will word processing benefit the organization?

– What are the objectives which will be addressed if word processing is implemented?

A feasibility study is just as important to complete if the

hypothesis at the beginning cannot be supported after the study has been completed. The evaluative exercise is an important management skill, valuable time was spent conducting it, and the report will speak for itself.

REQUIREMENTS DEFINITION

The data collected during the feasibility study will become the outline of the word processing system, should it appear that such an expenditure is justified. The specific applications can be elaborated upon and refined, and the blueprint of the system configuration, work stations, and peripheral interfacing devices will begin to evolve. It is at this point that the structure and placement of the equipment will be considered. Ordinarily there are three choices: centralized, decentralized, or a combination of both. Personal considerations, types of work stations, placement of printers, and the flexibility/expandability questions should be thought through at this step in the process.

Although idealistic, a word of caution about equipment selection is appropriate – remember who the buyer of the equipment is! It is desirable to conduct the feasibility study and requirement definitions independently. It is wise not to involve any vendor until one reaches this part of the process, because a vendor's objective differs from that of a buyer. During the first two steps, there is opportunity to investigate what is available on the market; but this should be done carefully, objectively, and, above all, competitively. An astute manager will avoid the soft sell, supportive sell, and other techniques of vendors until the purchasing activities begin sometime in the future, not in the study process.

The purchasing environment of today is competitive and bid-oriented. When the time comes to begin evaluating equipment, the requirements already outlined provide the basic checklist. The materials management or purchasing department of the hospital should be consulted and involved when sales representatives are consulted. They can coordinate and control vendor access to the department; and a good purchasing agent can lend an experienced, objective viewpoint to the sales arena. If the bidding process is standard to the hospital, a purchasing agent can also assist in preparing specifications tailored to the needs of the user rather than to a vendor's equipment. Many different equipment checklists are published in trade magazines and vendor brochures, and a literature search of consumer-oriented publications will lend direction to the method the manager may want to follow in evaluating competitive equipment.

SPACE PLANNING

As the blueprint of the word processing application is developed, some consideration must be given to space planning. What will be centralized? Can the area be ventilated and cooled properly? What is the traffic pattern? Are the office furniture and its arrangement suitable for the planned application? Where will the printers go? These questions and many related ones may be identified when the staff of the area are involved with the planning and feasibility study. They can help evaluate a proposal and are the best source when developing ideas for work-area planning and specific equipment configuration.

The justification of the cost and cost benefits must be considered in the requirements assessment. The impact of the equipment on staffing levels, productivity, additional services, equipment options, staff development, and related indirect costs should be identified and analyzed.

PURCHASING WORD PROCESSING EQUIPMENT

If the proposal for word processing contains a significant capital equipment investment, capital budget approval must be secured. Many times thorough preliminary work done up to this point will be enough for the materials management department to estimate the expenditure. For other proposals, the entire equipment selection process will have to be completed. There is often a 12-18-month lead time for capital equipment approvals, however, and equipment vendors can be very persistent in securing sales. Spending a great deal of time on equipment selection prematurely will not replace the prepurchase reviews. If the materials management estimates can be incorporated into the budget proposals, less time will be required for periodic "social" sales calls during the interim between capital budget and purchase.

Proposals for system changes are not only evaluated on their expressed and implied merit, but on the organization and conduct of the feasibility study, the thoroughness of the evaluation process, the logic of the option being proposed, and the presentation and clarity of the written report. The writer of the proposal should be prepared to defend the choices verbally, as most projects of this size will require open discussion.

GOING TO THE MARKETPLACE

Once approval has been secured, and the time frame of the purchase is established; the actual equipment available can be evaluated. At this point the clear definition of needs and objectives already prepared will be invaluable. These should guide the course of the equipment interviews, and never be too far away when the "bells and whistles" are displayed. Too much reliance on one particular vendor up to this point will severely limit the purchaser's ability to be objective and search out the best product. Vendor equipment terminology will vary considerably. Word processing software comes in many sizes and capabilities. Lack of industry standards will make comparisons difficult. To minimize the confusion of the equipment evaluation, several simple steps can be followed:

1. Always keep the plan and needs list handy.
2. Organize a survey team of personnel involved (materials management, plant engineering, supervisor, department or section head and an operator, etc.)
3. See the equipment in use preferably in a setting similar to the one planned.
4. Discuss each type of equipment with current users rather than just sales representatives. Obtain independent access to service representatives, if possible, to review the proposal and equipment configurations.
5. Investigate service and staff support thoroughly; because once the equipment is installed, the sales staff are no longer available.
6. Involve the hospital's data processing department to review compatability expansion and networking capabilities. The equipment selected should be the equipment which best meets the defined needs, at the best price.

A general checklist of considerations for equipment is found in Table 2. Purchasing agents involved in the evaluation process can be very helpful in negotiating prices.

Experienced practitioners report that even with the best

evaluation process there are always questions which are never asked. For example:

- What about service calls on weekends?
- What air filtering and dedicated electrical wiring will be needed?
- What related supplies have been overlooked (disks, backup equipment, ribbons, etc.)?
- Training not included with implementation: What is "advanced" and what will it cost?
- How will the room be kept cool in the heat of the summer?

TABLE 2
CHECKLIST FOR EQUIPMENT CONSIDERATION

Functions of Equipment

Safety and Error Handling
Losing material, backup, clarity of error messages, automatic verification sensitivity to environment.

Editing/Formatting
Word wrap, scrolling, blockmove and copy, global search, text insert, edit while printing, line spacing, headers and footers, centering, proportional spacing, underscoring, page numbers, etc.

Software Components
Dictionary, calculations, output, questions, productivity monitoring, etc., multifunctionality, upgradeability.

Equipment Hardware
Integration/Versatility
Programmability, data processing, capabilities, compatibility, expandability, storage capacity.

Peripherals
Modularity, specific features of printer and storage media, potential for expansion.

Human Engineering
Training/Staff Development
User friendly, ease of use to edit/format, training time.

Ergonomics
Tiltable screens, adjustable screens and keyboards, eyestrain, heat output, noise levels.

AUTOMATION IN MEDICAL TRANSCRIPTION

The nature of medical transcription lends itself easily to word processing automation. The large blocks of text in medical transcription are not often edited and revised after they are stored, but the ease in correcting general spelling errors, the dictator's change of mind in mid-sentence or paragraph, and the proofreading opportunities afforded by the word processor while the report is being transcribed, are strong and persuasive reasons to automate production. Transcribers also can enter more material into a word processor than can be entered in the same time at the typewriter, because the ball and element mechanics of the impact typewriter slow the process down. Since speed printers produce the printed material independently, most industry experts agree that word processing can increase a transcriber's output by 25-30 percent even before the merits and uses of general text editing and formatting are considered.

A manager must realize that productivity increases will vary in each application. If 30 percent more paper is generated in the transcription area, staffing the separating, processing, and distribution of the increased paper must be considered. Often the clerical duties added to the word processing operation are underestimated even if considered initially, because many operators expect these duties to be transferred to someone whose productivity is less scrutinized.

Traditionally the following reports have been produced in a centralized transcription center, usually located within the medical record department, with turnaround times specified as follows:

	Within
History and Physicals	24 hrs.
Consultations	24 hrs.
Reports of Operations	48 hrs.
Discharge Summaries	72 hrs.

Other traditional transcribed reports which may be centralized in the transcription center or may be the responsibility of the respective departments include:

	Within
Radiology	24 hrs.
Cardiovascular	
(Noninvasive)	24 hrs.
EKG	24 hrs.
Pathology	24 hrs.
Other Special	
Diagnostics	24 hrs.

Today's need for legible documentation has resulted in other reports, previously handwritten to become transcribed:

	Within
Emergency Department	24 hrs.
Clinic Notes	24 hrs.
Physical Therapy	24 hrs.
Pulmonary Function	24 hrs.
Industrial Medicine	24 hrs.

Whether a hospital is able to provide transcription services to departments which never used them before will depend upon the need for the service, legibility and continuity of care concerns, and the human and material resources available. As more transcribed material is added to the medical record, however, it is more likely that automated approaches to producing the output will be needed.

Standardization of portions of reports considered "routine" can be a time-saving factor for both the dictator and the operator. However, the processing of variable data into standardized reports takes time and usually becomes a duty of a transcription-support clerk because it interferes with the routine production of the individual operator. Controls must be instituted with this practice so a "standard" is individualized with specific patient variables to guard against "canned" reports.

DICTATION EQUIPMENT

Dictation equipment must be considered when word processing equipment is introduced into medical transcription because the input methods will have an effect on the manner in which output plans are made.

Convenience and proximity to nursing units, operating rooms, emergency rooms, clinics, and general patient intake areas will enhance the timeliness of dictation by physicians. If certain types of reports are to be transcribed centrally, the proximity of dictating equipment to work stations for radiologists, EKG readers, etc. is essential. Dictation formats guiding physicians through basic identifying information and outline headings for reports will assist in producing complete reports and save time for the transcriptionists in looking up case numbers and room numbers.

DICTATION MEDIA

The media on which medical transcription is recorded will be either self-contained or discrete. Discrete media include cassettes, minicassettes, microcassettes, and belts or disks which can be removed from the dictation equipment for transcription. Self-contained media such as endless loop, tape, or tanks are not physically handled by the operator. The advantages to discrete media are that they are all tangible, can be distributed quickly, have a visually measurable end, and can be counted. The disadvantages are that they can be more easily lost or misplaced, and forethought must be used to insure that ample supplies are available for dictation peaks and low staffed times.

The advantages of self-contained media are that there is no media handling, input priorities are well controlled, and lost dictation is minimal. Disadvantages include difficult access to stat work buried in a tank, volume recording cannot be distributed easily, and rerecording is necessary for some work distribution needs (particularly if certain work is being sent out to a service).

WORD MEASUREMENT IN TRANSCRIPTION

Turnaround standards will often be set in medical staff bylaws, rules, and regulations. They may also be affected by reimbursement, third-party payer, and personal preferences of dictators. It is essential, however, that the timely processing of dictated material be related to the needs of the patient care team for continuity of care and communication between practitioners. There are many demands today for instant transcription, and the hospital must evaluate the merits of this high level of service against the cost of such production and look at streamlining dictation practices as well as increasing transcription speeds. The organization of the dictation system must allow the identification of reports by turnaround standards in order to put first things first. Material promised in two hours cannot be buried with that which has a five-day turnaround. Since almost everything is desired the next day, even priorities within a 24-hour work period must be set. A single transcriptionist working the Friday afternoon shift, for example, must have clear guidelines on what to do first when EKGs, x-rays, and consults are awaiting transcription.

INPUT AND OUTPUT MEASURES

Volumes of transcription can be measured in terms of input or output. Input techniques count minutes of dictation, through the dictation equipment, and then utilize conversion formulas to represent work produced. Output techniques count printed lines produced and utilize the word processing equipment where counters can be found within the computer software or on the printers. In developing a method of work measurement, the key is the definition of a unit of measure. Transcription is most often measured in "lines." A line is designated to contain a certain number of keystrokes, i.e., 50, 55, 60, 78, 84, etc. (any number can be used). Commercial service agencies often use 50 characters to a line, which translates into a five-inch line of pica type (10 characters per inch) or slightly more than a four-inch line of elite type (12 characters per inch). Since a typed line of transcription is closer to seven and one-half inches long, a report of 10 typed lines can vary considerably in "line length" depending upon the definition of the line.

Once the department has agreed upon a "line," either output or input standards can be developed, depending upon equipment capabilities. Input conversion factors of 1:10, 11, or 12 (one minute of dictation equals 10, 11, or 12 lines) are commonly used. The choice of the conversion factor is then based upon time studies which can be conducted. The variable in input conversions is the speed of the dictator, and it will vary between dictators, but a representative sample in the study should result in an acceptable average. The variable in output conversions is how keystrokes are counted, and what portion of a line will be counted. Using either the printer or the word processor as the counter requires a software application; and if done on the printer, some additional capabilities are needed when a printer is shared by more than one transcriptionist.

STAFFING ESTIMATES

Because it is relatively straight production work, individual output measurements and requirements are common in medical transcription, i.e. the same type of work comes in and goes out each day and, therefore, is easy to count. When the definition of a line has been established, and an equitable method of keeping track of production is developed, gross personnel requirements can be estimated by dividing what has to be done by what one person can reasonably be expected to do. There are many published standards on minimum daily production targets for medical transcriptionists. Most, however, do not define the line equivalent; and because of this, comparisons are difficult. The most often mentioned are 800-1,000 lines per day on an IBM Selectric Typewriter and 1,000-1,500 lines per day on word processing equipment.

Other acceptable measurements which may be used are word counts, words per minute, cassettes typed, and number of reports or pages typed. See Table 3 for an estimate of gross staffing for one transcription department. This gross estimate of full-time equivalents must be qualified by turnaround expectations and paid time off before staffing patterns can be established. Tracking volumes by type of report, actual turnarounds (average but also worst examples) and dictation patterns will be necessary so staffing is organized for the best return. For example, dictation of history and physicals is often heavier on Sundays and late in the afternoons (dictation patterns); emergency department dictation is heaviest on afternoons and weekends; operative reports are usually dictated during the day, as are discharge summaries. More dictation with 24-hour turnaround is available for afternoon-shift production; consults may be evenly distributed throughout the seven days of the week.

Profiling dictation patterns in light of turnaround times will be necessary if limited staffing resources are to be used properly. There is staff resistance to weekend, evening, midnight and holiday scheduling, especially if it represents a change from current scheduling. But as faster service is demanded, more complex personnel scheduling is necessary.

The conclusion drawn from the example hospital in Table 3 reflects production in terms of working days. Paid days off are not accounted for in this example. Employees on vacation or using sick time and personal days are not contributing a workday of 1,000 lines when they are not there.

TABLE 3
ESTIMATE OF GROSS STAFFING

Community Hospital

Bed Capacity – 200 beds
Average Occupancy – 82%

Dictation Transcribed:

    History and Physical
    Operating Room Summaries
    Labor and Delivery Summaries
    Industrial Clinic Notes
    EKGs
    Consultations
    Other Reports

Average Lines per Month – 160,000

Daily Production Minimum Set – 1,000 lines

Minimum Workdays for Volume – 160 $\frac{160,000}{1,000}$

Number of Workdays in Month – 20

Minimum Number of Full-Time Equivalents (FTEs) to Handle Work – 8 $\frac{160}{20}$

To best estimate staffing requirements, a 15 percent adjustment factor should be added. In that case 9.2 FTEs would be a solid staffing target for the Community Hospital, provided 160,000 lines represent the average volume of transcription.

QUALITY CONTROL

Productivity management in medical transcription includes quality control programs which provide ongoing or periodic proofreading procedures; playout controls; and in-service training in new drugs, equipment, and surgical instruments. Standard formats should be in place, and examples of the reports generated should be filed in a central manual. Many transcription centers also file examples of routine dictations and specialized operative procedures for easy reference.

The institution of word processing equipment with continuous forms will standardize reporting; software programming will standardize report format. Training and orientation programs provide an excellent opportunity to monitor work production and should be in place as a routine process even for the most experienced newly hired transcriptionist. Between the microprocessed dictation equipment and word processors, the medical transcriptionist has become a sophisticated office-equipment operator. Because so much medical transcription is done on the second and third shift, each transcriptionist must be prepared to perform independently of a supervisor.

The quality control program should include methods to evaluate the independence of the medical transcriptionist both in work-priority selection, transcription production, and equipment usage and maintenance. Organized proofreading is a quality-control practice that is becoming more prevalent in transcription departments. Proofreading programs can vary from placing all the responsibility on the transcriptionist to hiring employees to proofread. An interim approach, if hiring proofreaders is prohibitive, assigns the supervisor or a team of transcriptionists to spot-check a certain amount of work from each employee on a regular basis. As the pressure for more production keeps building, measures to guarantee that the quality of the work is not suffering are required.

Acceptable error rates per completed page should be agreed upon by employees and management. Reports and summaries from the quality-control program in the department are a valuable component of work measurement plans such as incentive pay.

INCENTIVE PAY SYSTEMS

Because of the nature of medical transcription, incentive and bonus pay systems are often put in place where salary structure and work performance are based upon the quality and quantity of actual work produced. The following components should be included in the design of these pay systems:

- Equitable measurements of quantity of work produced
  - line counts defined
  - reliable methods of counting
  - procedures for recording production
- Equitable allocation/allowance for legitimate nonproductive time (in-service, department meetings, staff development, equipment down time, other employer demands)
  - adjust production up if nonproductive time is to be converted to equivalents of production
  - adjust work time down if nonproductive time is not to be credited
  - calculate production over longer periods of time where nonproductive time is spread evenly for all
- Competitive and reasonable pay policies
- Quality standards to counter speed problems
  - proofreading policies
  - standards for errors and error measurement

Incentive pay schemes can be organized to pay each employee in one of many ways:

- Strictly by the unit of measure (line, minute, page, etc.)
- A premium for units of measure over a minimum
- Utilizing a calculated average over a specified time period as a basis for determining an hourly rate

In the first application, using lines as the unit of measure, an employee would earn pay directly related to the work produced. In the second a minimum pay is guaranteed to the transcriptionist. Both of these methods offer immediate payoff to the transcriptionist. The first is most often found in independent transcription services, and the second is found in the hospitals. The nonproductive allocation allowance plus the necessity for daily bookkeeping are a few of the disadvantages of these two methods. A merit pay approach, where production totals are logged but averaged over longer periods of time, requires less bookkeeping and puts less pressure on the typist for a bad day or week. If the merit system is tied into annual or periodic hourly wage increases, the employees are rewarded for their production but not penalized for every reduction in output. For a merit system, the production targets are defined and correlated to step increases where the employee will merit a higher step increase depending upon average production. This third system is less threatening, requires less bookkeeping, and rewards employees for past work without the daily logging of nonproductive time.

GETTING THE WORK OUT

Word processing equipment also assists in finished work distribution as it is capable of being programmed to print on a distant printer. An in-house system can be configured so that reports are addressed to printers at nursing stations. Outside typing services can transcribe work off site and have it printed back at the hospital. Quality control and reporting can be set up automatically on the word processing equipment. Daily tallies of certain types of reports and error calculations can be programmed in to save many hours of manual counting and sorting. Proofreading dictionaries can be developed and applied to stored work before the work is printed.

OUTSIDE TRANSCRIPTION SERVICE AS AN ALTERNATIVE

If word processing is being evaluated to increase medical transcription production, the alternative of contracting with an outside service should also be investigated. In many areas, well-managed transcription companies which pick up the work or have it wired directly to their off-site offices are a viable and cost-effective option.

ADVANTAGES OF OUTSIDE SERVICES

Some of the advantages of off-site contracting are very attractive. The problems of personnel recruitment and retention are eliminated entirely, as are job orientations, training, and scheduling demands. Equipment purchase, maintenance, upgrading, downtime, and training on the transcription site are a thing of the past. Because the service agency has a vested interest in ease of dictation, equipment purchase and maintenance of dictating equipment becomes a shared responsibility. The requests for favors or other nonrelated typing projects, and problems with peak work, are also eliminated for the hospital. The contract with the service will specify turnaround times, and a well-negotiated contract should have financial or other consequences built in should turnaround times become a problem. A hospital which contracts all its work out will get production priority over a hospital which uses the service periodically, so a full-contract hospital usually gets the best service by the most experienced transcriptionists.

The quality of a report done by an outside company must be high in order to keep the customer happy, whereas the quality of in-house work often varies because of personnel, equipment and environmental pressures.

New facsimile, modem, and electronic equipment make it possible to receive instant printouts of work produced miles away. If the hospital wishes to limit its dictation equipment to in-house wiring, new speed recording devices allow for fast-forward recording from dictation equipment over telephone lines, thus eliminating the delivery and pickup delays. There are advantages to in-house transcription such as internal control, management experience and expertise, equipment availability for other word processing applications; responding to special requests, person to person contact for physicians, and confidentiality of in-house production, but space allocations and capital expenditure limitations often provide convincing reasons to investigate outside services.

When an evaluation of in-house and outside transcription production is undertaken, the existing program should be segmented into several components:

System Productivity – lines per productive hour, lines per paid hour, lines per full-time equivalent, etc.

System Responsiveness – actual turnaround times measured against standards, handling of priority work, personnel scheduling needs versus peak workload times, report transcription versus charting times, etc.

User Convenience – accessibility to dictator, user-satisfaction survey results, etc.

Report Quality – errors, error monitoring and proofreading needs, etc.

Employee Recruitment/Retention Potential – availability of experienced transcriptionists, on-the-job training capabilities, job satisfaction, competitive pay scales, programs or plans, scheduling of paid time off, etc.

Costs – direct and indirect cost schedules for internal production, price quotes for contracted services, overtime, and current contract costs.

Space – currently available space and future needs, feasibility of other uses if space were available.

Contract service may be interested in utilizing existing equipment (buying or leasing) and staffing the allocated space rather than sending the work to off-site offices if the hospital has some capital invested in transcription equipment, or there is significant objection to removing the work from the premises.

SELECTING AN OUTSIDE SERVICE

Many transcription services solicit business through direct mail campaigns, although a recommendation from another user is a much more reliable method of initial company identification. The company's reputation, user satisfaction, and financial stability are of primary concern. After the field has been narrowed down, the one or two companies in the running should be visited. Billing procedures, workflow, quality of reports, and employee morale can be observed. The company will become a direct extension of the medical record department, and it should exhibit a flexible and cooperative attitude in meeting the needs of the hospital.

Finally, a short term initial contract (three to six months) will provide the best opportunity to evaluate an outside service's ability to provide timely, quality transcription for the hospital.

OTHER WORD PROCESSING APPLICATIONS

There are other functions within the medical record department where word processing can be applied. Any function where a perfect copy is necessary should be evaluated if office automation capabilities are being considered.

The preparation and permanent storage of job descriptions and policy and procedure manuals can be greatly simplified when word processing equipment is utilized. Standard formats are designed, and the material is typed as it would be using an electric typewriter; but editing and revising it require only the retyping of the targeted segment, not the entire document.

DEPARTMENTAL FORMS AND FORM LETTERS

Standard routing forms, deficiency slips, form letters for correspondence, subpoena responses and certificates, new employee orientation checklists, employee skills inventories, outguide and sign-out forms (virtually any form used in the department) can be set up more easily with word processing equipment than on a typewriter.

INCOMPLETE RECORD PROCESSING

In addition to the setup of the deficiency form, all letters related to incomplete or delinquent records can be prepared on a word processor. Depending upon the other applications in use, the letters can be produced on the word processor; or the master form printed out and then copied or offset printed. If a dedicated word processor is used with list-merge software capabilities, the envelopes and original letters (with customized specifics related to each address) are an option to be automated. The only limits to these applications are those of the equipment and software in place.

TUMOR REGISTRY

The tumor registry utilizes forms for abstracting follow-up and reporting, both of which can be entered into a word processor. As with the suspension of privileges, correspondence such as follow-up letters and envelopes can be custom produced with certain software packages.

BIRTH CERTIFICATES

The error-free requirements of birth certificate processing make word processing an attractive solution. Some hospitals issue a birth verification form on special hospital stationery as a memento of the child's birth, and the correct data for the baby can be entered into the word processor where a perfect copy original can be produced. It is also possible to prepare the actual birth certificate on a word processor, but the time spent inserting the form into the printer may take longer than is justified. Other typing functions include lists for community welcoming agencies, newspapers, and local vital statistics offices.

MEDICAL STAFF ACTIVITIES

There are many applications for word processing in medical staff activity reporting:

Minutes – minutes preparation, setup and revision

Medical Record Committee – criteria

Review Committees – checklists and review forms

Correspondence – between and among committees, PRO responses, document preparation (Utilization Review and Quality Assurance plans)

Rosters, Call Lists, Committee Assignments

Many of the applications above can be done on in-house computer versions of word processing. Most of the time, the choice of dedicated word processing or mainframe computer programs will depend upon what equipment is in place. Utilizing hospital mainframe word processing may have some advantages, especially if terminals are already available, and software for computations on mainframe word processing is sometimes built in. But dedicated word processing allows the user much more freedom of design and lessens the dependency on mainframe computer programmers who may not be available to support word processing applications.

STATISTICAL REPORTS

Any type of statistical report can be entered into the word processor. The formats are memorized; and the new data is entered for the period, proofread, and then printed for copying. Monthly; quarterly; and annual statistical reports, and suspension summaries are typically prepared by medical record departments. If equipment is shared, or other departments have access to word processing terminals, financial reports, staffing reports and production monitors lend themselves immediately to word processing preparation.

SUMMARY

The information in this chapter covers the basic description of word processing systems and the five components of the equipment. Advances in office automation such as word processing have introduced changes in the work flow, work production, and employee orientation to the work. Because the medical record department is one of the largest offices in the hospital and because medical transcription is a logical function to automate, word processing will become as common in medical records as the electric typewriter and the computer. Many applications still remain to be automated, and newer and more sophisticated equipment will continue to move the medical record department forward toward the automated office of the future.

WORD PROCESSING GLOSSARY

Automatic Carriage Return – A feature that lets you type without slowing down at the end of the line. If a word extends into the right margin, it is automatically moved to the next line. Also called word wrap.

Backup – To make copies of important documents or files on either diskettes or tape. This enables recreation of the files if the originals are lost, stolen, or damaged.

Bidirectional Printing – A means of increasing printing speed by printing odd lines going from left to right and even lines from right to left.

Blockmove – The electronic equivalent of "cut and paste," this feature allows you to mark a block of text and move it anywhere you want in a file. It is also possible to block copy (the block stays in its original position as well as appearing in the new place) and block delete.

Board – A piece of fiberglass or pressboard on which chips are mounted. The connections between the chips can be wires or metallic ink printed on the board.

Boiler Plate – Portions of text stored on disk that are used continually with little modification to create standard documents containing customized information.

Bold Print – The overprinting of a portion of text to cause it to stand out from the rest of the page.

Bundled – Said of a system sold together as one package, rather than each component separately.

Burst Speed – The top speed of a printer, usually the speed at which it can repeatedly print one letter.

Byte – Unit of computer storage equivalent to one character or eight bits.

Capacity – The number of characters that can be stored on a diskette or the document size that can be worked on in the machine. Capacity is usually expressed in bytes or characters of storage.

Carriage Return – The key on the keyboard that indicates the end of a line and causes cursor movements to the left margin of the next line.

Center – The equal positioning of text on both sides of a center-line between two margins.

Character – A single piece of printed information. The character alphabet consists of letters (A-Z), numbers (0-9), and special symbols (:,/[]--).

Character Oriented Word Processor – A word processor capable of printing a variable number of different characters on a line. Character oriented word processors will do proportional printing.

Clear Key – The key used to cancel an operation that has already been started, to cancel a delete operation, or to stop printing.

Column – A horizontal space. An 80-column screen displays 80 characters on each line.

Compatible – Able to work together.

Computer – An electronic machine that can be converted into a useful tool by a program. It's also the physical machine used for word processing.

Continuous Form Paper – Perforated paper normally fan-folded to facilitate automatic paper feed to a printer. (After printing, the pages can be easily separated.)

Control – A character that initiates a machine operation (it doesn't print).

Copy – The process of copying a file from one physical disk to another.

CPS (Characters per Second) – The speed at which a printer can print.

CPU (Central Processing Unit) – The heart of a computer, it controls the interpretation and execution of instructions.

Create – The process of telling the system that a new document or data base will be entered. The system creates space for it on the disk.

CRT (Cathode-Ray Tube) – The TV-like screen used by the word processor to display information as it is typed and the means by which the system writes messages to you.

Cursor – The means of indicating the present position on the CRT, usually a blinking square or underline. It is moved around the screen by the directional arrow keys.

Cursor Arrows – Keys with arrows printed on them that move the cursor to the direction indicated.

Cut-Sheet Feeder – A machine that fits on top of a printer and feeds separate sheets of paper into it.

Daisy Wheel – The print element used in letter-quality printers. The daisy wheel has a raised character on each "petal" and is rotated to print letters.

Dedicated Word Processor – A computer designed specifically to do word processing, usually with limited ability to be used as a general-purpose computer.

Delete – The editing operation to remove characters, words, lines and paragraphs from text. Once the section is deleted the rest of the text closes up.

Dictionary – A program used to help you correct spelling errors while editing a document.

Directory – A list of all files and programs stored on disk.

Diskette (or Floppy Disk) – Magnetic-coated flexible plastic disk able to store 100,000 to one million characters of information. Disk sizes are standard 8″, mini 5¼″, and micro 3″ to 4″.

Distributed Logic – Independent "intelligent" terminals which can also access a common larger computer and storage unit.

Document – The name given to any text material written and stored on a word processor.

Dot Matrix Printer – A printer which fires pins against a print ribbon to create a character made up of dots.

Double Spacing – Skipping a blank line after each line of text, used often for draft copy printing because it leaves room to write in corrections.

Down – Not working (as opposed to up).

Dumb Terminal – A terminal that can only send and receive information. A "smart" terminal has processing and storage capability as well.

Edit – Changing the contents of a document by adding, removing, or rearranging text.

Electronic Mail – The transfer of documents over an electronic network to another word processor or computer.

Elite Type – A type face printed in 12 characters per inch. Also called twelve pitch.

Enter – A key on the word processor that instructs it to carry out an instruction. Also, to type in information on the keyboard.

Ergonomics – Design of equipment for user comfort and safety.

Error Message – Text that appears on the screen to tell you something is wrong.

Field – A unit of information within a record.

File – A collection of documents stored on a disk.

Fixed Disk – A hard disk that can't be removed from its drive.

Floppy – See Diskette.

Flush Left – Text lines aligned on the left margin. Also called left justified.

Flush Right – Text lines aligned along the right margin. Also called right justified.

Footer – A line of information printed on the bottom of each page of a multipage document.

Format – The complete printed form that a document will take.

Formatting – The "initializing" of a disk for use by a computer system. Formatting a disk erases all information that was on a disk.

Friction Feed – A means of feeding single pages to a printer by friction rollers, in contrast to a sprocket drive.

Full Page Display – A CRT display of a full page of material, normally 66-100 characters wide by 54-66 characters long.

Function Keys – Additional keyboard keys for carrying out special word processing functions.

Global Editor – That part of the editor that makes changes everywhere in a document, not just where the cursor is.

Hard Copy – Text printed on paper.

Hard Disk – A high capacity data storage device capable of storing megabytes of information.

Hardware – Physical computer equipment. The stuff you can touch: VDT, computer disk drives, printer, etc.

Head – The actual device that magnetically stores information on a disk or reads it from one.

Header – A line of information printed at the top of each page.

Home – The upper-left corner of the screen.

Horizontal Scrolling – Ability to move text horizontally across the screen to work on documents whose width is greater than the screen width.

Impact Printer – Any printer that forms a character by forcing an imprint mechanism (such as a key) against a ribbon and onto the paper.

Information Processing – Combining word processing and data processing into a single system.

Ink Jet Printer – A nonimpact printer that shoots small droplets of ink on the paper to create characters.

Insert – An editing operation in which additional text elements are added into a document.

Insert Mode – When a word-processing program is in this mode, it inserts text at the cursor, pushing all text after the cursor right and down.

Intercharacter Spacing – The spacing between characters, a fixed value for all printers except proportional ones in which the spacing varies with the size and shape of the character printed.

Interword Spacing – For justified printing, the spacing between words on a line is varied to ensure that the characters align with both the left and right margins.

Justification – The alignment of all text lines so that they are flush with both the left and right margins. See also flush left and flush right.

Keyboard – Part of a word processor that looks like a typewriter containing electronic keys for entering information. Word processor keyboards usually contain more keys than a typewriter keyboard.

Letter Quality Printer – High quality printer that creates printed copy as good as that produced on an electric typewriter.

Line Editor – An editor that requires you to specify the line (and word) you want to make your changes on, rather than letting you just move the cursor there. As opposed to a screen editor.

Line Oriented Word Processor – The standard word processor that lets you create text having a typewriter look. It is not capable of proportional printing.

Magnetic Media – A generic name for floppy disks, hard disks, tapes, and any other object or substance that stores data in the form of magnetic impulses.

Mainframe – The largest kind of computer, bigger than a minicomputer. Mainframe is also another name for a computer box.

Margin – The border around a printed page: left, right, top, and bottom.

Mega – One million. Ten megabytes of storage can hold 10 million characters of information.

Memory Mapping – A system for transmitting information to a screen in which it's read directly from the *memory* or the *bus* of the computer, as opposed to terminal mode.

Menu – A means to choose between available alternatives. Usually displayed as a numbered list.

Merge-Print Program – A program that lets you produce personalized form letters, and the like, by combining information from various sources during the actual printing of each document.

Microcomputer – A small-scale computer that can be used for word processing. The most popular and least expensive are the 8-bit and 16-bit machines.

Mini Diskette – A 5¼" diskette capable of storing 100,000 to 1 million characters of information.

Motherboard – A slotted board in the computer box that other boards are mounted into.

Multitasking – A computer or word processor with an operating system capable of running multiple programs at the same time.

Multiuser – A multitasking system working with several people at the same time.

Nondisplay (Screenless) Word Processor – External memory storage device (tape or disk-drive system).

One-Line Display – A single-line display setup usually found on electronic typewriters.

Orphan – The first line of a paragraph sitting alone at the bottom of a page.

Page – The amount of text on a single sheet of paper. Generally estimated as 1,500 characters.

Page Scrolling – A feature that lets the system move forward or backward through a document one page at a time.

Paragraph – A section of text usually set off by an entered carriage return, with indentation or extra line space before its first line.

Peripheral – Any device that is attached to the word processor. Printers, disk drives, and modems are peripherals.

Personality Area – The memory area of the computer that holds the application program. If the application program is a word processor, the machine assumes the personality of a writing machine.

Pica Type – A print size of 10 characters per inch. Also called ten pitch.

Pin Feed – Printer paper movement relying on special holes in the paper that fit a turning ring of pins on the machine.

Pitch – The number of printed characters per inch. Ten pitch is called pica: twelve pitch is called elite.

Plotter – A computer peripheral that draws things.

Preview – The display of text on the CRT as it will appear on paper.

Print Element – The piece of a printer that actually puts the characters on paper.

Print Wheel – See Daisy Wheel.

Printer – A device used to print text on paper.

Program – A set of instructions, stored in the program storage memory area, which establishes the system "personality." It converts a computer into a useful tool.

Program Storage Area – The portion of the computer's memory that holds and runs the application program.

Proportional Printing – The width and spacing of characters result in hard copy that is very printlike. Both the software and the printer must support this feature.

Protocol – The formal control information required to make it possible for two word processors or computers to communicate with each other. It's a set of rules for the exchange of information.

Ragged Right – Printed output with the type aligned flush with the left-side margin only. An alternative to justified text.

RAM (Random Access Memory) – A measure of the internal computer storage space available for the word processor program and text. Specified in kilobytes, otherwise known as thousands of characters.

Record – An item of stored information composed of a series of fields.

Reformat – The process of reestablishing margins, etc., after changes are made to a document.

Rename – To change the name of a stored document on a disk.

Replace – Replacement of characters or words of text with new text.

Revision – Making changes to a document stored on a disk file.

Ribbon – Inked cloth or carbon film used to create the printed image on paper.

Screen Editor – An editor that lets you move the cursor all around the screen (as opposed to a line editor).

Scrolling – Means of viewing more of a document than will fit in the CRT "window" at one time. The text is scrolled both horizontally and vertically.

Search – To locate a character, word, or series of words in the document. The search starts from the current position and will move toward the end of the document, stopping when a match is found.

Search and Replace – The process of finding indicated text and replacing it with alternate text.

Shannon Test – A piece of text designed to approximate the speed of a printer in actual use, as opposed to its burst speed.

Shared Logic – A word processing setup where more than one person is using the same computer system from different video display terminals.

Shared Resource – A word processing system where several terminals or word processors share peripherals (noncomputer parts) such as the printer and disk storage.

Sheet Feeder – A printer attachment to feed single pages to a printer.

Software – Programs that establish the machine personality. Programs are kept on the system's disk and loaded into the computer program area or personality area for use.

Spelling Checker – A program that goes through a file and checks for spelling errors.

Stand-Alone System – A complete word processor containing a VDT, small computer, printer, and word processing program.

Surge – A very sudden and very sharp increase in voltage.

System – A computer plus its peripherals – terminal, printer, keyboard, monitor, disk drives, etc. Sometimes system also includes software.

System Disk – A disk that has the operating system (and often other programs) on it. If a disk isn't a system disk, you can't boot it.

Telecommunications – Communication between word processors using the telephone lines.

Text Editing – A program for working with written text. Originally it referred to programs for revising computer programs but recently has become synonymous with word processing.

Text File – A file that contains text (rather than, say, a program).

Thermal Printer – A nonimpact printer which uses heat-sensitive paper.

Thimble – The print element used on NEC Spinwriter formed-character printers.

Thin-Window Display – A non-CRT display that shows just one line or part of a line. Typically, it runs across the top of the keyboard.

Time Sharing – The sharing of power and cost of large computer facilities among a number of word processing or computer terminals.

Tractor Feed – A lightweight, mechanically simple paper-feeding device that attaches to the top of a printer and engages sprocket holes in the paper with pins. The distance between the pins can be altered to accommodate papers of different widths.

Up – Working (as opposed to down).

User-Friendly – Another name for friendly.

Utilities – Program used to perform support operations for auxiliary disk functions. Copying disks for backup is a utility function.

VDT (Video Display Terminal) – A combination video display screen and keyboard.

Vendor – A company that provides equipment or supplies.

Widow – The last line of a paragraph sitting alone at the top of a page.

Winchester Disk – A rigid, nonremovable sealed magnetic disk unit, more compact and reliable than floppys. Capable of storing 5-100 megabytes of information.

Word – The machine word size is the amount of information that can be transferred in one chunk. It is usually a whole number of bytes.

Word Processing Systems – The hardware, software, and procedures used to carry out writing, editing, and filing text.

Word Wrap – The automatic movement of the text exceeding the right margin to the next line during typing. Increases typing speed since margin decisions are made automatically by the system.

Work Station – An individual work area for carrying out word processing, consisting of the word processor, desk, chair, and peripheral equipment.

STUDY QUESTIONS

1. What is word processing? List five components of word processing.
2. Distinguish between the three types of word processing systems, giving advantages and disadvantages of each.

3. Discuss the steps which should be followed:
   a. In evaluating the potential use of word processing equipment in the medical record department.
   b. In evaluating in-house and outside transcription production.

4. Discuss the advantages and disadvantages of discrete and self-contained dictation media.

5. Describe the various components of an equitable production pay system in medical transcription.

6. List some of the applications of word processing (other than medical transcription) for medical record departments.

REFERENCES

BEACH, LINDA. "Software Primer: Word Processing: Alive and Well." *Information Management*. August, 1984.

BIFANO, JAMES L. "A Cost Justification: Word Processing in a Medical Transcription Environment." *Journal of the American Medical Record Association*. October, 1983.

CHIRLIAN, BARBARA. *The Tenderfact's Guide to Word Processing*. Beaverton, Oregon: Dilithium Press, 1982.

DEMSTER, GLADYS. "Outside Transcription Services: a Cost-Effective Alternative to In-House Word Processing." *Topics in Health Record Management*. September, 1983, pp. 73-81.

GLATZER, HAL. *Introduction to Word Processing*. Berkeley, California: SYBEX Inc., 1981.

KAHL, KEN, VLAZNY, JIM, and CASEY, DENNIS. "Word Processing Eliminates Use of Outside Transcription Service." *Journal of the American Medical Record Association*. October, 1980, pp. 74-78.

KONKEL, GILBERT J., and PECK, PHYLLIS J. *The Word Processing Explosion*. Stamford, Connecticut: Office Publications, Inc., 1976.

———. *Word Processing and Office Automation*. Stamford, Connecticut: Office Publications, Inc., 1982.

MASENCUP, BONNIE. "Ergonomics: The People Factor." *Topics in Health Record Management*. September, 1983.

MERONEY, JOHN W. "Laying the Foundation for a Successful Word Processing System." *Information and Records Management*. June, 1982.

————. "Word Processing – A Link Between Data Processing, Records, Communications." *Information and Records Management.* June, 1982.

NAIMAN, ARTHUR. "Word Processing Buyer's Guide." *BYTE.* Peterborough, New Hampshire: McGraw Hill, 1983.

PAYNTER, DAN. *Word Processors and Information Processing, A Basic Manual on What They Are and How to Buy.* Santa Barbara, California: Pars Publishing, 1982.

PIKUKARIC, JOANNE M. "Transcription Incentive Plan." *Journal of the American Medical Record Association.* October, 1980, pp. 84-90.

ROTWEIN, SUZANNE. "The Word Processor – A Transcription Quality Assurance Mechanism." *Journal of the American Medical Record Association.* June, 1981, pp. 70-74.

SOLOZAR, RAELENE. "Word Processing for the Medical Record Department and Beyond." *Topics in Health Record Management.* September, 1983, pp. 51-62.

STERN, FRED. *Word Processing and Beyond.* Santa Fe, New Mexico: John Muir Publications, 1983.

STREMGREN, BONNIE. "Contract Transcription Services – Cost Containment Decision." *Journal of the American Medical Record Association.* October, 1980, pp. 79-83.

TEGEN, ANNE VOSS. "The Word Processing Evaluation Process." *Topics in Health Record Management.* September, 1983.

chapter *17*

THE LEGAL ASPECTS
OF MEDICAL RECORDS

GENERAL PRINCIPLES

OVERVIEW

A study of the legal aspects of medical records requires a general understanding of the way in which our legal system operates, as well as specific knowledge of the particular statutes, judicial decisions, and administrative regulations which affect medical record practice in the individual states.

In the United States, laws come from the three branches of government: legislative, executive, and judicial. Each exists at the federal, state, and local levels. Each has defined functions, but simply stated, the legislative branch enacts statutes; the executive branch enforces and administers the law, and the judicial branch interprets the law and settles disputes.

Hospitals and other health care institutions are required to maintain medical records. These requirements are found either in statutes or administrative regulations in every state. However, understanding the legal aspects of medical records also requires a knowledge of standards produced by nongovernmental sources, such as those set by hospitals themselves, accreditation groups, and professional organizations. It is important to recognize that the law does not and cannot provide answers to all of the questions which arise in the operation of hospitals or departments within the hospital.

Medical records would be maintained even if no statutes or regulations imposed the requirement. We need medical records in order to provide the best health care possible.

The medical record is in demand by a growing number of disparate groups. Patients and attorneys, physicians and insurance carriers, governmental and other accrediting agencies, the hospital itself, and portions of the community at large are all interested in the contents of the record or the data abstracted from the records. It is the responsibility of the medical record practitioner to evaluate the needs of each of these sometimes competing groups. He will be immeasurably aided by sensible standards or guidelines developed by the hospital, which take into account the existing laws and acceptable practice standards.

Beyond direct patient care, health information provides a sound base for a variety of legitimate activities. Therefore, patient care information from the original medical record may be transferred to a wide variety of secondary records. Secondary records include all indexes or other medical information which is individually identifiable by patient or health care provider. The medical record director and staff are generally responsible for the aggregation and control of this information.

This chapter defines some of the legal principles which affect the maintenance, handling, and disclosure of medical and secondary records. While it is true that there is no individually identifiable body of law governing medical records, medical record practitioners must know about the laws that affect their professional activities in order to make the judgments required of them in day-to-day operations.

REQUIREMENTS FOR KEEPING MEDICAL RECORDS

The requirement that hospitals maintain medical records, including data relating to the admission, diagnosis, treatment and disposition of patients, is found most often in state licensing regulations. Such regulations set forth minimum requirements for the information to be contained in the record, and many states' laws cover a wide range of record-related subjects. For example, the Indiana state law mandates in part that:

> (16-10-1-12)-A9. Medical Records – 1. Accurate and complete records shall be written for all patients. A computerized record shall be considered the same as a written record, and these rules and regulations shall apply.
>
> a. An inpatient hospital record shall include identification data, chief complaint, present illness, past history, family history, physical examination, progress notes, reports on consultations, copy of transfer form, reports on laboratory, x-ray and operative procedures, special reports, doctors' orders (signed and dated), notes and

observations, treatment records of nurses, dietitian, therapists and other personnel, reports on vital signs, final discharge summary, and summary sheet giving final diagnosis, complications, operative procedures, and signature of the attending physician. Readmissions within reasonable time and with the same diagnosis may require only a readmission note on patient's condition and reason for readmission.

Hospitals must maintain a variety of other records. Public health laws in every state require hospitals to keep certain statistics relating to patients. Reports of contagious diseases, births, deaths, fetal deaths, autopsies, and child abuse may be required to alert proper authorities and for state vital statistics.

Hospitals must conform to the requirements of state regulations and statutes. Many hospitals also aim to comply with voluntary standards set by the Joint Commission on Accreditation of Hospitals or the American Osteopathic Association. Hospitals not accredited by JCAH or AOA must be reviewed using the "Conditions of Participation," promulgated by the Secretary of the U.S. Department of Health and Human Services as a condition for receiving Medicare and Medicaid reimbursement.

RESPONSIBILITY OF THE MEDICAL RECORD PRACTITIONER

The medical record department director has the responsibility to maintain medical records, to ensure they are accurate, and to handle the information in accordance with laws and standards. Physicians, nurses, allied health practitioners, and others provide accurate and timely information that becomes the chronicle of the patient's hospitalization or treatment. If patient care data is not documented accurately and appropriately, the medical record director must see to its proper completion in order for the record to serve its medical, legal, and administrative functions. The medical record director must assure that the records and related information are available and accessible to those persons authorized to use them, and that the information is protected from those not authorized access. The tasks involved should be guided by written policies understood by all users and contributors to the medical record.

OWNERSHIP OF THE RECORD

The medical record is the physical property of the health practitioner or facility responsible for its compilation. In most states, legislation specifically provides that hospital medical records are the property of the hospital.

Usually ownership of property carries with it the right and power to control the use of the property. But in the case of the medical record, there is increasing recognition of the patient's right to control the information contained in his hospital record.

The fact that the hospital owns the pieces of paper upon which the record is written does not prevent certain others from submitting legitimate claims to see and copy the information therein. Real problems arise when there are competing interests for, and claims on, the information in medical records.

The American Medical Record Association supports the right of the patient to have access to his own medical record, unless there are specific contraindications, and to give express consent to the release of information for uses other than his own health care.

In most states, legislation gives the patient, his physician, or his authorized agent the right to examine or copy the hospital medical record. Where no specific state statute has given the patient a right to see his medical record, state judicial decisions related to this question should be taken into consideration.

Other issues of access to information contained in the medical record are addressed later in this chapter.

CONFIDENTIALITY OF MEDICAL DATA

The primary purposes of the medical record are to document the course of the patient's health care and to provide a medium of communication among health care professionals for current and future patient care.

In order to fulfill these purposes, significant amounts of data must be revealed and recorded. The patient must be assured that the information shared with health care professionals will remain confidential; otherwise, the patient may withhold critical information which could affect the quality of the care provided.

Economic issues, social issues, and technological advances have eroded the traditional relationship of confidentiality which exists between the patient and a health care professional. The desire of third-party payers to substantiate services provided has generated an increasing number of requests for information from patient health records. At the same time, the increase in the amount of computerized health data poses a threat to the privacy of medical information. The public is increasingly aware of this threat and the consequences of a loss of confidentiality in the health care system. Adequate measures to safeguard medical privacy must be established and followed.

Health care facilities receive and respond to numerous requests for information from the medical records in their custody. Requests may be made in writing, by telephone, or in person, from a broad spectrum of users. The responses are usually written; but in emergencies, they may be given by telephone upon verifying the authenticity of the caller as the patient, his representative, or another party permitted access by hospital policy.

TYPES OF DATA

Health care facilities ordinarily consider medical record information to fall into three categories:

Identification Data — Consist of entries in the record which do not specifically relate to the patient's care or treatment in the facility. Examples of identifying information are the patient's name, sex, spouse, and marital status. These items are often found on the admission record or face sheet of the health record and are frequently not considered confidential.

The increased emphasis on patient's rights and personal privacy, however, has led many institutions to take a more cautious approach and declare all data in the medical record confidential. Such a policy requires the patient's authorization to release health data in response to any request, except subpoenas, court orders, and those prescribed by law.

Clinical Data — Include all items entered in the medical record relating to the patient's diagnosis and treatment. Reports generated by physicians, nurses, allied health personnel, and results of tests and therapies fall under this category. Individually identifiable clinical information in medical records is confidential, because information obtained through the physician-patient relationship (and extended to other direct providers of care) is privileged and thus protected from disclosure. This privilege is supported in the Hippocratic oath and the law.

Secondary Medical Information – Includes all indexes or other medical information maintained by the institution which is individually identifiable by patient/provider. The increase in the amount of computerized health data, the advancement of record linkage techniques, the merging of clinical and financial data for billing, and the development of large data bases all pose new threats to confidentiality in the health care system. Secondary health information should be protected with the same diligence as clinical data.

STATUTES AFFECTING CONFIDENTIALITY

It is the policy in most states to regulate, to some degree at least, the ability of the physician to disclose information relating to his patients. He is prohibited from revealing medical information by licensing laws and regulations in some states, and generally by professional ethics and by the prohibition against his testimony in court.

Physician/Patient Privilege – A statutorily created prohibition found in the laws of most states which prevents a physician who attended a patient from testifying in a court or similar proceeding about the diagnosis, care, or treatment that he rendered to the patient unless the patient consents to such testimony or waives the protection by his conduct. The privilege belongs to the patient, thus protecting communications between patient and practitioner. These communications are called privileged and are confidential.

The privilege exists and is justified legally and ethically because society has determined that patients ought to be secure in disclosing information to their physicians so the physicians will be able to treat them fully. Indeed, there are several other special relationships which the law protects: lawyer-client, clergyman-parishioner, journalist-informant, and accountant-client.

A majority of the states now have statutory provisions or rules of court procedure designed to protect the confidential information between a patient and physician by prohibiting the physician's testimony in court. The protection varies considerably. A majority of the states with such statutes limit the privilege in regard to the nature of the information protected and the kind of legal proceeding in which it applies.

The great majority of litigation involves actions to recover damages for personal injury or wrongful death; to collect proceeds under life, accident, or health insurance contracts; for malpractice; for matters involving wills and trusts; in divorce proceedings; for workers' compensation; lunacy; criminal prosecutions involving assaults; abortions; sexual offenses; and homicides. In many of these cases, testimony of a physician, nurse, or other health professional is essential to aid the judge and jury in finding the facts.

The physician-patient relationship and its protection may be waived by the patient voluntarily or as a result of his actions. If the patient introduces his medical condition into legal proceedings, the door is opened for the opposing party to discuss it.

> In Collins v. Bair (256 Ind. 230, 268 N.E.2d 95 (1971)), the Indiana Supreme Court admitted testimony in a suit for back injuries from an automobile accident because "a party-patient impliedly waives his physician-patient privilege as to all matters either causally or historically related to the condition he has voluntarily put in issue by way of claim, counterclaim, or affirmative defense, and which have a direct medical relevance to the legitimacy of such claim or defense."

Calling the physician as witness for the patient in a trial typically voids the silence imposed by privileged information. Also, if a patient brings legal action against his physician, in many states he automatically relinquishes his right to confidentiality of medical information during court proceedings.

While state laws vary in their definitions of privileged communication and to whom it applies, there are some typical elements. Obviously, in this context, the communication must involve medical information.

> The Indiana law (Ind. Code S 16-14-I.6-8) says "all information obtained and maintained in the course of providing services to a patient or client is confidential and shall be disclosed only with the consent of the patient or client, unless otherwise provided in this section."

Likewise, the California Confidentiality of Medical Information Act applies exclusively to any individually identifiable information which is in the possession of or derived from a provider of health care regarding a patient's medical history, mental or physical condition, or treatment. The scope of the state laws varies as well; some include nurses along with physicians. The California Confidentiality of Medical Information Act includes, generally, any licensed practitioner, health care facility, or group practice prepayment plan.

With reference to the nature of the information, most states limit the protection to that which is acquired professionally and is necessary to enable the physician to treat the patient. Other states limit the protection even further. In Pennsylvania, for example, the privilege applies to information which would tend to "blacken the character" of the patient. With reference to the kind of proceeding, many states limit the privilege to civil actions, thereby leaving testimony in criminal action unrestricted.

It is important to remember that the privilege is not absolute, and it is not uniform. Each medical record practitioner should know the language of the privilege in his particular state and the extent of its application.

Other Statutes and Protections – It is also necessary for the director of the medical record department to know the language of other statutes and regulations which, independent of the privileged communication provision, make certain health records confidential; for example, any statutes relating to institutions for the mentally disabled which may make the records of those institutions confidential. On the other hand, the medical record director must also know of the statutes which require that certain information be made available. Hospital lien laws may permit records to be examined by persons against whom action has been brought for personal injuries. The hospital itself may use the records to provide better patient care, measure the effectiveness of its medical staff, undertake educational programs and research, and protect itself from suit. In developing internal rules and regulations for disclosure, the hospital may be strict or lenient; but such rules must recognize that, as a general rule, the patient has an interest in the information which is enforceable in a court of law. This interest is enforceable in two ways. The patient may use the courts to obtain access to his record, or he may resort to the courts because information from his record has been improperly revealed.

PATIENT'S RIGHT TO PRIVACY

The spread of consumer awareness in the health care field has spawned increased interest in patients' rights. The Privacy Act of 1974 mandated specific rights of persons wishing to gain access to individual records kept by federal agencies, including federal government hospitals. This legislation also established the Privacy Protection Study Commission, which undertook a three-year study of privacy provisions needed in other areas of the country. The recommendations of the Commission are contained in their report "Personal Privacy in an Information Society," submitted to Congress in July, 1977. With regard to medical record-keeping practices, the report concludes, in part, that the use of medical record data is growing rapidly, with the data being used by more persons and organizations with less control than ever before. At the federal and state levels, legislation to provide stricter controls on the flow of patients' medical information is slow in its formulation; and many of the concerns identified in 1977 still exist and have even been heightened by increased data collection and dissemination facilitated by computerization.

Various organizations in the health care industry have taken major steps to ensure patients' civil rights. Issues of concern include such areas as equal access to medical care, the right to dignity and privacy while patient care needs are being met, the right to confidentiality of medical information, and the right to be fully informed of one's condition and treatment methods. The U.S. Department of Health and Human Services requires attention to patients' rights as part of the Medicare requirements. A similar position is taken by the Joint Commission on Accreditation of Hospitals in the *Accreditation Manual for Hospitals.* Likewise, the American Hospital Association promulgated, as early as 1973, comprehensive ideas on the preservation of patients' rights in its "Patient's Bill of Rights." This statement says, in part:

> The patient has the right to every consideration of his privacy concerning his own medical care program. Case discussion, consultation, examination, and treatment are confidential and should be conducted discreetly. Those not directly involved in his care must have the permission of the patient to be present.
>
> The patient has the right to expect that all communications and records pertaining to his care should be treated as confidential.

One of the standards of the American Medical Association's *Principles of Medical Ethics* states: "A physician shall respect the rights of patients, of colleagues, and of other health professionals, and shall safeguard patient confidences within the constraints of the law." (AMA House of Delegates, 1980.)

Consumer awareness has focused in part on the medical record professional as the hospital's delegated representative to protect patient information from unauthorized access or disclosure.

Patient Access to Records

As stated earlier, the hospital owns the record, but the patient has a legitimate interest in the information contained therein. Conflicts most often appear and legal questions are raised when the hospital denies access to information in the record to the patient or his authorized representative. In several states, statutes give the patient, his attorney, or authorized agent the right to examine and copy the patient's record. The California statute is illustrative:

> . . . any adult patient of a health care provider, any minor patient authorized by law to consent to medical treatment, and any patient representative shall be entitled to inspect patient records upon presenting to the health care provider a written request therefor and upon payment of reasonable clerical costs incurred in locating and making the records available; provided, that a patient who is a minor shall be entitled to inspect patient records pertaining only to health care of a type for which the minor is lawfully authorized to consent. A health care provider shall permit such inspection during business hours within five working days after receipt of such a written request. The inspection shall be conducted by the patient or patient's representative requesting the inspection, who may be accompanied by one other person of his or her choosing.
>
> Additionally, any patient or patient's representative shall be entitled to copies of all or any portion of the patient records which he or she has a right to inspect, upon presenting a written request to the health care provider specifying the records to be copied, together with a fee to defray the cost of copying, which shall not exceed twenty-five cents ($0.25) per page or fifty cents ($0.50) per page for records that are copied from microfilm and any additional reasonable clerical costs incurred in making the records available. The health care provider shall ensure that the copies are transmitted within 15 days after receiving the written request. (AB610, 35252 (a)(b))

Where there are no statutes, judicial authority should be followed. Cases arising in several states have held that a former patient, his attorney, or other authorized person may obtain an order compelling the hospital to permit inspection and copying of records. These courts have said that the patient has a right to the information in the record, and if he shows a legitimate reason for seeing the information he must be served.

In the absence of state laws, the medical record practitioner may wish to establish an access policy based on the model policies from the American Medical Record Association's position statement on "Confidentiality of Patient Health Information."

POLICIES FOR HANDLING MEDICAL RECORDS AND SECONDARY MEDICAL RECORDS

The administration of each hospital, after due consultation with legal counsel, the medical record director, and the medical record committee, should adopt definite policies and regulations governing the release of information from medical records. These should cover not only situations involving outside interests, but also those situations involving the use of information for hospital purposes. The regulations should be disseminated in the hospital, and copies should be made available to the individuals and organizations frequently calling upon the medical record department for release of information.

Each health care facility should establish and enforce a confidentiality policy to protect secondary records. The policy should include confidentiality statements to be signed by all employees and data users prohibiting the release of data to unauthorized users, with penalties stated for violation of the agreement. The policy should identify specific persons and departments authorized to obtain secondary data, and should delineate legitimate purposes for which patient or health care provider identifiable information may be used. Further, the policies should specify that data with patient or provider identifiers will be released only for the purpose specified and only to those authorized by law or by patient consent to receive such data.

The American Medical Record Association's published model policies can serve as valuable guidelines for the development of individual facility policies. They may not all be adaptable because of individual state statutes or regulations which prohibit their implementation, but they reflect the trend toward increased vigilance in safeguarding patient care information.

Release to Authorized Persons

When medical record practitioners speak of release of information, it is often with a sense of recognition that the line between patient privacy and society's right to know is not always clear. The record is maintained precisely, because the information it contains is valuable to the individuals and organizations having a legitimate need to know its contents. The majority of requests comes from third-party plans which need information on those they insure. Attorneys present a large number of requests. Moreover, patients and their relatives, members of the medical staff, other physicians and hospitals concerned with the care of patients, and governmental and other agencies also request information.

There are several common problems associated with authorizations to release information:

First, in "blanket" authorizations, patients or guardians sign releases which allow facilities to disseminate "any and all" identifiable information to the bearer. The patient is not himself "informed" as to the full extent of the record's content, which segments of it will be open to third-party access, or what will happen to the information once it is in the third-party's possession. "Blanket" authorizations do not serve to instill a sense of responsibility in the collectors, holders, and users of patient data.

Second, difficulty arises from the common third-party practice of requesting "prospective" authorizations or consent to the release of information prior to treatment. This means the patient is consenting to the dissemination of information which is not yet collected, a practice which precludes any intelligent decision-making on the part of the patient.

Third, most insurance companies employ a form of consent which could be construed as "perpetual" authorization, since there is no time limit set for validity of the authorization. With other requesters, health care institutions vary in the time limits within which they accept patient authorizations as valid. In some cases, health care institutions are adopting more stringent time limits; but there is no uniformity of policy in this area.

Fourth, in most authorizations there is no provision against rerelease of the information by the recipient.

Fifth, there are questions as to who has the right to consent. In the case of minors, this right is exercised by the parent or guardian until the minor reaches the age of majority or becomes emancipated (released from the control of his parents). The definitions of majority and of emancipation differ from state to state. In addition, many states grant minors the right to seek treatment without parental knowledge for certain specific conditions. In such instances, the parent or guardian cannot be informed as to the record's content. Yet another insurance-related problem is when the patient is not the party who signed the insurance contract prospectively authorizing release of information.

Sixth, special consideration must be given to the rights of the person considered incompetent. Such persons fall into two categories:

1. Those patients who have been deemed incompetent by court decision. In this process, a guardian has been appointed by the court and will exercise the consent.

2. Those persons suffering from medical conditions that prevent them, temporarily or permanently, from acting knowingly or effectively in their own behalf but have not been adjudged incompetent. In these instances the consent is exercised by the next of kin when one is available, as long as the patient's condition warrants. In the absence of next of kin, there is an obligation for the medical care facility to act in the best interests of the patient.

AUTHORIZATION TO DISCLOSE DATA

CONTENT OF AUTHORIZATIONS

A patient may authorize disclosure by giving written authorization. Standard forms may be obtained from commercial companies, or the facility may find it preferable to design its own in accordance with applicable laws. A properly completed and signed authorization to release patient information shall include at least the following data:

a) name of institution that is to release the information

b) name of individual or institution that is to receive the information

c) patient's full name, address, and date of birth
d) purpose or need for information
e) extent or nature of information to be released, including inclusive dates of treatment
   Note: An authorization specifying "any and all information . . ." shall not be honored.
f) specific date, event, or condition upon which consent will expire unless revoked earlier
g) statement that consent can be revoked but not retroactive to the release of information made in good faith
h) date that consent is signed
   Note: Date of signature must be *later* than the date of information to be released.
i) signature of patient or legal representative
   Note: In the case of treatment given a minor without parental knowledge, the institution shall refrain from releasing the portion of the record relevant to this episode of care when responding to a request for information for which the signed authorization is that of the parent or guardian. An authorization by the minor shall be required in this instance.

New forms designed to authorize release of information should be reviewed by the facility's legal counsel prior to implementation. A letter from the patient directing the hospital to release certain information to a specified recipient will suffice as a proper authorization and may be honored by the facility if it contains the elements required by law or by hospital policy.

Care should be taken not to honor generally worded patient authorizations to release "any and all" information from the record. The American Hospital Association's *Institutional Policies for Disclosure of Medical Record Information* states that "one of the purposes of a well-drawn authorization for disclosure of medical record information is to indicate to the patient, or persons acting on his behalf, what subject matter is being authorized to be disclosed, the person or organization that will receive the information, and any applicable time limit." Medical record department personnel should attempt to ascertain exactly what items are required to adequately fulfill the needs of the requester and only that information should be sent. If there is some question regarding the legitimacy of the patient's signature on the authorization, comparison should be made with other signatures on the admission record and consent forms contained in the medical record.

If the record contains no other signatures for comparison or if there is reasonable doubt as to the validity of the signature, a notarized signature is recommended. Policies and procedures may be developed by the medical record department to deal with cases where other factors have affected the patient's signature, such as use of a married versus a single name.

Some hospitals submit photocopies of an entire medical record when an abstract or summary is requested. While such a practice may take less time to prepare than an abstract, it may be more costly; and in addition may furnish information not authorized by the patient. A summary, on the other hand, usually contains only excerpted and pertinent information.

GOVERNMENT AGENCY REQUESTS

Government agencies frequently request confidential information concerning a patient. Some requests are made in person by representatives, and others are received through the mail. Unless a statute specifically gives government agencies the right to receive such information, they are not entitled to it without the written authorization of the patient, as is the case with private agencies. The most common example of a law specifying the release of information to a governmental agency is that governing workers' compensation cases. The Iowa statute regarding workers' compensation reads in part as follows:

> Any employee, employer, or insurance carrier making or defending a claim for benefits agrees to the release of all information to which they have access concerning the employee's physical or mental condition relative to the claim and further waives any privilege for the release of such information. Such information shall be made available to any party or their attorney upon request. Any institution or person releasing such information to a party or their attorney shall not be liable criminally or for civil damages by reason of the release of such information. Code of Iowa, chapter 85.27, paragraph 2.

The medical record department director should verify the existence of the Workers' Compensation claim. If the case is alleged but a claim not filed, patient authorization should be obtained. (*Medical Records and the Law,* Illinois Medical Record Association.)

A hospital will receive many inquiries from welfare agencies, veterans' bureaus, and other organizations. Such inquiries are usually for the benefit of the patient; and it would seem that in such cases, release of information without written authorization of the patient would not meet with criticism. However, for the patient's protection, the medical record department director should always require proper authorization from the patient for release of information. The authorization should be filed in the record with a note identifying the information released.

Health departments are increasingly interested in the control of disease and have expanded the scope of their interests to include means of disease prevention and promotion of health. In these activities, the hospital, while not bound by law in many states, has an ethical responsibility to the public's welfare and should cooperate to the fullest extent. But if a state or federal agency requests information which individually identifies the patient, a signed authorization should be obtained from the patient; or the record must be subpoenaed.

Unless state law prohibits release, information may and should be given to the police only to the extent that such information would be found in the police register, such as the nature of an accident, whether automobile accident, industrial accident, etc. Representatives of law enforcement must present proper identification, and the medical record department director should ascertain that the office is acting in the line of duty and not as a private person. No specific medical data should be given without authorization of the patient, court order, or other legal process.

DRUG AND ALCOHOL ABUSE INFORMATION

The sensitive nature of medical data compiled for drug and alcohol abuse patients became the subject of increased government concern; so on July 1, 1975, a law went into effect to protect "records of the identity, diagnosis, prognosis, or treatment of any patient which are maintained in connection with the performance of any drug or alcohol abuse prevention function." (42CFR, Part 2.)

Release of all patient-related information for these persons is left to the patient's discretion. Even the fact that the person is a patient in the facility may not be disclosed if this would indicate the reason the person is hospitalized. Release of any patient information, whether during or after treatment, is forbidden unless the patient has signed a special authorization form with specified items of information.

As the hospital's designated custodian of health information, the head of the medical record department generally is responsible for seeing that the information on alcohol and drug abuse patients is not released in an unauthorized manner. A thorough understanding of the regulations and their implementation is necessary for the performance of these duties. In-service training for medical record personnel is advisable to ensure that no violations occur. The medical record professional may also be responsible for training other hospital departments' personnel in proper procedures for maintaining the privacy of alcohol and drug abuse patients.

THIRD-PARTY PAYERS

There are many types of third-party insurance plans concerned with sickness or injury. Among them are Blue Cross and Blue Shield plans and commercial insurance companies providing health and accident insurance, medical and surgical insurance, workers' compensation, and others. In the past, each third-party payer had different claim forms and requested different information regarding the insured's hospitalization. In 1982 a National Uniform Billing Committee, composed of representatives from the Medicare and Medicaid agencies, insurance and hospital associations, and the American Hospital Association, agreed to a claim form designed to meet the needs of the various third-party payers. Many of the payers, including Medicare and Medicaid, require hospitals to use the uniform bill called "UB-82," for filing claims.

Before paying claims for the insured, insurance companies frequently ask for more detailed information from the medical record. The hospital should have a properly signed authorization before releasing the information.

ATTORNEYS

Requests from an attorney outside the hospital must include the patient's written authorization, whether he represents the patient or the opposing side. This holds true if the requester desires a copy of the record or an appointment to view the record in the medical record department. If a patient's authorization cannot be obtained, legal proceedings are available as an alternative.

The medical record is used to protect the patient, the physician, and the hospital. Because hospital employees are allowed access to patient records necessary to complete their work, the hospital's own attorney may have access to records in cases where his counsel is required, such as legal action against the facility.

HEALTH CARE PROVIDERS

Medical information from the patient's record is often necessary for continuing care of the patient by other health care professionals. In nonemergency situations, a patient authorization should be requested as a matter of policy. However, emergencies may dictate releasing information immediately, after assuring the authenticity of the caller's request. Transfer of patients directly to another facility, such as a skilled nursing facility or rehabilitation center, for continued treatment should automatically include transfer of appropriate information. Special transfer forms may be used, or a copy of the medical record or portions thereof may be sent. (See Chapter 5.)

The mobility of today's population places additional demands on the medical record department to scrutinize requests for patient information from distant physicians and health care facilities. If a patient moves to another city or area, he should send a written request or authorization asking that a copy of his records be forwarded to his new doctor.

THE MEDICAL RECORD IN COURT

ADMISSIBILITY AS EVIDENCE

The presentation of information from medical records as evidence in a court or other duly constituted tribunal, agency, or commission is quite proper. The record is an unbiased chronological report of the patient's treatment in the hospital, and it is made in the hospital's regular course of business.

As a general proposition, any information from the record can be admitted into evidence; because the record is a business record. If the court can be assured that the record is reliable and trustworthy, it will allow all or part of the information to become evidence subject to rules relating to privilege, relevancy, materiality, and competency. Several state statutes relate specifically to the admissibility of medical records into evidence. The New York statute provides an example:

> (a) Generally. Any writing or record, whether in the form of an entry in a book or otherwise, made as a memorandum or record of any act, transaction, occurrence or event, shall be admissible in evidence in proof of that act, transaction, occurrence or event, if the judge finds it was made in the regular course of any business and that it was the regular course of such business to make it, at the time of the act, transaction, occurrence or event, or within a reasonable time thereafter. All other circumstances of the making of the memorandum or record, including lack of personal knowledge by the maker, may be proved to affect its weight, but they shall not affect its admissibility. The term business includes a business, profession, occupation and calling of every kind. (New York Civil Practice Law and Rules, Section 4518)

SUBPOENAS

When one of the parties involved in litigation desires to present hospital medical record information to the court, he will cause an order of the court to be sent to the hospital as custodian of the records. When the hospital or medical record director receives such an order, there is no recourse but to obey it. Of course, if the subpoena is unclear, proper inquiry may be made; but the subpoena is a court order designed to cause a witness to appear and give testimony. It commands the witness to come before a specified court or officer at a specified time.

Court rules in the federal judicial system and in many state systems provide for the use of notary or deposition subpoenas in order to obtain information before the actual trial of a case. These pretrial discovery procedures and the rules for examinations before trial vary widely from jurisdiction to jurisdiction (territorial range of authority or control). It is necessary to become familiar with local practice, but the subpoena used in pretrial discovery is also generally enforceable and should be obeyed.

A subpoena requires the presence of the witness. A subpoena duces tecum requires the witness to come with certain specified records. In several states the practice has been to allow the custodian of business records to certify a copy of the records and to send them to the clerk of the court. The requirement to appear personally is thus removed. A statutory example of such practice can be seen in the language of the New York statute, which says that any person may comply with a subpoena duces tecum by appearing with the requisite books, documents, or items, identifying them, and testifying respecting their origin, purpose, and custody. (New York Civil Practice Law Article 23, Section 2305(b).) The person to whom the subpoena is issued may be considered in contempt of court if he does not honor it, or present a satisfactory explanation of the reasons why it was not honored.

The admissibility or exclusion of testimony of the witness or the records of the custodian is governed by the rules of evidence. These rules are complicated, varied, and outside the scope of this chapter. One should note, however, that in any case, none, part, or all of the information in the record may be actually admissible. Admissibility will be governed by the particular rules of the state and the issues and subject matter of the case. The judge and opposing counsel have the responsibility to resolve controversy dealing with the rules of evidence. The responsibility of the medical record practitioner is to be an objective witness as a representative of the facility. As noted previously, the New York statute expects the judge to determine whether the record was made in the usual course of business. The medical record practitioner will be asked questions regarding his position in the facility, whether he has the record and whether it was made in the usual course of business.

While the server of the subpoena is still present, or upon first inspection of a subpoena received in the mail, the subpoena should be checked for the type of subpoena, the name of the person or organization upon whom the subpoena is served, the name and location of the court, the date and time the witness must appear, signature of the court clerk, and the seal of the court. Subpoenas for civil cases should be accompanied by payment of any fees authorized by court rules. If the subpoena is a copy, it should be checked with the original, which the server should have with him, to ensure they match and that the original bears the seal of the court. If the subpoena lacks any of the above information, the attorney who caused the subpoena to be issued should be notified that the subpoena was improperly served. The attorney's name may be obtained from the clerk of the court if not listed on the subpoena.

It is not possible to predict which hospital records will be subpoenaed. Therefore, each medical record must be regarded as potentially subject to courtroom scrutiny. Consequently, a careful quantitative analysis by the medical record practitioner of the medical record of every discharged patient is of utmost importance. For example, entries that have been erased or not corrected according to the rules of the hospital should have been rejected and sent back for proper correction. The position of the medical record department director is one of special trust; it is, therefore, his duty to ascertain that the record is properly completed.

PREPARING SUBPOENAED RECORDS FOR COURT

After a subpoena duces tecum is accepted, the requested records must be found and prepared for use as follows:

1. Log in subpoena according to hospital policy.
2. Determine whether the patient has a record at the facility and where it is located; e.g., inpatient, ambulatory care, emergency service, etc.
3. Check the record to make sure it is complete, that signatures and initials are identifiable, and that each sheet contains the patient's name and number.
   a. If the record is incomplete, take steps to expedite its completion.
   b. If the record is on microfilm, notify the attorney who caused the subpoena to be issued so he can arrange for either a microfilm reader to be in court or pay for having the record reproduced in hard copy. Microfilm records are admissible as primary evidence in place of the original record under the provisions of Public Law 129.
4. Become familiar with the contents of the record, in case you are called to read from the record on the witness stand.
5. Read the record to be sure it is not a potential malpractice suit against the facility or physician. If you believe

it is, or might be, notify the administrator and the attending physician.

6. Obtain additional records specified in the subpoena; e.g., x-ray films, bills, etc.

7. Remove all correspondence, duplicate copies of reports, copies of medical records from other facilities, insurance reports, and social service histories unless the subpoena specifically calls for such documents.

8. Number the front and back of each page of the record in ink, and record the total on the record folder.

9. Photocopy the record (or make a paper copy of microfilm) and complete a statement certifying that the copy is an exact duplicate of the original. If only portions of the record were subpoenaed, prepare a copy of the whole record as it may be required by the court to admit the subpoenaed portion into evidence.

10. Prepare an itemized listing in duplicate of the record contents which can be used as a receipt if the record is left in court. The copy of the listing should be retained at the facility.

11. Record the type and number of the patient record and the number of pages in the log. If no medical records exist on the patient specified in the subpoena, submit a "no record" statement to the issuer of the subpoena. You may be required to testify in court as to this fact.

CONDUCT AS A WITNESS

Before going to court, it would be well for the medical record practitioner to familiarize himself with the following counsel given in *Legal Aspects of Health Care Administration* by George D. Pozgar:

1. Do not be antagonistic towards the plaintiff's counsel. The jury may already be somewhat sympathetic toward the injured party; your antagonism may only serve to reinforce such an impression.

2. Be organized in your thinking and recollection of the facts regarding the incident.

3. Do not use the witness box to show how knowledgeable you are. What you think is harmless may be the downfall of the case.

4. Explain your testimony in simple, succinct terminology.

5. Do not overdramatize the facts you are relating. The witness box is not the place to make your stage debut.

6. Do not allow yourself to become overpowered by the cross-examiner.

7. Be polite, sincere, and courteous at all times.

8. Dress appropriately, and be neatly groomed.

9. Pay close attention to any objections your attorney may have as to the line of questioning being conducted by the opposing counsel.

10. Never deny discussing the case with your attorney when questioned about such practice.

11. Be sure to review any oral deposition you may have participated in during examination before trial.

12. Be straightforward with the examiner. Any answers designed to cover up or cloud an issue or fact will, if discovered, serve only to discredit any previous testimony you may have given.

13. Do not show any visible signs of displeasure regarding any testimony with which you are in disagreement.

14. Be sure to have questions that you did not hear repeated and questions which you did not understand rephrased.

The presiding judge at the trial determines whether all or portions of the hospital record should be received in evidence; and, if he so rules, the record, according to the general practice of the courts, must be identified by the person representing the hospital. The medical record practitioner is qualified to testify that the record was kept in the hospital's regular order of business, to the component parts of the record, and to identify who was responsible for the compilation of each part of the record. For this reason he should be the person to answer a subpoena duces tecum. His testimony on such facts, however, is the extent of his responsibility as a witness.

The record is usually marked for identification and then offered in evidence and may be later used by the doctor, resident, intern, or nurse to refresh his memory.

When the medical record practitioner is called to the stand, he is usually sworn before being questioned and then asked to identify himself and answer certain questions to lay the foundation for the introduction of the record in evidence. Subject to objection from opposing counsel, he may be asked to read portions of the record. On the other hand, the attorney may merely ask for the medical record; and the medical record practitioner may be excused from the stand. The medical record department director should obtain a receipt for the record if the original must remain with the court, so he may return to his duties at the hospital. The judge may permit photostatic copies to be substituted for the original record.

To obviate the necessity for leaving the original record, many medical record directors photostat the record and take the photocopy together with the original medical record when answering a subpoena. Many trial judges will accept the photocopy in lieu of the medical record after the latter has been properly identified.

While a receipt may be accepted from the court in case the medical record is retained, there is the possibility that the court may keep the record for an indefinite period; therefore, it is advisable to have the photocopy of the medical record substituted, or to remain during the entire court procedure and recover the medical record whenever possible. For obvious reasons, the original record should be returned to the hospital. If it becomes necessary for the court to retain the record for a long period during court procedure, permission will generally be granted to have a photocopy substituted after comparison with the original. The court or the lawyers for the litigants will usually permit the records to be received promptly in evidence if the medical record director requests it. Then it will not be necessary for the medical record practitioner to remain in the courtroom for any great length of time.

ACCEPTANCE OF MICROFILMED RECORDS

Statutes and rules of procedure in most if not all the jurisdictions authorize the use of microfilmed medical records as primary evidence. When a subpoena duces tecum has been received in the proper form and it is found that the medical record which must be produced has been microfilmed, the roll of film or the individual card or cards into which the microfilmed copy of the record has been processed or inserted must be produced at the stated time and place in lieu of the original medical record. The medical record practitioner can cooperate with the attorney by notifying him upon receipt of the subpoena that the record requested is on film so he can make preparation to have the record read at the proper time. The attorney who had the subpoena issued is responsible for providing the means for reading the film, because the hospital has complied with the order of the court by producing the record.

If the subpoena has been issued for the microfilm in sufficient time prior to trial, the attorney who issued it will often request the director of medical records to have photographic prints of the same size as the original record made before court convenes. Otherwise, the medical record practitioner informs the court when he arrives that since many other records are a part of the film roll, the roll cannot be released except upon order of the court. He can also state that if the party desiring the record would pay the expense incurred, he would have photographic prints made of the pertinent sections of the roll. The prints will then be used in lieu of the original record. The medical record practitioner should take the roll of film to the processing laboratory himself and indicate to the photographer which parts of the film are to be printed. He will probably have been instructed by the court to bring both the film and the photographic prints of the record back to court, where, after the proper foundation has been laid, the prints made from the microfilm of the original record (made in the hospital's usual order of business) will be admitted as evidence.

Photographic prints of microfilmed records can be made as easily and as quickly as photostatic copies and are usually made by the same processing companies.

The question of privilege with respect to the records of other patients does not arise in hospitals which have their microfilmed records processed into or inserted into unit cards containing the record of only one patient. However, it is customary even with this type of microfilmed record to have prints made rather than to use a projector in the courtroom.

LIABILITIES

Potential liability for mishandling medical records may arise in three broad areas. First, the possibility exists that the hospital's accreditation, licensure, or eligibility for participation in governmental hospitalization insurance programs may be jeopardized by failing to comply with state regulations or the "Conditions of Participation" promulgated by the Secretary of Health and Human Services.

Next, the maintenance of incorrect records or the failure to read records correctly may cause harm to patients, resulting in liability for negligence. Finally, the unauthorized disclosure of information from medical records may lead to liability for invasion of privacy. Each of these liabilities will be briefly discussed.

LOSS OF ACCREDITATION, LICENSURE, OR ELIGIBILITY

A remote possibility exists that one or more of the state regulatory or licensing agencies which have the power to license hospitals may actually suspend a license or censure a hospital for failure to maintain medical records properly. Medical record deficiencies, when coupled with deficiencies in other departments, may also give rise to withdrawal of accreditation. Loss of accreditation severely restricts the ability of the hospital to participate in numerous state, federal, and nongovernmental programs, and would mean the hospital loses its "deemed status." (Hospitals accredited by JCAH are "deemed" to have met the federal Conditions of Participation for the Medicare and Medicaid Programs.)

For non-JCAH accredited hospitals, a state agency is utilized by the Secretary of Health and Human Services to determine "substantial" compliance with the "Conditions." If, after a survey, the state agency finds a hospital is not in compliance with the "Conditions," it is likely that attempts will be made to bring the hospital into substantial compliance with the standards by means of negotiation. Of course, if there is repeated and continual failure to meet the standards and no showing of an attempt to bring the institution into substantial compliance, then the hospital's eligibility to participate as a provider of services might be withdrawn. It is unlikely that eligibility will be withdrawn at the first instance of failure to comply.

NEGLIGENCE

The record itself may be negligently prepared or interpreted, and it thus may be the instrument through which harm is caused to the patient. In simple words, negligence is careless-ness. We have a duty to act with due care under all cir-cumstances. To determine what is or is not careless, that is, whether the duty has been obeyed, the law has developed a measure called the *standard of care.*

The standard of care is determined by finding what a reason-ably prudent person would have done under similar cir-cumstances. The jury makes this determination. The reasonably prudent person is fictional, a creature of the law, a hypothetical character, used to indicate what should be done under similar circumstances.

After determining what the reasonably prudent person would have done, the actual performance of the person charged with negligence is measured against this standard. If his actions meet or surpass the standard, there has been no negligence, just an unavoidable occurrence. But if the act of the defendant failed to meet the standard, there has been negligence; and the jury must determine whether negligence was the proximate cause of the harm. If this is determined to be so, then liability will follow.

Thus, the essential elements of negligence are: (1) the duty to use due care under the circumstances, (2) a breach of that duty by an act or failure to act, and (3) the breach proximately causing harm to another.

This duty applies to all of us as we drive our cars, maintain our homes, and live and act in society. When we act in a special capacity, such as when we practice a profession, the law im-poses a higher standard upon those actions, a standard commen-surate with our special qualifications.

The duty applicable to health care practitioners is that they use reasonable care under the circumstances and perform acts with the degree of skill and knowledge ordinarily used by mem-bers of their profession in good standing.

Note that we are no longer talking about the ordinary pru-dent man. We have gone to a fictional average person who has skill, training, and experience similar to the physician or other professional person who may be charged with a careless act. We cannot expect the jury, judge, or attorney to know or guess at this standard; so expert witnesses tell us what the general stan-dard of practice for the profession is in the community. Expert witnesses perform a service for the court. They aid the judge and the jury by providing information upon which a reasonable judgment can be made.

The medical record gives us information about what actually occurred, and the testimony of expert witnesses gives us information about the standard by which the trier of fact can judge the acts as shown in the medical record and in the testimony of witnesses to the event.

The medical record itself can be negligently prepared and thus be a contributing cause to injury. Illustrative of this is Favolora v. Aetna Casualty and Surety Co., 144 So. 2d 544 (La. App. 1962). In this case, the patient sued the radiologist and hospital for injuries sustained as the result of a fall during an x-ray examination. The judgment was rendered against the radiologist due to his failure to secure the patient's medical history prior to the x-ray during which the patient collapsed and was injured. The radiologist was found negligent; because the history would have disclosed that one of the purposes of the exam was to determine, if possible, why the patient was subject to fainting.

UNAUTHORIZED DISCLOSURE

The three legal theories which may be employed to support a suit for damages for the unauthorized disclosure of information from a medical record without consent, are: (1) the theory of defamation, (2) breach of a confidential relationship, and (3) invasion of privacy.

Under the theory of defamation, that is, libel or slander – the complaining party sues because of a written or oral communication of false statements which tend to injure his character or reputation.

In one case involving this theory, Berry v. Moench, 331 P.2d 814 (Utah, 1958), a physician responded in writing to questions a second doctor asked about a former patient. The second doctor had made his inquiry on behalf of the parents of a girl who contemplated marriage with the former patient. The court held that the doctor who answered the inquiry could be held liable because of statements made in the letter (which indicated the plaintiff was mentally unfit, had trouble in school, had had difficulties with the authorities during the war, did not have a successful first marriage, and had not paid his bill).

The defendant doctor based these statements on his treatment of the patient seven years prior to the writing of the reply and upon the unverified statements made at that time by persons who might not have been objective about the patient. After receiving the reply, the inquiring doctor showed it to the parents of the girl; and the parents then actively attempted to stop the marriage. The daughter married the plaintiff, however, and she was disowned by her parents.

The defendant claimed that his statement was privileged, but the court said the privilege was exceeded by the use of information that was unjustified.

This case shows there is a limit to the privilege a physician has in revealing information to third parties. Further, it shows the need for care – extreme care – in formulating answers to inquiries even when there is a qualified privilege.

The second basis upon which a claim for damages can be made for disclosure of information without consent is that based upon a breach of a confidential relationship. It arises in an existing physician-patient relationship when a physician discloses, to a third party, nonpublic information about a patient which he acquired in the course of treating the patient.

Some cases on this point have indicated that the physician or therapist will not be held liable if he reveals the information in response to a superior duty. In fact, in a well-known California case, the court imposed a positive duty upon a psychotherapist to disclose confidential information to the extent necessary to avert danger to third parties. Tarasoff et al. v. Regents of the University of California et al., 131 Cal. Rptr. 14, 551 P.2d 334 (1976). In Tarasoff, the parents of murder victim Tatiana Tarasoff alleged that the killer had confided his intention to kill Tatiana to a psychologist employed by the university. At the psychologist's request, campus police briefly detained the killer but released him when the psychologist's superior so ordered. No one warned Tatiana of the threat, and she was killed. The court ruled that although public policy favors protection of the confidential character of patient-therapist communications, that privilege must end where public peril begins. The duty to disclose confidential information is limited, however, to that information necessary to avert danger to others. Even then, the disclosure must be accomplished in such a way as to preserve the privacy of the patient "to the fullest extent compatible with the prevention of the threatened danger."

The third theory, invasion of privacy, has given rise to most of the suits for liability for disclosure. In an action for invasion of privacy, if the information is disclosed and a person is held up to ridicule, scorn, or humiliation in the community, or if one unreasonably intrudes upon the seclusion of another, liability will follow.

In a case in Oregon, Humphers v. First Interstate Bank, 684 P.2d 581 (Or. App. 1984), a physician revealed an ex-patient's name to the patient's natural daughter, who had been given up for adoption more than 20 years previously. The physician instructed the hospital to allow the daughter to review the mother's medical records so the daughter could determine the mother's whereabouts and contact her regarding her use of diethylstilbestrol during pregnancy. The hospital allowed the daughter to view and copy the mother's records, and the daughter thus discovered the mother's identity. The court ruled the physician's actions had substantially interfered with the seclusion which the mother had deliberately placed over a portion of her life, and thus constituted an invasion of privacy.

There is, therefore, possibility of liability for disclosure of information when the nature of the disclosure falls in any of these theories. Although medical record practitioners have not figured in any of these theories due to their diligence and strict adherence to the rule of confidentiality, it is always possible for a suit to be brought if the medical record department should become careless in handling medical information.

The degree of damages awarded in such disclosure cases will be related to the humiliation, scorn, and public ridicule suffered by the person whose privacy has been invaded, who has been defamed, or who claims that breach of the confidential relationship has occurred.

OTHER LEGAL ASPECTS

The following legal issues affect the medical record department primarily indirectly. They are discussed here to provide information to aid in the operation of the department. Other hospital personnel have the primary responsibility in the areas discussed.

INFORMED CONSENT

Each patient has the right to decide for himself (or through his authorized representative) what treatment, therapy, or procedures will be performed on his person. Consent for treatment may be express or implied. A patient gives express consent by agreeing, orally or in writing, to the treatment. Because it is difficult to prove that oral consent was given, most express consent is expected to be in writing and documented in the medical record. Consent for emergency treatment is implied unless the provider has reason to believe the patient would not consent.

In order for the consent to be valid, the patient must be informed regarding the treatment to which he is consenting. The Veteran's Administration defines informed consent for care under their jurisdiction:

> "The freely given consent that follows a careful explanation by a practitioner to the patient or the patient's representative of the proposed diagnostic or therapeutic procedure or course of treatment." Further, Veteran's Administration regulations specify that the "patient should be given the opportunity to ask questions, to indicate comprehension of the information provided, and to grant permission freely and without any coercion for performance of a procedure or course of treatment, as well as the opportunity to withhold or revoke such permission at any time without prejudice."

While the patient must be given sufficient information to be informed, the question arises of how much information is sufficient. Certain states have enacted legislation regarding informed consent; but in the absence of legislation, it is generally the practice to inform the patient (or his authorized representative) of the nature of the proposed treatment; the expected benefits; reasonably foreseeable risks, complications or side effects; reasonable alternatives; and anticipated results if the treatment or procedure is not performed.

It is generally held that the physician, not the hospital, has the responsibility for obtaining informed consent, unless the physician is employed by the hospital. Failure to obtain consent to a medical or surgical procedure may result in an action against the physician for battery – unlawful touching. Battery is distinguished from negligence in that negligence is carelessness which causes harm, whereas battery is a touching to which the patient has not consented.

Some hospitals use a blanket consent to medical and hospital treatment, signed when the patient is admitted. However, these general forms may provide no more legal protection than the implied consent inherent in admission to the hospital.

For major procedures, more detailed and specific consent forms are generally used. The medical record should contain all consent forms signed by the patient.

An adult patient may consent to his own treatment, unless he is physically unable or declared legally incompetent to handle his own affairs. Most states have enacted statutes which clearly specify who is entitled to act on behalf of such persons. If there is doubt as to a person's ability to act on his own behalf, the doctor should obtain consent from the patient and the patient's nearest relative.

A spouse's consent, in addition to the patient's, may be requested by a facility as a matter of policy for procedures affecting the patient's sexual or reproductive functions, or those procedures which may result in the death of an infant. It must be remembered that these consents are not essential to treating the patient. Rather they are often obtained as a public-relations effort to avoid misunderstandings which could surface at a later time.

MINORS' CONSENT TO TREATMENT

In most states, a person is considered a minor until he has reached the age of 18 or 21 or is emancipated from his parents as defined by the law. The facts and circumstances of emancipation vary from state to state. In some states, laws provide guidelines for establishing emancipation; in others, the terms are strictly spelled out.

Children under the age of majority or who are not considered emancipated by law cannot generally consent to their own treatment. The parent or legal guardian should sign the consent.

In some cases, whichever parent accompanies the minor patient may consent to his care. Should a dispute arise, however, between legally separated or divorced parents, the final authority for treatment rests with the parent who has legal custody of the child.

It should also be noted that many states have enacted legislation providing that minors may consent to treatment for venereal diseases, drug and alcohol dependency, and some have specific provisions allowing married or pregnant unmarried minors to give consent for their own care and that of their child.

The medical record practitioner should become familiar with the applicable state provisions, since most laws governing a person's ability to consent for treatment apply equally to his right to authorize release of information from the medical record.

AUTOPSIES AND CORONER'S CASES

An authorization for autopsy is as important as an authorization for operation. By statute in most states and by custom in the others, a consent must be obtained. The accepted theory is that there is a quasi-property right in dead bodies vested in the nearest relative of the deceased and rising out of their duty to bury their dead.

In many states the order of responsibility for burial is set forth in statutes, and the right to authorize the hospital to perform an autopsy is given to the person who has assumed custody of the body for burial.

> In the absence of binding directions by the deceased, the surviving spouse is recognized as the person who controls the disposition of the remains. However, in some states, if the surviving spouse has abandoned and is living apart from the deceased, the right is waived. If there is no surviving spouse or if the surviving spouse fails to act or waives the right, then control passes to the next of kin. Unless statute or common law precedent in the jurisdiction establishes a different order of kinship, the priority is generally recognized to be adult child, parent, and adult sibling.

The great majority of autopsy consent statutes can be classified into two groups: those that establish an order for obtaining consent to autopsy based on the nature of kinship to the deceased, and those that require a consent from enumerated persons without an order of priority. In addition, every state has legislation and procedures defining the authority of persons to donate organs or authorize autopsy after death.

All states provide for investigation of certain deaths by specified officers, usually called the coroner or medical examiner.

In most states, coroner's or medical examiner's cases include deaths suspected as being due to suicide, homicide, or any criminal or wrongful act including late effects of injury or poisoning; when a body is found lying dead or unattended (those occurring without medical attendance); and cases where the patient dies in the operating room. In such cases, the coroner or medical

examiner takes charge of the body; and he may or may not authorize an autopsy. In any event, an authorization is not
needed; and the coroner or medical examiner completes the
death certificate. All states have statutes empowering the
coroner or medical examiner to perform an autopsy where death
occurs suddenly, or under suspicious circumstances, or without
medical attendance, or where the manner of death is in doubt.

VALIDITY OF PHYSICIAN SIGNATURES

The medical record practitioner often thinks of a signature as
a name written by a physician, resident, intern, nurse, or other
health care provider, intended to signify that the person agrees
with the data which precede. However, in the broader sense, a
signature is any distinguishing sign, stamp, or mark. The
courts have held that any form of authorized signature, such
as that made with a rubber stamp, typewriter symbols, or initials, may be held to be valid, providing the person affixing the
signature was authorized to do so.

However, if thought is being given to the acceptance of
rubber-stamp signatures or initials, four points should be considered: (1) the Joint Commission on Accreditation of Hospitals
does not accept rubber-stamp signatures unless there is a signed
statement in the health facility administrator's file to the effect
that the physician is the only one who has the stamp and is
the only one who will use it; (2) it may be very difficult to identify initials at a later date; (3) regulations in many states require the signature of the physician in language which precludes the interpretation that a facsimile will be an adequate
substitute; and (4) rubber-stamp signatures are unacceptable in
Medicare attestation statements.

In view of the standards of the Joint Commission on Accreditation of Hospitals, in light of state licensing regulations, and
in consideration of the general requirements of system security
and system reliability, hospital policy with regard to signatures
should be carefully formulated.

If the attending physician is not required to affix his signature by his own hand on the records of his patient, the hospital
has no assurance whatsoever that the physician evaluated the
record's content before the stamp was affixed. Medical evaluation of the medical record is very necessary for the welfare and

protection of the patient, the hospital, the physician, and to meet the requirements of accrediting agencies.

AMENDING OR CORRECTING THE MEDICAL RECORD

Both minor and serious errors may occur in the record. For minor errors, such as errors in transcription and spelling, persons authorized by hospital policy to make record entries may correct them when discovered soon after the original entry was made. Errors of a more serious nature, such as correcting erroneous medication orders or supplying important progress notes after the fact, must be corrected by the health professional involved, if possible, and recorded in acceptable fashion. Careless alterations create the appearance of tampering. Writing over an entry, eradicating, erasing, or adding marginal notes all cast suspicion on a record. The following procedure should be followed:

- Draw a single, thin line through each line of the inaccurate material, making certain it is still legible.
- Date and initial the error.
- Add a note in the margin stating why the previous entry has been replaced.
- Enter the correction in chronological order.
- Authenticate the correction, and record the date and time the correction was made.
- Make certain to indicate which entry the correction is replacing.

AMENDMENTS TO RECORD BY PATIENT

Some patients request modification of medical records. The AMRA's "Position Statement on Confidentiality of Health Records" states "in the event that the patient wishes to correct data, it shall be done as an amendment, without change to the original entry." When a patient requests that his record be amended, hospital staff should advise the patient's attending physician of the changes requested. The physician should discuss the matter with the patient if the physician considers the requested amendment inappropriate.

If the physician concurs with the appropriateness of the amendment, some hospitals permit the physician or nurse supervisor to make amendments in the same manner as corrections of substantive errors as previously described. If the record is amended, the physician or nurse supervisor should add an entry to document that the change was made at the request of the patient, who will, thereafter, bear the burden of explaining the change.

Instead of changing the original entry, some hospitals permit the patient to add a letter of amendment to the record. If the staff concurs with the statement, the concurrence may be noted on the letter.

HOSPITAL LIEN LAWS

A lien law gives a hospital the right to file its claim for payment for services which it has rendered to a person injured by negligent or tortious conduct of another.

In some states the lien is operative against the person who causes the injury, as well as against the insurance company which insured the person causing the injury. Some states provide in their lien law that a hospital claiming a lien must permit all defendants in the damage suit to examine all records of the care and treatment of the injured person without signed authorization of the patient; other states require the patient's consent. The Texas law is illustrative:

> The records of any such association, corporation, or other institution or body maintaining such hospital records in reference to such treatment, care, and maintenance of such injured person shall be made available as promptly as possible for examination to any party's attorney by, for, or against whom a claim shall be asserted for compensation for such injuries, under such reasonable rules and regulations such hospital may require, except that access shall not be denied on the basis of such records being incomplete. The records are admissible as evidence in any civil suit based on those personal injuries subject to applicable rules of evidence. (Vernon's Annotated Texas Statutes, Article 5506(a).)

INCIDENT REPORTS

An incident or occurrence report is an important administrative tool used for the following purposes:

- to notify hospital administration and medical staff that an incident has occurred.

- to notify the hospital risk manager, attorney, and insurer that a possible claim against the hospital exists.
- to use in conducting loss-prevention activities to attempt to prevent future incidents.

An incident report becomes especially valuable in cases of legal action at a later date, because it is written at the time of the occurrence while the incident is fresh in the minds of those who report it.

Because of the potential value of such reports, the American Hospital Association, some years ago, urged hospitals to establish a reporting system. At that time, they defined an incident as "any happening which is not consistent with the routine operation of the hospital or the routine care of a patient."

However, hospital management is increasingly concerned about the possibility that reports which reconstruct the factual details of incidents involving patients, visitors, or employees may be obtained by attorneys and become the basis of lawsuits. The concern is valid. As in many other aspects of administration, the law plays a secondary, but very influential, role in the decision-making process. Hospital management must seek a balance among several considerations.

Occurrence reports are routinely kept and evaluated to provide important information which can direct the hospital's loss prevention programs. However, if they are routinely made a part of the hospital's record-keeping system, they may be subject to subpoena. If incident reports are especially prepared for use by hospital attorneys and insurers, other attorneys may not be able to obtain copies under subpoena. Access to incident-report regulations varies from state to state and is an important consideration when the hospital's incident-reporting system is developed.

There are administrative judgments that have to be made which balance the value of an incident-reporting system with the possibility of damage to the hospital if the information becomes known to an inquiring attorney.

Routinely, incident reports should be filed in the hospital administrator's, attorney's, or risk-manager's office. They should not be filed in the medical record. However, any incident affecting a patient's care should be noted in the physician's progress notes or in the nurses' notes. It is to be remembered that the incident report is a factual report, and it should not attempt to fix or avoid blame or negligence. If an incident-report system

Incident Report

An incident is any occurrence which is not consistent with the routine operation of the institution or the routine care of a particular patient. It may involve an injury or damage to property. It may involve visitors, in-house staff, or patient.

CONFIDENTIAL REPORT OF INCIDENT
(Not a part of Medical Record)

—USE ADDRESSOGRAPH IF PATIENT—

Hospital　　LARS Loc. Code

PERSON INVOLVED: (Last Name) (First Name) (Middle Initial)
☐ Child ☐ Male ☐ Female Age:

Exact Location of Incident | Date of Incident | Time of Incident ☐ A.M. ☐ P.M.

EMPLOYEE: Department | Job Title

VISITOR: Home Address | Home Telephone

OTHER: Home Address | Home Telephone

PATIENT: Room Number | State Cause of Hospitalization
Patient's condition before incident ☐ Normal ☐ Senile ☐ Disoriented ☐ Sedated ☐ Other
Were Bed Rails present ☐ Yes ☐ No ☐ Up ☐ Down ☐ Ordered | Other Restraints

Name, Address and Telephone Number of Witness(es)

Describe exactly what happened. (Facts, no opinions):

Date of Report | Person Preparing Report

Form used with permission of Hartford Insurance Group, Hartford, Connecticut.

FIG. 1 – INCIDENT REPORT

is maintained either as a routine or in special cases only, a form similar to that shown in Figure 1 may be considered.

Some cases have indicated that if incident reports are routinely made, they are subject to subpoena; but if they are specially prepared for the hospital's attorney or insurance carrier, they may be protected from disclosure as part of the attorney's "work product."

There are strong reasons for maintaining incident reports. As indicated, a factual report written at the time of the incident is a valuable document not only because the memories of witnesses and participants will be fresh, but also because periodic review and analysis by the facility's safety committee can lead to corrective measures which will benefit the hospital and the patient.

The incident report is not an indictment. It will not necessarily lead to the conclusion that someone has been negligent. The report, in fact, may show the patient was careless; or that the occurrence was unavoidable. However, the possibility of suit is present; and even if the outcome is favorable to the hospital, the suit will be time-consuming and costly. On the other hand, hospitals are now sued with greater frequency than in the past; but this has not come about because incident reports have been maintained.

The hospital medical record committee, along with legal counsel, should make a review of the facility's incident-reporting procedures and practices. A policy should then be developed to meet the needs of the hospital in light of the legal climate in the state.

HOSPITAL AND MEDICAL STAFF COMMITTEE REPORTS

Ongoing review of the quality and appropriateness of medical and hospital care is the responsibility of various hospital and medical staff committees such as Tissue Review, Pharmacy and Therapeutics, Medical Record, Blood Utilization, Quality Assurance, and Utilization committees. The purpose of these committees is to provide ongoing review of care to identify, assess, and resolve patient care problems.

Statutes have been enacted in most states which limit the applicability of the subpoena process to the minutes and records of these committees. Some statutes make the information inadmissible. On the other hand, several courts have permitted the use of subpoenas in pretrial discovery. If the plaintiff can show that the information sought is relevant to the subject matter or reasonably calculated to lead to the discovery of admissible evidence, he is on more solid ground. There is growing recognition that plaintiffs in malpractice cases have difficulty in obtaining relevant information which may be in the sole possession of the physician and his colleagues or in hospital records other than patient records. It is to be noted that even when documents are expressly inadmissible in evidence, they may be subject to discovery in the pretrial process.

It is important that the hospital administrator and the medical record director obtain information from hospital counsel on the applicability of the discovery process to all hospital records. The practice varies from state to state, and within each state the federal rules may differ from the state rules.

SUMMARY

The medical record as an order of business is the property of the hospital, while the personal data contained in the record are considered a confidential communication in which the patient has a protectable interest. The record is compiled, preserved, and protected from unauthorized inspection for the benefit of the patient, hospital, and physician as required by law in some states and by administrative practice in others.

Since the medical record frequently is used as legal evidence of the patient's hospitalization, it can serve as a protection to the hospital, physician, and patient only when it clearly shows the treatment given the patient, by whom given, and when given. It must show that the care and service given by the hospital and by the physician were consistent with good medical practice. By the same token, the record may prove to be a potent weapon against the hospital or physician in an action by the patient.

The medical record must be maintained to serve the patient, the health care providers, and the institution in accordance with legal, accrediting, and regulatory agency requirements. The health facility should have a provision for making its procedures regarding disclosure, access, and amendment of health record information known to patients upon request; and the release of information should be closely controlled. A properly completed and signed authorization is required for release of all health information except:

a) as required by law

b) for release to another health care provider currently involved in the care of the patient

c) for medical care evaluation

d) for research and education in certain situations

The medical record practitioner who wishes to serve his hospital, the patient, and the community properly must be familiar with the statutes, regulations, and cases governing medical records in general, and those which apply to his state and community in particular. In addition, he must take an active role in the development and enforcement of the policies of his hospital regarding the proper release of information, whether it be in answer to a subpoena, in response to requests from governmental agencies, from the individual patient, from relatives of patients, or others.

STUDY QUESTIONS

1. Specify the recommended items to be included in a form for authorization of release of patient information.

2. List the steps to be taken in preparing a patient's medical record for entry into court proceedings in response to a subpoena duces tecum.

3. Describe the circumstances in which the patient may intentionally or unintentionally waive the privilege of consenting to release of his medical record.

4. Differentiate between medical records and secondary records.

5. Discuss the rights of insurance companies and law enforcement agencies to confidential patient information.

6. Define negligence, and explain how the concept "standard of care" is used in potential medical liability cases.

7. Discuss potential conflicts that may arise over the hospital's property right to the medical record and the patient's right to control the information contained in it.

REFERENCES

"A Patient's Bill of Rights." American Hospital Association, 1975.

Accreditation Manual for Hospitals. Joint Commission on Accreditation of Hospitals. Chicago, Illinois, 1985.

BROCCALO, BERNADETTE MULLER. "The Importance of Proper Medical Record Entries." *Topics in Health Record Management.* September, 1981.

BRUCE, JO ANNE CZECOWSKI. *Privacy and Confidentiality of Health Care Information.* Chicago, Illinois: American Hospital Publishing, Inc., 1984.

CHRISTOFFEL, TOM. *Health and the Law.* New York, New York: The Free Press, 1982.

"Conditions of Participation, Hospitals." United States Department of Health and Human Services.

"Confidentiality of Patient Health Information." A Position Statement of the American Medical Record Association. Revised, 1985.

Consent Manual. 11th Edition. California Hospital Association, 1984.

CUSHING, MAUREEN. "Informed Consent, an M.D. Responsibility?" *American Journal of Nursing.* April, 1984, Vol. 84, pp. 437-440.

Health Record Information Manual. Texas Medical Record Association, 1979.

Medical Record Guidelines. Iowa Medical Record Association, 1981.

Medical Records and Michigan Law. Michigan Medical Record Association, 1974.

Medical Records and the Law – an Illinois Guide to Medicolegal Principles and Release of Information. Illinois Medical Record Association, 1977.

Medicolegal Manual. Medical Record Association of New York State, Inc., 1981.

MILLER, ROBERT D. *Problems in Hospital Law,* 4th Ed. Rockville, Maryland: Aspen Systems, 1983.

Personal Privacy in an Information Society. The Report of the Privacy Protection Study Commission. July, 1977. U.S. Government Printing Office, Washington, D.C.

POZGAR, GEORGE D. *Legal Aspects of Health Care Administration.* Rockville, Maryland: Aspen Systems, 1979.

Principles of Medical Ethics. American Medical Association, 1980.

Release of Information Guide. Indiana Medical Record Association, 1981.

The Record That Defends Its Friends. Chicago, Illinois: Care Communications, 1979.

The Right of the Patient to Refuse Treatment. American Hospital Association, 1975.

"Topics in Health Record Management, Legal Issues, Part I and II." Rockville, Maryland: Aspen Systems. June/September, 1981.

"Veteran's Administration Final Regulations" (on Informed Consent). *Federal Register*, Vol. 49, No. 49, March 12, 1984, pp. 9171-9173.

chapter *18*

MEDICAL RECORD DEPARTMENT MANAGEMENT

INTRODUCTION

OVERVIEW OF MANAGEMENT

Basic Components – Management has been defined as the process of getting things done through and with people. It is the effective utilization of resources toward the accomplishment of specific objectives. Four basic components emerge from any definition of management: effectiveness, functions, resources, and objectives (see Figure 1).

First, the term "management" should be synonymous with effectiveness. Effectiveness ensures that the utilization of resources accomplishes the objectives. In general, an organization will define its objectives in terms of producing a certain number of products or services at a specified level of quality with a specified amount of resources. Effectiveness embodies productivity, performance, and efficiency. Productivity is the quantitative aspect – the number of items created or the number of services accomplished. Performance is the qualitative aspect – the number and types of errors or defects in the products, or the sensations and perceptions created in the person for whom a service is rendered. Finally, efficiency is the appropriate utilization of the specified resources.

The process of utilizing resources toward accomplishment of an objective is generally defined as the combined functions of planning, organizing, directing, and controlling. *Planning* is the definition of objectives and the plotting and devising of a course of action to accomplish the objectives. *Organizing* brings together resources in an orderly manner and arranges people in an acceptable pattern so they can perform activities to accomplish the objectives. *Directing* deals with stimulating members of a work group to perform work in such a manner that the ob-

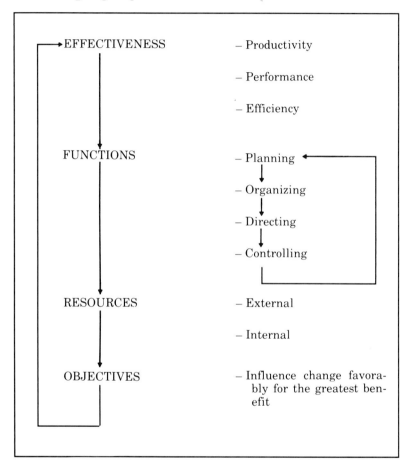

FIG. 1 – MANAGEMENT DEFINED

jectives are met. *Controlling* is the feedback mechanism to the planning function. It is guiding operations in accordance with plans and ensuring that desired results (objectives) are achieved.

The third component of management is resources, which are both external and internal to a manager. External resources include manpower, money, materials, methods, and machinery. Internal resources include the managerial traits of creativity, coordination, cooperation, communication, common sense, and many other behavioral characteristics.

Finally, objectives exist because underlying all of management is the existence of change. Objectives direct an organization in the face of change – in human attitudes, technology, legislation, and all aspects of the environment. A manager is one who monitors an organizational environment to anticipate change and to bring about the necessary adaptive responses to ensure that the organization's objectives are met.

As can be seen by its definition, management is a complexity of interrelated conceptual, human, and technical components. The management challenge is a demanding one. The abilities needed to become a manager must be developed not only through study but through experience and the cultivation of one's own innate talents. A single chapter in a text designed to define the roles and functions specific to medical record practice cannot fully cover every aspect of management. Thus, this chapter identifies pertinent aspects of management which the medical record practitioner uses to achieve a medical record department's objectives. To gain a full knowledge and understanding of the concepts and techniques presented, the reader is expected to study additional references, such as those provided at the end of the chapter.

THE PLANNING FUNCTION

It has been suggested that planning is "something you do before you do something, so that when you do it, it's not all mixed up" (A. A. Milne, *Winnie the Pooh*). Planning is the process of determining a desired outcome and defining a course of action to achieve the outcome.

Planning is the most important management function, yet often the most neglected. Managers may not take the full time required for planning or may procrastinate over its decision-making component with the result causing "crisis" management. The "crisis" manager takes action on problems only when the efficient operation of all or part of the department is significantly hampered. By the time this has occurred, problems have to be solved rapidly; there is no time for thorough investigation of their causes or careful consideration of alternative solutions. While planning cannot foresee or prepare for all problems which may arise, it can certainly contribute to their reduction.

Planning may be simple and informal, such as in scheduling the day's activities; or it may be complex and very formal as in implementing a new computer system. At whatever level planning occurs, there are two major activities in the planning process – problem analysis and decision making. Problem analysis is the identification and understanding of deviations from defined objectives.

PROBLEM ANALYSIS

Components

1. Identify objectives in which change is causing a deviation.
2. Collect complete data about all factors surrounding the problem.
3. Analyze data fully to understand the problem and how it came about.

DECISION MAKING

Components

1. Identify planning premises – requirements and constraints surrounding the objective.
2. Develop alternative solutions to the problem to meet the objective.
3. Select the best alternative which meets as many requirements and constraints as possible in accomplishing the objective.
4. Define how and when the alternative will be accomplished.
5. Develop a system for follow-up to evaluate the progress of the objective's accomplishment.

Various types of plans are formulated for medical record departments to meet their varied objectives, and various techniques may be used in the planning process.

TYPES OF PLANS

Objectives are the targets which provide scope and direction to the department manager. The departmental objectives should complement and supplement overall organizational goals, and they should be understood by all. Objectives are usually further elaborated upon and documented in three, not necessarily mutually exclusive, types of plans – operational, programmatic, and financial.

Operational

Operational planning addresses objectives relating to the ongoing activities of the medical record department. These identify specific categories of services to be performed, such as "provide medical record retrieval service daily" or "transcribe basic reports for inclusion in the medical record within two days of their dictation."

Operational plans are frequently developed through a technique called management by objectives (MBO). Originally designed as a participative management tool in which the flow of planning moves from the bottom of the organizational hierarchy up; MBO is frequently practiced in reverse – where objective setting begins with top management and filters down through the organization. MBO can be very effective in having everyone in the organization take part in defining its future and thereby developing a commitment to the objectives. One of the primary disadvantages of MBO, as it is frequently practiced, is that it can become an exercise in short term objective setting for the benefit of the organization as a whole.

Operational plans are frequently embodied in policies, procedures, standards, and rules. Policies are plans for decision making. A policy defines the area in which decisions are made but does not necessarily provide the specific decision. An effective policy requires judgment but not complex interpretation. Policies within an organization should also be consistent. An example of a policy is "promote from within whenever possible." The phrase "whenever possible" allows the manager to look outside the organization for a qualified candidate if, in the manager's judgment, none exists within.

Procedures are plans for action. They are a series of related steps designed to accomplish a specific task. Procedures are developed for repetitive work in order to specifically define the task, to achieve uniformity of practice, and to facilitate training. An example of a procedure is displayed in Figure 2.

A standard is a measure established to serve as a criterion or level of reference for determining the accomplishment of an objective. Because standards are so closely tied to the controlling function, they will be fully described under the topic of controlling later in this chapter.

PROCEDURE: _Assembly of Medical Records_   PAGE: ___1___ OF: ___1___

PREPARED BY: _Mary Martin, RRA_   REVISION: ___7-7-85___

PURPOSE: Arrange the contents of the medical records of discharged patients to facilitate later review and permanent filing.

RESOURCES: Medical records from Discharge Area
Hole punch, black pen

DETAILS: 1. At 9:00 am and 1:00 pm visit the Discharge Area to obtain medical records of discharged patients to assemble.

2. Assemble all sheets pertaining to the hospitalization period in accordance with the Filing Arrangement of Medical Records (see Appendix A).

3. Each group of like forms (e.g., all progress notes) should be filed in date order, from admission date to discharge date.

9. Attach all sheets in the correct order to the top set of prongs in the medical record. Punch holes if necessary.

10. Deliver assembled records to Analysis Work Station immediately.

FIG. 2 – SAMPLE PROCEDURE

Rules are plans that delineate a required or prohibited course of action. Rules allow for no decision making or interpretation but, rather, require or limit specific action authoritatively and officially. Examples of rules include "sign in when work is begun" and "no smoking except in designated areas." Within an organization, rules should be reasonable, known to all, and applied equally to all.

Programmatic

The second major type of plan, the programmatic plan, addresses objectives relating to special projects or programs, such as "install a medical record monitoring system on a personal computer." The organization may contract with an independent consultant to design and implement a program or project, in which case the program or project will be defined by the organization in a request for proposal (RFP). The consultant will then draw up a programmatic plan which the organization accepts or rejects. When programs or projects are to be accomplished internally, without outside assistance, the organization draws up the programmatic plan. A programmatic plan is highly formalized, explicitly documenting each step of the planning process. Depending on the scope and nature of the project or program, any number of planning techniques may be utilized, such as interviews, forecasts, decision trees, schedules, and audit trails.

Financial

Financial plans are the third major type of plan. Financial plans are plans expressed in monetary terms. The most common financial plan is the budget. It outlines the objectives for a specific period of time and the resources required to achieve those objectives. For a health care organization as a whole there may be four elements comprising the budget: the revenue and expense budget, the cash budget, the capital budget, and the pro forma (projected or estimated) statements. In a hospital the revenue and expense budget includes estimates of gross patient revenue; allowances for cost-based payers and uncollectible accounts; expenses for personnel, supplies, depreciation, interest, and insurance; and other nonpatient care operating and nonoperating revenue and expenses. This budget is based on statistical estimates for occupancy, patient or case mix, ancillary services, and other level-of-activity projections. The cash budget is a projection of cash balances at the end of each month throughout the budget year, based on operating cash receipts and disbursements, receipt or payment of loan principal, and capital expenditures. The capital budget is a plan that shows major expenditures and sources of funds for plant and equipment which are expected to last longer than a single budgeting period. The pro forma statements are projected or forecasted statements of a future period. The most common pro forma statements include the pro forma balance sheet showing the financial condition at a future point in time and the pro forma income statement describing the financial results of operations for a future period.

The budget may be developed in a number of ways. For health care facilities, the two most common are the standard budget (by responsibility or function), and zero-based budget. A standard responsibility budget is one that is organized by cost center or group of cost centers over which a single manager is responsible. A separate budget is prepared by each manager and defines accountability for specific portions of the organization-wide budget. A standard functional budget is organized along functions, services, or departments in order to identify such functional costs as nursing, housekeeping, and medical records. One advantage of this type of budget is that service costs can be compared among different facilities.

A zero-based budget is one which is created as if all activities were entirely new. Each activity is evaluated for funding or elimination. Appropriate funding levels are determined by priorities and ranking established by top management according to the overall availability of funds. This type of budget instills accountability into the manager, for all activities must be completely justified, not just increases over the previous year's appropriation as in the standard type of budget. These two budgets are not mutually exclusive, and a health care facility may develop a zero-based functional budget. The steps in the budget process are outlined in Figure 3.

Another financial plan common in hospitals is a cost analysis, sometimes termed cost-finding analysis. This is the process of allocating all costs of operating a hospital to cost centers or departments which produce revenue. The result of cost-finding analysis on revenue-producing departments is the issuance of a budgetary policy describing each department's expected revenue contribution. For nonrevenue producing departments, such as medical records, the result is an apportionment of funds to finance its operations. Cost-finding analysis is a complex process due to the nature of a hospital's sources of revenue. The hospital's primary source of revenue is third-party payers paying for services rendered. The major third-party payers are Blue Cross and the federal government (principally Medicare and Medicaid), which pay on a wholesale "cost" basis. Furthermore, these costs may be paid under a periodic interim payment (PIP) plan in which the hospital receives interim payments at least monthly, based on estimated costs with retroactive adjustments at the end of each accounting period. Other payers are commercial insurance companies and the patient who pay at retail rates, higher than "cost" or "cost-plus." With concerns over health care costs and the recently introduced prospective payment system paying predetermined average rates, cost-finding

ACTIVITY	RESPONSIBILITY
1. Determine long range objectives.	Senior Administration Governing Board
2. Develop budget format. Develop guidelines for range increases.	Budget Committee
3. Forecast volume of work.	Department Managers
4. Approve forecasts.	Budget Committee
5. Develop preliminary revenue and expense budgets; prepare proposals for special programs and positions.	Department Managers
6. Review department budgets.	Individual Senior Administrators
7. Consolidate cost center or department budgets into tentative hospital-wide budget.	Budget Director
8. Determine desired net income, rate increases, scale and merit salary increases, and funds available for new programs and positions. Review, rank, and recommend approval for requests for new programs and positions.	Budget Committee
9. Approve final operating budget.	Budget Committee Senior Administration Governing Board
10. Distribute budget to managers and administrators.	Budget Director

FIG. 3 – STEPS IN THE BUDGET PROCESS

analysis has become an even more complex planning process. Cost-accounting techniques have also begun to be used where exact unit costs are determined for all supplies and services (instead of cost finding, which groups all costs and spreads them over the various supplies and services).

While performed for the organization as a whole, every department should be aware of the cost-finding process and understand its position relative to it. The medical record department, in particular, while nonrevenue producing, has a significant impact on a hospital's accounts receivable. Well-planned systems in the medical record department mean prompt and accurate flow of information for billing, which in turn means improved cash flow for the hospital.

THE ORGANIZING FUNCTION

Organizing is the management function of distributing or allocating resources toward the accomplishment of the objectives defined in the plans. Organizing requires an understanding of the concepts of staffing and work distribution. Organizing, however, also includes the allocation of material, machine, and space resources.

STAFFING AND WORK-DISTRIBUTION CONCEPTS

The allocation of work among staff has both horizontal and vertical components (Figure 4). The horizontal components of organization include the concepts of departmentation, line-staff responsibility, and coordination, since they involve dividing work into departments, assigning tasks to departments, and coordinating these departments. Levels and span of control, authority, and delegation make up the vertical components, explaining how authority is delegated downward within the organization.

DEPARTMENTATION AND COORDINATION

Departmentation is the efficient and effective grouping of jobs into meaningful work units to coordinate efforts. The major means of departmentation are by purpose or process. Purpose departmentation is most common in the industrial/product sector, where work is divided by specific products, customers, or geographic locations. This type of departmentation emphasizes an external, "market" orientation, one which the health care industry is now considering as it begins to be reimbursed for services according to product lines (e.g., cases, DRGs, etc.), to differentiate specific customer groups (i.e., acute care, long term

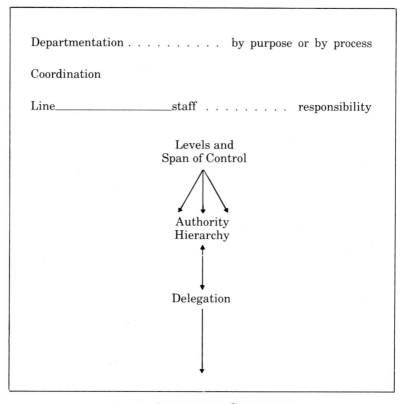

Departmentation . . . . by purpose or by process

Coordination

Line_____staff . . . . responsibility

Levels and
Span of Control

Authority
Hierarchy

Delegation

FIG. 4 – ORGANIZATION COMPONENTS

care, ambulatory care, intensive care, etc.), and to provide its services in alternate locations (in mobile units, shopping centers, etc.). The more traditional means of departmentation for health care organizations has been by process. Process departmentation focuses on building departments around functions. Thus a hospital would have a medical record department, dietary department, finance department, pediatric department, etc. Departmentation also occurs within a department, where subdepartments or subunits are formed by purpose or process. Within the medical record department, process subdepartmentation might result in a transcription area, filing area, discharge processing area, etc.

Departmentation, especially by process, results in units that are highly differentiated, in that they develop different goals, points of view, and organizational structures within themselves. Yet no organization can meet its overall objectives without all departments working together. Coordination is the process that integrates the differentiated, yet interdependent, departments. Organizations use rules, plans, and the authority hierarchy to coordinate work units; but as problems facing the organization become more numerous and complex, then the rules, plans, and referral up the organizational hierarchy become insufficient. A manager then must create lateral relationships to reduce and solve problems.

Formal coordinating mechanisms include committees, liaison roles, and independent integrators. Committees, task forces, or teams are the most common means of trying to achieve coordination, where members meet to discuss and resolve problems common to several departments. Less commonly, a liaison (a person from one department, such as medical records, who works with or in another department, such as billing) is used to handle communication between two departments where problems are frequent but can be resolved quickly with the liaison's expertise. An independent integrator is still another coordinating means in which an individual or department coordinates activities which cross several departmental lines. An example is the patient representative in a large hospital who frequently must work with several departments, as well as the patient, to see that the patient's needs are met. Formal means of coordination, however, have limited effectiveness without a cooperative spirit on the part of the respective departments. Developing informal coordination is difficult and frequently depends on the personalities involved.

RESPONSIBILITY AND AUTHORITY

Dividing work into departments and then coordinating the departments is but one aspect of organizing. Each department must also be assigned responsibility for certain tasks and be given the authority to see these tasks to their completion. Responsibility is the obligation of an individual to carry out assigned activities to the best of the individual's ability. Within an organization, responsibility is usually defined by the relationship of the position to the accomplishment of the organization's objectives. In an organization there are two major types of relationships – line and staff. Line positions have direct responsibility for accomplishing the objectives of the organization. Line positions form a hierarchy within an organization with each position reporting to the level above. Span of control refers to the number of immediate subordinates who report to a manager. Proper span of control is determined by a number of factors. The type of work is the most important factor. In situations where the work is essentially simple and repetitive, the manager may have a wide span of control (as many as eight to fifteen immediate subordinates); whereas in highly dynamic and complex activities a more narrow span of control (four to eight immediate subordinates) is customary. Thus, at lower levels of the organization where day-to-day operations occur, managers generally have wider spans of control than at higher levels of the organization where they must deal with more strategic issues. Other factors which can influence the span of control are the necessity for frequent and involved communication, the amount of subordinate training, and the level of planning which can anticipate and propose solutions for subordinate problem solving. Staff positions are those which assist and advise the line manager in accomplishing the objectives. Staff positions are sometimes considered "less important"; however, these positions usually are ones of a high degree of specialization and are afforded esteem for their level of expertise.

In addition to the relationship between a position and its responsibility for accomplishment of the organization's objectives, each position must have a degree of authority commensurate with its responsibility. Authority is the right given to each position holder to command the behavior for which the position is responsible. It gives managers the right to carry out their tasks by giving orders to their subordinates and to expect compliance. Equally important, but sometimes overlooked, authority also gives subordinates the right to carry out their duties as assigned and to expect support from their superiors when those activities are carried out within their scope of authority.

DELEGATION

The conveyance of responsibility and authority from superior to subordinate is delegation. Delegation involves determining the results expected, assigning the tasks, granting the authority for accomplishment of the tasks, and holding the subordinate responsible for their accomplishment. Delegation is critical to an organization, for one individual cannot accomplish an organization's objectives single-handedly. Most managerial failures result from poor delegation, and much of the reason for poor delegation lies in personal attitudes toward delegation. There are many reasons why managers do not delegate, among them a desire to dominate, a sense of indispensability, an unwillingness to accept risks, and an insecurity in their own positions. But a manager who is receptive to a subordinate's ideas, willing to let go of the right to make decisions within the scope of delegated authority, able to let others make mistakes, trusting of subordinates, and who establishes broad controls as a means of feedback, will find success in accomplishing the organization's objectives through delegation.

INFORMAL ORGANIZATION

A final prerequisite to organizing staff and distributing work is awareness of the informal organization. Whenever people work together, informal groups based on various interests will form. Such informal groups have both advantages and disadvantages. The informal organization affords its members status which, especially in a large organization, may provide a sense of belonging and contributes to personal satisfaction, resulting in a happier, more productive employee. Social values of the informal group, however, may work against the objectives of the formal organization when restrictive membership makes individuals feel outcast or when perpetuation of social values creates resistance to change. The informal organization also promotes communication among members, which, with members helping one another, may lighten management's workload and may act as a safety valve for members to relieve their frustrations. When such communication includes unfounded rumors, or when frustrations become self-fulfilling, the informal organization can undermine morale. The informal organization also provides social control by influencing and regulating members' behavior. Such conformity may keep members in line with formal organizational goals or may stifle initiative and creativity.

STAFFING AND WORK DISTRIBUTION TECHNIQUES

In staffing and work distribution, the organizational structure is usually depicted in an organizational chart (see Figure 5). Each position is shown, most typically, from the top of the authority hierarchy down. Line relationships are shown as solid lines and staff as dotted lines. An organizational chart shows employees and others the limits of each position's authority and responsibility. An organizational chart also aids the manager in discovering confused lines of authority, duplication of functions, inefficient allocation of personnel, too large a span of control, and lack of intermediate supervisory levels. Separate charts may be drawn in an attempt to depict informal or coordinating relationships, although their volatile nature makes them become out of date quickly. Organizational charts should be drawn carefully so authority relationships are not confused with status. For instance, if a secretary reporting to the department head is shown closer to the department head than the assistant department head, there can be confusion over who actually is at a closer level in terms of authority.

The organizational chart contains job titles or functions of one or more individuals. A job is made up of tasks and responsibilities which, when considered together, are regarded as the regular assignment of an individual. To ensure that tasks and responsibilities are organized properly, a manager may perform a job analysis. Jobs are analyzed to determine the content of a job, including the skills, knowledge, abilities, and responsibilities required of the worker. Job analysis provides the manager the opportunity to clarify lines of responsibility and authority. Job analysis can ensure that tasks are grouped and responsibilities are assigned appropriately, resulting in efficiency and quantifiable standards of performance. Wage and salary administration is also facilitated by job analysis. Comparing tasks within jobs across organizations can provide a basis for establishing or realigning a salary structure. A job description is the written result of job analysis and is a listing of duties and responsibilities of a particular job as an average incumbent might fulfill it (see Figure 6).

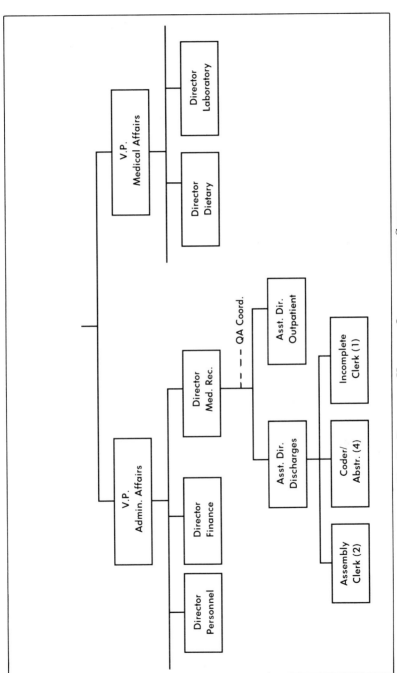

Fig. 5 – Portion of Hospital Organizational Chart

Job descriptions facilitate personnel selection and placement. The personnel department can use them in recruiting job applicants. On the job, descriptions can enable the supervisor to pre-

---

DEPARTMENT: *Medical Records*

POSITION: *File Clerk*   GRADE: *I*

HOURS: *8:00 am – 4:30 pm*   DAYS: *M–F*

JOB SUMMARY: *Files and retrieves medical records; receives, sorts, and files clinic appointment slips, sends and receives medical records to and from Outpatient Department and Admitting Office.*

JOB DUTIES:

    1. Retrieves, as requested, from straight numerical file, medical records for OPD and Admitting Office.

    2. Retrieves and sorts medical records for OPD by appointment slips.

    8. Performs other duties as assigned.

EXPERIENCE: *No experience required, will train on job. High school diploma preferred, but not essential. Must be able to arrange numbers in numerical sequence.*

PHYSICAL: *Standing, stooping, walking 90%; sitting 10% of time. Must be of physical build to permit travel through closely aligned files.*

ENVIRONMENT: *Works in clean, moderately lighted, well-ventilated room.*

REPORTS TO: *File Area Supervisor.*

Fig. 6 – Sample Job Description

pare job orientation plans and training manuals. Job descriptions are necessary for an effective performance-evaluation system and good labor relations as formal documentation of the standards against which an employee will be rated. The list of duties can also be used in investigating grievances regarding the nature of the employee's responsibilities.

An effective tool which can be used to analyze the various tasks within a work unit or department in order to group the tasks into jobs is the work distribution chart (see Figure 7). It records the work activities performed, the time it takes to perform them, the individuals who are working on the activities, and the amount of time spent by each person on each activity.

Activity	Total Hours	MARY SMITH	Hours	SUSAN JONES	Hours	
Chart Assembly	10	Assembly	9	Assembly	1	
Chart Analysis	50	Analysis	20	Analysis	20	
Chart Controls	5	Secure All Charts	2			
Maintenance and Filing Activities on Recent Discharges	8	Chart Repair Filing Loose Reports Chart Location	1 4 1	Chart Repair Chart Location	1 1	
Phone	1	Answer	1			
Statistics	12	Fill Out Work Sheets	2	Fill Out Work Sheets Daily Re-Sort	3 4	Fill Out Daily
Coding	12			Coding	3	Cod
Indexing	23			Indexing	6	
Total	121		40		39	

FIG. 7 – WORK DISTRIBUTION CHART

A work distribution chart is prepared by having each employee keep daily task lists of the various major activities performed throughout each day for several days. (The number of days will depend on the cyclical nature of the unit's work, but usually a week is adequate.) At the end of the data collection period, the manager summarizes the time spent on all activities by each employee on the work distribution chart. Each employee's time may not add to the total number of hours in the work day. Allowances need to be made for fatigue and unavoidable interruptions. A 10 to 15 percent margin of discrepancy is often reasonable.

The work distribution chart lays out work assignments in a form that facilitates critical questioning of the existing situation. It does not provide solutions, but it makes finding them easier. Analysis of the work distribution chart will answer questions such as what activities take the most time? Are unnecessary activities being performed? Are employee skills being properly utilized? Are employees doing too many unrelated tasks? Are tasks being spread too thinly throughout the department or unit? And is work in the unit being distributed evenly?

ORGANIZING THE WORK ENVIRONMENT

The most common means to physically arrange the work environment is to use a layout. This is an architectural chart, drawn to scale, which depicts the location of furniture and equipment within available space. Constraints in designing a layout include permanent physical structures such as walls, posts, and windows, and the location of electrical outlets, water, and drains. Environmental factors such as lighting, color, air conditioning, heat, and sound must be considered when designing a layout. The nature of the furniture and equipment itself puts constraints on their placement. Finally, the policies of the department or organization with regard to private offices, space commensurate with position or tenure, and other elements play a part in the layout. The ideal layout provides for an effective work flow, space that is ample and well utilized, employee comfort and satisfaction, ease of supervision, favorable impression on visitors (if applicable), ample flexibility for varying needs, and balanced capacity of equipment and personnel at each stage in work flow and safety.

One of the greatest problems in designing a layout where work is performed in a sequence of steps passing from one employee to another, or where one employee must move to different work stations, is planning an efficient work flow. Much time can be wasted in backtracking and crisscrossing throughout the work area. A movement diagram (Figure 8), which is an overlay of the flow of work through the layout, is a simple tool which can check that furniture and equipment are placed effectively.

Important points in layout include:
1. Equipment should be near the user.
2. Employees' desks should face in the same direction with two and one-half to three feet between desks.
3. A supervisor should be placed at the back of the group of workers supervised.

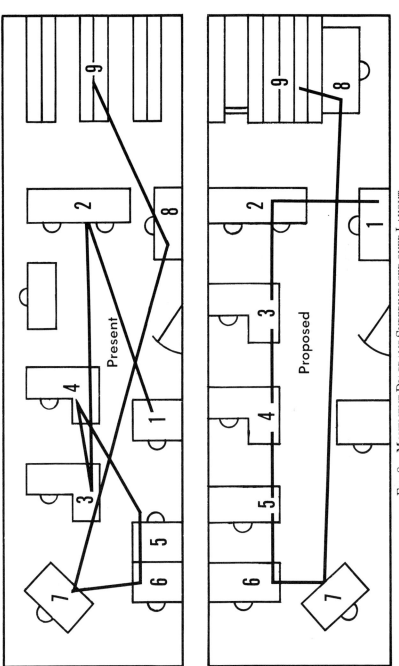

FIG. 8 – MOVEMENT DIAGRAMS SUPERIMPOSED OVER LAYOUT

4. As a general guideline, each clerical employee should be allowed 60 square feet, including space for filing cabinets, additional work area and aisles for each employee.
5. It is best not to place the file room near the main office entrance, in order to reduce the accessibility of medical records to unauthorized personnel.
6. Since medical transcription is one of the noisier activities, it should be confined to one area. Soundproof booths or partitions help to reduce the noise from typewriters.
7. Employees who most often deal with patients or other hospital personnel should be placed near the entrance of the department.
8. Main aisles should be at least 5 feet wide; secondary aisles should be at least 3 feet wide.

In addition to architectural charts to aid in organizing the environment, there are also tools which aid in organizing equipment. Such a chart is a configuration chart, which is a specialized tool for depicting equipment. The need for a configuration chart arises when there are many pieces of interrelated equipment, located in several physically separate areas. The configuration chart helps to keep track of the location and type of equipment and how each is connected. Standard symbols or pictures are used to depict the equipment. Lines connecting the symbols or pictures delineate the flow of data, materials, or work through the equipment. The configuration chart can be effectively used to show computer system equipment, or dictation and transcription equipment.

THE DIRECTING FUNCTION

The directing function of management involves getting all members of a work group to contribute effectively and efficiently to the achievement of the organization's objectives. The terms "directing" and "actuating" are sometimes used synonymously. The dictionary definition of direct is "to set straight, to show or point out, to regulate the activities or course of." The definition of actuate is "to move to action." The slight but distinct difference in these two terms relates to two, often-competing aspects of management – the scientific approach of directing, using tools of work simplification or methods engineering, and the humanistic aspects of actuating, including leadership, motivation, communication, appraising employee performance, developing employee skills, and appropriately compensating productivity and performance.

WORK SIMPLIFICATION

Work simplification is commonly referred to as the organized use of common sense to find easier and better ways of doing work. Work simplification, however, is not a speed-up system, or a new way of working harder or faster. It means doing a better job with less effort, in less time, without hurrying, with greater safety, and with lower costs. This is accomplished by eliminating unnecessary parts of the work, combining and rearranging other parts of the work, and simplifying the necessary parts of the work. Work simplification does not imply changing the basic tenets of a procedure, but changes the methods employed to accomplish it. This may involve new supplies, equipment, a new arrangement of materials, or new operations.

Several tools are available to gather facts, question these facts, and consider the alternative ways to do the work. A flow process chart is the most common tool (Figure 9). While it is possible to simplify without a formal chart, a chart ensures that as much data as possible about the work have been recorded. It permits the analyst to see the whole task at one time. It is useful in comparing alternatives, and it provides written information for others who will be implementing and evaluating the task. The flow process chart is prepared by listing every step in the work in the sequence performed; classifying each step according to type; and recording distance, time, and/or quantity related to each step. Then, every step is challenged – asking why the step is done, why at that location, at that time, by that person, and in that manner. Finally, an improved method should become apparent – one that eliminates or combines; changes places, sequences, or persons; and simplifies.

The result of work simplification is change. Yet most people tend to resist change. Change disturbs complacency and disrupts habits. One of the most critical reasons for resistance to change is that change implies criticism. Every way of doing something was devised by somebody; so when someone else tries to recommend a change, persons related to the previous method

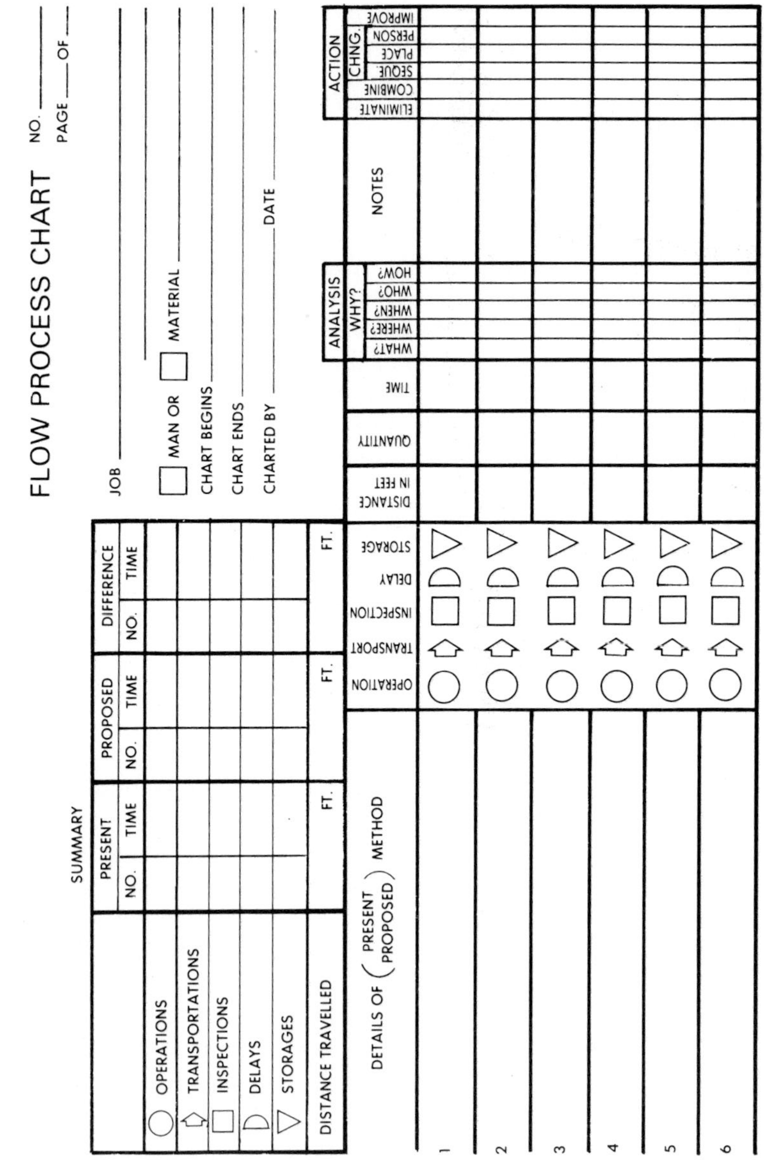

Fig. 9 – Flow Process Chart

often feel their ideas and efforts are being criticized. Another factor related to work changes is the feeling of insecurity which often results. People may feel they will be unable to perform as well with the new method or machine or may not be able to learn the new method. A major goal of work simplification should be to develop open-mindedness toward work methods in everyone – managers and employees alike. The manager's role in work simplification should be one of guidance and assistance, while it is the employee's role to initiate the improvements. Such an atmosphere in which work simplification is a team effort requires a manager who is an effective leader, who understands factors which motivate people, and who can develop a climate conducive to action.

LEADERSHIP

Leadership is important to all kinds of groups. Leadership is the interpersonal influence directed toward attainment of a specific goal or goals. Influence infers power; and, indeed, power is necessary for influence. But power comes in several forms, some of which are more desirable in managerial leadership than others. French and Raven, in a classic work on power, suggest six sources of power:

1. Coercive Power – Based on a follower's perception that an influencer has the ability to inflict punishment.
2. Reward Power – Based on a follower's perception that an influencer has the capacity to administer some reward.
3. Legitimate Power – Based on a follower's internalized values which convince the follower that an influencer has the right to influence and the follower is bound to accept. This base of power is at the core of a traditional influence system, which endows leadership positions with formal authority.
4. Referent Power – Based on a follower's desire to identify with a charismatic leader, who is followed out of blind faith. This is maintained only so long as the follower behaves as the leader directs.
5. Expert Power – Based on a follower's perception that the leader has special knowledge or expertise which can be useful in satisfying the follower's needs.

TITLE	CHARACTERISTICS				
	LEADER'S POWER BASE	LEVEL OF CONFIDENCE IN EMPLOYEES	MOTIVATION TECHNIQUE	DIRECTION OF COMMUNICATION	LEVEL OF PARTICIPATION
SYSTEM 1 Exploitive – Authoritative	Coercive	Little	Fear and Punishment	Downward	Decision Making at Managerial Level
SYSTEM 2 Benevolent – Authoritative	Reward Legitimate	Patronizing	Some Fear and Punishment, Some Reward	Permit Upward	Some Delegation with Close Control
SYSTEM 3 Consultative	Referent Expert	Substantial	Reward with Occasional Punishment	Up and Down	General Decisions at Top–Specific at Bottom
SYSTEM 4 Participative – Group	Representative	Complete	Reward and Involvement	Up, Down and with Peers	Encourage Decision Making

FIG. 10 – LIKERT'S SYSTEMS OF MANAGEMENT

6. Representative Power – Based on followers democratically delegating power to the leader for the purpose of representing their interests and making decisions on their behalf.

A manager's source of power often determines the type and effectiveness of leadership. Rensis Likert, one of many researchers in the field of leadership theory, is a proponent of participative management. He believes an effective manager is one who is strongly oriented to subordinates and relies on communication to keep the organization running. In order to clarify his concepts, Likert has defined four systems of management (see Figure 10). These form a hierarchy, with the fourth system the one which Likert believes describes the manager who is the most successful leader. A manager might study these systems and perform some self-appraisal to determine the need to move into a higher system.

Another approach to understanding one's leadership style has been proposed by Robert Blake and Jane Mouton. Blake and Mouton's primary concern was that interest in people must be coupled with interest in production. They displayed this concept on a managerial grid (Figure 11). The grid is a useful tool for classifying managerial styles, although the underlying cause of a classification is not directly evident. Personality, training, environment, and other situational factors influence the manager's position on the grid, and must be considered before a manager attempts to alter personal style.

MOTIVATION

In addition to understanding one's personal style of management, an effective leader must also understand motivation and what factors motivate other people. Motivation can be described as a desire within an individual for satisfaction of a need, which stimulates action. Motivation can be looked upon as a series of events: (1) there is an initial need, (2) there is the desire to satisfy the need, (3) the individual is disturbed because of the unsatisfied need, (4) the individual's unrest becomes a motivator, (5) the individual takes action as a result of the motivation, and (6) the action results in satisfaction of the need. Motivators, then, are those things which induce an individual to take action, i.e., something which influences an individual's behavior.

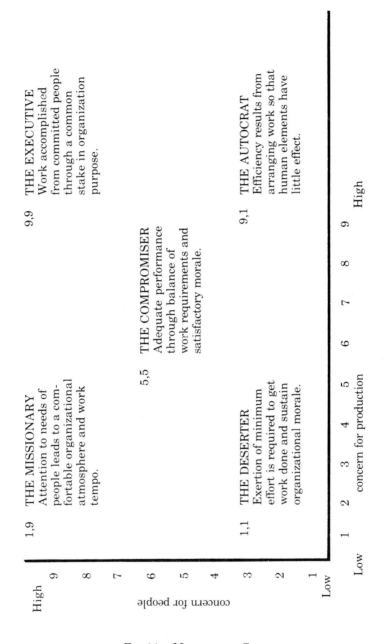

FIG. 11 – MANAGERIAL GRID

Need satisfaction and motivation, however, are highly complex things. One of the most well-known psychologists in the area of motivation, Abraham Maslow, defines a needs hierarchy. This hierarchy begins at the lowest level with basic physiologic needs, such as hunger, and moves through security, acceptance, esteem, and self-actualization. The last four depend on the environment, and thus may suggest their utility to managers as motivators. Maslow's hierarchical theory has been the subject of much research without very much support; but the needs themselves are widely accepted, and the suggestion that there are two groups of needs – biological and other – seems to have been borne out by others in their research.

Frederick Herzberg and associates also define two categories which they call maintenance factors and motivators and propose within each category those things which might satisfy the needs, i.e., serve as motivators or maintenance factors. These, and Maslow's hierarchy, are shown in Figure 12.

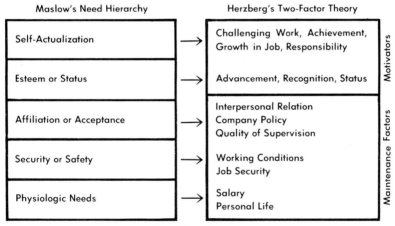

FIG. 12 – MOTIVATION

Any one researcher's theory cannot totally be relied upon to fit every situation. In practice, managers must be aware of their employees' needs, study motivational factors, and then decide for themselves what might actually motivate an employee at any given time in any given situation. Common motivational techniques can be identified, but they are not guaranteed to motivate in any given situation. The following are some of these:

1. Money has traditionally been considered a motivator. However, it appears that money itself may not be the motivator, but that it can be used to buy things which satisfy needs may actually be the motivator. Money in an organization is usually looked upon as a means to ensure an appropriate staff complement. It can also be suggested that money is not so much a motivator when most organizations try to pay employees at the same rank similar salaries.

2. Positive reinforcement, also known as behavior modification, is a technique made famous by B. F. Skinner. In this technique, specific goals are set with employees, regular feedback is provided, and other recognition and praise is awarded. Even where performance does not meet the goal, the action on the part of management is a positive one – coaching and finding something about the employee to praise. While it has had many doubters who suggest it is too simple or perhaps even morally wrong, research conducted in several organizations has found the approach beneficial.

3. Participation is another technique which has enjoyed strong support. A relatively new vehicle for participation is the quality circle. A quality circle is a group of employees that meets voluntarily and regularly to solve problems affecting the work area. Members receive training in problem solving, statistical quality control, and group process. A facilitator, usually a trained member of management, helps train the members and ensure that things run smoothly. Quality circles recommend solutions for quality and productivity problems which management may then implement.

4. Finally, job enrichment is a technique which is believed to make work challenging and meaningful, and thereby satisfy some of the higher level needs. Job enrichment must be distinguished from job enlargement, which serves to add jobs to make one employee's work more varied and less dull and routine. Job enrichment gives the employee more opportunities for decision making, participation, responsibility, and involvement without more work.

COMMUNICATION

Creating a climate in which motivational techniques will be successful, and thus reducing resistance to change, depends on effective communication. Frequently, a manager talks to employees or sends a written report to administration; and then is surprised that the employees do not follow the message, or the administrator does not understand the message. The manager has communicated but not necessarily what was desired. The Hay's communication model in Figure 13 is commonly used to depict the communication process. The significance of this

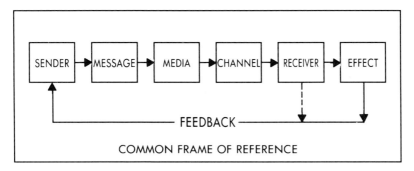

FIG. 13 – HAY'S COMMUNICATION MODEL

model is that it displays communication as an interaction between two parties which takes place by means of several factors and within a common frame of reference. In addition to the manager simply speaking or writing words, the manager must be aware that there are factors which can alter the intent of a message or even block a message totally. For instance, a reprimand given to an individual orally in front of a group has a different effect on the individual than if it is given in private and face-to-face, and still different than if it is given in writing. Effective communication is that which comes closest to conveying the intended message and no other.

The first factor that may alter or block the intended message is the way in which the message is conveyed. Communication media are spoken words, written words, pictures, and graphics. A second factor in conveying a message is the channel through which it is conveyed. Spoken words may be conveyed face-to-face; in person in front of a group; or over telephone, television, or radio.

Channels vary for written messages as well, from letters, memos, and computer screens, to billboards. The message sender selects the medium and the channel and in so doing has some control over the ability to convey the intended message. Other factors over which the message sender has varying degrees of control include the frequency, accuracy, completeness, and timeliness of the message.

For there to be effective communication, the sender and receiver must also have a common frame of reference. It is not enough to speak the same language; the background, education, emotional state, and other aspects of both the message sender and receiver make a difference in how effective communication will be. For instance, one person who is embraced by the manager may feel very uncomfortable, while another of a different culture may feel satisfied or consoled by the same gesture. The message sender has little or no control over the frame of reference of the receiver; so instead he must attempt to understand the receiver's frame of reference and adjust the communication in view of it.

Because communication is an interaction between sender and receiver, it is possible to obtain feedback on the message by observing the effect of, or reaction to it. It should be understood, however, that the nature of the feedback frequently depends on the communication medium and channel used by the sender, with less immediate feedback from some. Also, feedback is essentially another communication; so it also goes through a medium and channel and depends on the frame of reference. For instance, the effect of a message of good news may be happiness for two different people, but one may be very open about the happiness and another more quiet and reserved.

A manager should constantly monitor the effectiveness of communications in order to take steps to improve it. Some symptoms of communication problems in the work environment include increased rumors, unaccountable increases in mistakes, confusion in the implementation of decisions, increased demands of subordinates for personal contact, and the need to repeat communications frequently. Some steps which the message sender may use to improve communication include:

1. Gain a positive self-concept. If the sender is insecure, timid, or is convinced that no one wants to hear the message, these factors will be manifest. Monitor feedback for ways to improve.
2. Form a clear idea of what, where, when, and how you want to communicate. Also communicate not only the content of the message but its context – explain as concisely as possible why it is being delivered, where it fits in, and what its implications are likely to be.
3. Invest some of yourself in the message. Effective communication requires courage to reveal one's honest thoughts and feelings. Hold the receiver's attention through the character of the message.
4. Balance self-disclosure with a sense of propriety and courtesy that maintain a positive image. Maintain control over the communication – check that the message has been received, understand its effect, and make adjustments for different frames of reference.

Listening (or concentrating on the written communication) is as important in communication as is the conveyance of the message. Every message sender is ultimately a receiver. Steps which improve listening (or reading) improve the effectiveness of the overall communication. The receiver should avoid distractions; hear or read the full message before making judgments about it; evaluate the sender and make adjustments for a different frame of reference; seek to sort out the major theme and key points of the message to cut down the amount of information that must be remembered and thus aid memory; consider the factors surrounding the message to learn its full meaning; reflect on what is being heard or read; seek further clarification if necessary; and then respond to the message thoughtfully.

PERFORMANCE APPRAISAL, DEVELOPMENT, AND COMPENSATION

Performance appraisal, development, and compensation are the tangible results of the human relations aspect of the directing function. Performance appraisal is the official, periodic evaluation of work performed by an employee. It is done primarily to ensure that organizational objectives are being met; and, therefore, depends on information from the planning function of management (what are the objectives?), the organizing function (what objectives is this job designed to fulfill?), and the controlling function (how well did this employee meet these objectives?). Performance appraisal, however, is also a means of motivating employees by clarifying expectations and improving communications and mutual understanding of organizational problems. The formal evaluation of work provides a basis for determining salary increases, bonuses, promotions, or other rewards or punishment. The assessment of the employee's strengths and weaknesses during performance appraisal should result in a plan for employee development.

Performance appraisal is often done on the anniversary of the employee's hiring, though it may be done at any time; and it may be done more often than once a year. Because this is a formal evaluation of work, however, it should not be done so frequently as to lose its impact. The completion of a performance appraisal form usually initiates the evaluation. This may be done by the manager or by both the manager and the employee. When both participate in the form's initial completion, the nature of the form and the process of its final completion should be made clear to all concerned prior to the start of the performance appraisal. The form usually describes various attributes such as attitude and behavior (as measured by attendance, interpersonal relations, etc.), knowledge and skills (demonstration of technical competence in meeting productivity and performance standards, ability to learn new tasks, etc.), personal impression (such as appearance, poise, etc.), and, if for a supervisory employee, supervisory traits (including leadership, communication skills, decision making, etc.). Performance appraisal sometimes is conducted without the use of a form. However, forms identify for employees the factors to be evaluated. They are also used to document the appraisal function and serve as a reference for comparison over time. Discussion of the performance appraisal form with the employee is the second step in the process. Both strengths and weaknesses should be evident from the initial completion of the form. If a management-by-objectives program is in use, it is appropriate to evaluate the employee's achievement of objectives and to discuss new objectives. The final completion of the form involves the employee commenting on the appraisal and acknowledging, in writing, that it has been discussed with the employee; or the merging of the employee's performance appraisal form with the manager's.

Performance appraisal is an art as well as a tool. Many managers and employees alike are uneasy about performance appraisal. For the manager, it requires a strong understanding of human relations, complete information about the employee's productivity and performance, and, above all, objectivity. For the employee, it requires maturity, an honest appraisal of one's self, and the conviction to state one's own viewpoint. If appraisal is done regularly and in good faith, it can be an effective human relations tool.

One of the major purposes of appraisal should be an employee development program: a formal effort on the part of the manager to assist employees in maintaining and improving their work. Not all performance problems are developmental problems. In some cases, the problem is one of training, or resources, or even organizational and managerial ineptness. Finding out why there is a performance problem is sometimes more difficult than just identifying the fact of its existence. In addition, employee development should not be limited to where there is a problem; but it should be used to enrich or enhance already acceptable performance. Employee development may include all manner of means, including coaching, counseling, formal in-service lectures or seminars, job rotation, games, task forces, and others.

Finally, performance appraisal is often associated with compensation. Unless the organization makes across-the-board adjustments in compensation to all employees, which is rare, performance appraisal is the basis for changes in compensation. Compensation includes base pay, bonuses, fringe benefits, etc. The various types of compensation are often given in a mix depending on a number of factors. Compensation factors, in addition to the performance appraisal, include such considerations as salary range for the job, length of employee's service, cost-of-living, shift differential, and many others. While it has been shown that money is not necessarily the primary motivator, compensation is an extremely important issue and presents one of the greatest challenges for a manager.

THE CONTROLLING FUNCTION

While all of the four functions of management are interrelated, the functions of controlling and planning are more directly related to one another than any other functions. Controlling is the feedback mechanism for planning. Controlling is determining whether planning has been effective: whether objectives have been met, and taking steps to ensure that objectives are met. Controlling can be viewed as detecting and correcting significant variations in the results obtained from planned activities.

Controlling requires an understanding of what is necessary to meet the standards defined in the objectives. It requires monitors to determine and compare actual performance with the expected. It also requires mechanisms to ensure that adequate resources exist to meet standards (staffing and budgeting) and that corrective action is taken so performance will meet standards.

STANDARDS

Standards are embodied in the objectives set in the planning function of management. Frequently, however, standards are not so explicitly defined in objectives that they are easily usable as controls. For instance, the objective "transcribe basic reports for inclusion into the medical record within two days of their dictation" does not define how many lines of transcription a transcriptionist is expected to type, the number of transcriptionists required for the volume of dictation, or the level of transcription quality expected.

Standards are developed for a particular task by measuring all aspects of the work, and evaluating the results for their reliability and validity for use as a standard. Once the most reliable and valid measure possible is found, it becomes the official criterion or reference point for staffing, budgeting, and ensuring that performance meets the standards. While setting standards can be a complex process, it is extremely important that standards be set with, if not by, the employees to whom the standards apply. Working together to set standards will contribute to the reliability and validity of the standards and ensure that they are realistic. The employees will also feel they are controlling their own destiny, which will improve their compliance with the standards.

Measuring work in order to define a standard first requires the definition of a unit of measurement. For example, "basic hospital reports" is quite vague when discharge summaries, operative reports, and history and physical examination reports differ greatly in their length and complexity. A measurement unit for quantity must define the precise item which will be counted – number of reports by type, number of lines, or number of lines by type of report. A measurement unit for quality must also be defined – number of errors or number of omissions. A unit of measurement is important not only for consistency but for ease in subsequent use of the standard. The unit of measurement, however, should not be too cumbersome to use continually (for example, hand counting keystrokes transcribed may be very precise but not practical over time).

Once the unit of measurement is defined, there are several ways to accomplish the measurement. These include primarily the use of scientific method, simulation, and production and performance records.

Applying scientific method in measuring work results in the highest degree of accuracy. Scientific method refers to the study of different workers in different organizations performing essentially the same task to arrive at a "normal" quantity and quality level. Unfortunately, most of the work in this area has been done for setting time standards in factory work. One recent study done for medical record services is the *Productivity Standards Manual*, developed by the California Medical Record Association.

Another method for measuring work in order to define a standard is simulation. This method is frequently used when attempting to define a standard for new work. In simulation, one person performs the task several times as if it were actual work and (the same person or preferably another person) records the time it takes to complete the task and the number and types of errors made. The "someone" to perform the task for the simulation is difficult to choose. Persons generally available for this are the manager, an "average" employee, the "best" employee, or an outsider. With each person there are problems which may influence the reliability of the standard, including how well the person knows the task, how comfortable they are in performing the task, and their attitude about what they are doing. In addition to these problems, until the standard is instituted, there is no means to verify it against actual practice.

Using past production and performance records is the third, and most common method of work measurement. These records refer to data collected, by a variety of means, on actual work performed previously. Several problems with this method exist. Standards set by production and performance records will not be valid if a change in procedure, methods, or qualifications of personnel takes place. If procedures, methods, and personnel qualifications remain the same and the intent of defining standards is to institute them where none previously existed, or where only the volume and frequency of work are expected to change, then the only caution about using production and performance records is their reliability. One would not want to base future standards on poor productivity or performance.

MONITORS

Production and performance records are used not only to define standards but also to monitor production and performance. Although production and performance have been defined as quantity of work done and quality of work done respectively, there are elements of quantity control in quality assurance (e.g., the quality of timeliness of transcribed reports depends on whether the transcriptionists are meeting quantity standards) and elements of quality assurance in quantity control (e.g., meeting the quantity standard is not significant if the quality standard is not met). Thus many monitors may be adapted for either quantity control or quality assurance, even though they are, in general, either a production or performance type of record. The following is a description of several records:

1. One of the most widely used production records is the employee-reported log, which collects data on how much work comes in and how much work is produced. To collect data on "input," a log might be set up where each type of work entering the work unit is represented by a hash mark. The input log may be combined with an "output" log to demonstrate backlogs (see Figure 14). Such logs are

quite reliable because their data can usually be verified against other records. However, these records are generally only useful for identifying trends in workload.

CORRESPONDENCE PRODUCTION REPORT (Workload and Backlog)			MONTH: _April_ EMPLOYEE: _Sue_
DATE	INCOMING FORMS	FORMS MAILED	DIFFERENCE (Note exceptions)
4/2	3 4	3 0	− 4 (mail Late today)
4/3	TTHL HLL HHH HHHTHL I	2 6	0
4/4	HHL HLL HH HHHH HHL HHL II	2 9	− 8
4/5	18	2 2	− 4

FIG. 14 – EMPLOYEE-REPORTED LOG

2. A time log is another means for monitoring productivity. In this record, the employee notes on a time sheet the time spent on each activity (see Figure 15). Such a time log is used with other pertinent data such as the daily census or employee-reported logs to produce information on how much time is spent on each function. This is not the most accurate means of determining productivity, since the time log can be disruptive to work. Employee cooperation in reporting all work as well as personal time must be obtained in order for this type of record to be reliable. However, time logs serve a useful purpose in pointing out such things as constant interruptions or where adjustments could be made in work duties or procedures so the employee can accomplish the work expected.

3. Stopwatch time study, another production monitor, is a more accurate method of studying productivity. This study involves observing work and timing each element with a stopwatch (see Figure 16). Such a study may be performed where one wants to determine if the employee is performing a given task at an acceptable speed, or it can replace

the time log to determine time spent on all activities. As a quantity control device the stopwatch time study can pinpoint problems, such as too much time spent on one component of the task, wasted time in not performing components uniformly, proving to an employee that a task can be performed in the established time, or finding that a

TIME LOG	Name: *JANET*					Date: *4-2*	
TIME	DUTY	TIME	DUTY	TIME	DUTY	TIME	DUTY
8:00		11:00	*B*	1:00	*LUNCH*	3:00	
8:05		11:05		1:05		3:05	*A*
8:10		11:10		1:10		3:10	*A*
8:15		11:15		1:15		3:15	
8:20		11:20	*A*	1:20		3:20	*D*
8:25		11:25	*C*	1:25		3:25	
8:30		11:30		1:30		3:30	
8:35	*ARRIVE*	11:35	*D*	1:35		3:35	*B*
8:40		11:40		1:40		3:40	
8:50	*C*	11:45		1:45		3:45	
8:55	*A*	11:50		1:50		3:50	
				1:55			
				2:00			
		12:05				4:05	

SUMMARY:

DUTY	CODE	TOTAL	PERCENT
A =	*answer phone*	*1 HR 10 min*	*20%*
B =	*Write requisitions*	*2 Hr 5 min*	*30%*
C =	*Personal time*	*20 min*	

FIG. 15 – TIME LOG

task cannot be done as originally expected. Stopwatch time study, while being very precise, is the weakest technique psychologically, for having someone watch your every move is quite unsettling to most people. While it may seem truer with the time log, both techniques allow for the same amount of employee manipulation. In the time log the employees are on their own to record whatever they feel is "right," but employees can also pace themselves in front of a stopwatch analyst. Other problems with the stopwatch time study relate to the analyst. The supervisor performing this function can instill feelings of insecurity or defensiveness. An outsider will need explanation as to what is being done, thus automatically slowing the employee. To be effective as well as precise, this tool must be used with a great deal of employee cooperation and, perhaps, is only reliable in its use as a technique for establishing standard time data where employees understand that their results will be pooled with others' results.

STOPWATCH TIME STUDY								
Employee JANET – WARD CLERK				Date 4-3				
Task POSTING ORDERS				Analyst MA				
ELEMENT				CYCLE				
		1			2			3
	Start	Stop	Total	Start	Stop	Total	Start	Stop
1. FIND ORDER	8:46	8:52	6					
2 PULL KARDEX	8:53	8:54	1					
3. POST	8:55	9:07	12					
4. CHECK	9:08	9:10	2					

NOTES: (interruptions, irregularities, other)

SUMMARY:
    Allowance for P F & D 12 %
    Unit time standard (time + allowance) _____ min./unit
    Work standard   _____ units/hr.

FIG. 16 – STOPWATCH TIME STUDY

4. Work sampling is spot checking work and drawing conclusions from it. Work sampling is based on probability – that a sample taken at random will tend to resemble the actual work. The key to accuracy in work sampling is in the number of observations made and how they are made. Elements in determining the number of observations which will make the sample statistically significant are:

a. Population – The full range of activities from which a sample will be drawn should be defined. For instance, if sampling the file area functions, the population may include filing medical records, pulling medical records, answering the phone, filing loose sheets, and miscellaneous activities performed by all file clerks on the day shift.

b. Sample – The part of the population to be studied. The sample must contain a large enough number of observations to be valid and small enough to be cost effective. Statistical formulas are available to calculate sample size for a desired degree of accuracy. An alignment chart may also be used. In using an alignment chart, the percent of activity constituting the work and the desired degree of precision are decided upon; then the result of alignment through these points on the chart is the number of observations. In Figure 17, the element of work being sampled constitutes 80% of a job and the degree of precision is 7% (i.e. the probability that the sample will not represent the population is ± 4% from 80%). Thus, 400 observations must be made. Note that if it were desired to be twice as precise, (± 2% from 80%) 1,500 observations would have to be made.

c. Random – The condition that every activity has an equal chance of being observed. In order to ensure randomness, a random number table found in most statistics textbooks can be used. Tables of random observations, such as displayed in Figure 18, can either be designed from a random number table or found in some management textbooks. Such a table identifies times for making observations.

Once all observations are made, the percentage of each type of observation out of the total number of observations is applied to the volume of work and hours in a workday to determine the standard time. For instance, if in the total 400 observations, 140 observations were made of one employee filing records, this would represent 35% of the employee's time. If the employee works 7 hours a day (420 minutes), then the employee spends 147 minutes filing per day. If during the day the employee averages filing 100 records, then it took 1.47 minutes per record to file.

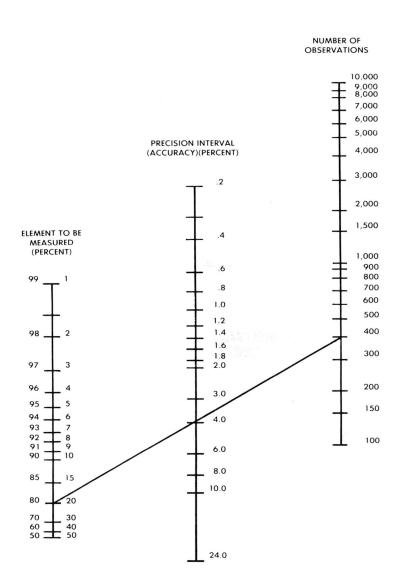

NUMBER OF
OBSERVATIONS

PRECISION INTERVAL
(ACCURACY)(PERCENT)

ELEMENT TO BE
MEASURED
(PERCENT)

Reprinted with permission of Aspen Systems Corp. *Managing Health Records* by Joan G. Liebler, 1980.

FIG. 17 – ALIGNMENT CHART

While observations would probably be best made if they were unannounced, this is not suggested because most employees would discover the observation some-

TABLE OF RANDOM OBSERVATIONS

Employee _MARY_   Job _CLERK_   Time Period _April_

	Week 1		Week 2		Week 3	
Monday	8:20 A	1:00 B	8:05	1:20	8:40	1:23
	8:25 B	2:45 A	8:40	1:30	9:20	1:40
	9:15 B	2:47 D	8:43	3:50	11:15	2:12
	11:07 B	3:06 D	9:20	3:55	11:16	3:56
	12:13 C	4:08 D	10:50	5:00	12:19	4:20
Tuesday	8:30 D	1:20 A	8:15	1:01	8:12	1:05
	8:35 D	1:30 B	9:00	2:15	9:12	2:20
	9:35 A	3:19 D	10:00	4:49	10:02	3:46
	10:15 A	4:40 D	11:43	4:50	10:30	4:08
	12:09 A	5:00 D	11:50	5:17	12:00	5:10

SUMMARY: TASK   CODE   PERCENT OF TOTAL OBSERVATIONS

A = _FILING_   MR
B = _PULLING_   MR
C = _ANSWERING PHONE_
D = _FILING LOOSE SHEETS_

FIG. 18 – WORK SAMPLING

time and would rightfully be more upset than if informed from the start. Employees do not need to be notified every time an observation is made, but must be told that they will be observed and the purpose of the observation. An effective manager should be able to put employees at relative ease with work sampling. All work measurement depends on the rapport between the manager and employees, but work sampling can easily become the most deceptive and thus the most disliked.

5. Direct inspection is the quality assurance technique of actual verification of all or selected work done by an employee to determine its accuracy. In inspection, the man-

ager, or another employee, either retrospectively performs or concurrently observes the work in its entirety. If the work is such that it cannot be repeated, inspection must be done concurrently with the work, making this monitor very similar to the stopwatch study for recording production. Direct inspection is most useful when quality can be quantified, either as a single generally accepted practice, or as a range of normal values. For instance, this monitor would be used to count the number of typographical errors in transcription, the number of diagnoses coded incorrectly, etc.

6. The checklist is a monitor for direct observation of the quality of work performed when the quality is less easy to quantify. The checklist provides a specific listing of factors which will be observed. The factors may be evaluated as simply "yes" or "no," or on a rating scale. An example of an application for the checklist monitor is in defining standards and evaluating the work of the insurance clerk – observing factors such as "did the clerk greet the patient respectfully?" The American Medical Record Association's *Professional Practice Standards* are another example of a checklist.

7. Audit is a formal quality assurance technique patterned from the production industry. Generally, the audit is tailored to fit the area being studied and involves a comparison of the present operations against the intended. The primary objective of an audit is to reveal variations in any of the elements examined and to identify areas for corrective action.

8. Questionnaires are an indirect method of evaluating quality of work performed. A questionnaire is completed by the persons who receive the service, rather than by those who manage it (for example, physicians may be asked questions about medical record department personnel). Questionnaires should not be used as the only quality assurance monitor, but they can provide information about performance which is not observed by the manager or cannot be evaluated directly in an audit.

9. Reports are records of work or work characteristics made by persons other than the manager (but not the consumer of the service as in the questionnaire type of monitor). Reports may be anecdotal, describing an incident, in the form of letters of commendation, complaints, or requests that reflect on the work of the department or employees. Reports may also be regular records that demonstrate level of work and variations from planned activities. Such reports include department budget variance reports, personnel statistics (such as sick time, vacation, and overtime usage, etc.), results of the Medicare Peer Review Organization's DRG validation, feedback on abstracting errors from the abstracting computer service, and many others.

In selecting the monitor or monitors to use for the various quantity control needs in the medical record department, several points should be kept in mind. First, monitors should measure significant tasks. It may not be appropriate or necessary to establish standards and evaluate certain types of tasks, for instance, those which are done infrequently. Monitors should not only aid in setting standards and comparing actual work but should also aid in analyzing the cause of deviations from the standards so preventive as well as corrective action can be taken. Monitors should be objective – this is especially true of those which attempt to measure less quantifiable aspects of performance. Monitors should be flexible in the face of changed plans – there should be room to identify and explain variations when this is the case. Monitors should be cost effective. They should be evaluated to determine that the cost of their implementation does not exceed the benefit of their implementation.

VARIANCE ANALYSIS

Once standards are established, monitors are used to determine variances from the standards. Variances from standards should be regularly analyzed for their rate of occurrence, severity, and cause.

A minor variance that happens infrequently probably can be ignored. Alternatively, a major variance should be investigated immediately, and corrective steps taken so it will not be repeated. Minor variances that are frequent, or that follow a pattern of occurrence, should also be investigated so their cumulative effect is minimized. In order to analyze the rate of occurrence of variances, data collected from productivity and performance records should be plotted on a table or graph. For instance, in the graph displayed in Figure 19, during the first

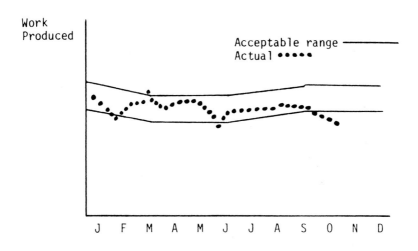

FIG. 19 – VARIANCE ANALYSIS

three quarters of the year, variance from the range of acceptable productivity occurs three times, twice slightly below range and once slightly above. These are probably not significant. However, during the fourth quarter, all production is below range and there is a downward trend which should be investigated. The rate of occurrence of variances can also be evaluated by comparing productivity and performance. If performance deteriorates when productivity increases beyond the standard, it may be that workload has increased and work simplification or additional staffing may be necessary. Yet if performance remains the same as productivity increases, the standard may be too low, or the employee may be demonstrating improved productivity.

The severity of the variance depends on the nature of the task for which the standard is set and the degree of deviation from the standard. A small deviation in a very critical task may be very important, whereas a moderate deviation in a less critical task may not be as important. Defining standards within an acceptable range is useful in evaluating the severity of deviations.

Analysis of variance also includes the determination of the cause of the deviation. It is necessary to evaluate the data from monitors with respect to the procedure, job description, or work method in order to determine the cause of a variance. For instance, the procedure may be out of date, the employee now performing the task may not be qualified, or the employee may have changed the work method. Aggregate production and performance records may also have to be separated by employee, or by smaller units of time to determine the specific attributes of the problem deviation.

CORRECTIVE ACTION AND FOLLOW-UP

Viable solutions to the problems that are identified in variance analysis should be developed and implemented. Solutions are many and varied, depending on the problem. In finding solutions, however, increases in staffing and budget should be a last resort. Too often, more staff and more money have been used to attempt to solve problems, yet the problems remain because their real cause has not been determined. Instead of more staff and money, procedures may need to be revised or updated, methods may need to be improved, work may need to be redistributed, employees may need additional training or counseling, and, of course, management is never exempt from the need to improve.

Controlling does not end with corrective action taken on a problem or set of problems. Corrective action must be followed up to ensure that it was appropriate and effective. A new set of monitors must also be implemented for ongoing quantity control and quality assurance. As with all the functions of management, controlling is a continual, integrated process.

SUMMARY

Efficient management of the medical record department is an important factor in the effective functioning of health care facilities. The health facility exists for the benefit of the patient; and the medical record department is responsible for the completeness, accuracy, safekeeping, and availability of the medical record at all times. The department can discharge these responsibilities only when it is well managed.

Management is the effective utilization of resources toward the accomplishment of specific objectives. Good management is facilitated by carefully made plans, a chart of organization, proper analysis of each job, a study of the work flow with simplification when necessary, adoption of necessary internal controls, and adequate written procedures for each individual job and for the medical record department as a whole.

The medical record department director must not only create and supervise the organization but must also provide the leadership to ensure that all functions are properly executed. Cooperative and responsive personnel are essential for effective management.

Because of higher educational and professional standards during the past few years, registered or accredited medical record practitioners have earned recognition as trusted and responsible partners in the successful administration of health care facilities. As department heads they are responsible for certain functions which support the proper care of the sick and injured. To be successful in one's position, the medical record practitioner must unceasingly analyze the procedures, delegate duties, supervise personnel, and encourage an enthusiasm for work while keeping the department in step with the ever-changing health care environment.

STUDY QUESTIONS

1. What are the four components of management?
2. What are the steps in the planning process?
3. Explain the process of management by objectives.

4. Distinguish between policies, procedures, standards, and rules.
5. Describe a programmatic plan. What types of techniques would be used in its development?
6. How are budgets used as both planning and controlling tools?
7. Describe the impact management of the medical record department has on the hospital's accounts receivable.
8. Define the six components of departmental organization.
9. Why is it important for the manager to delegate authority?
10. Describe tools used in analyzing and developing staffing patterns, work distribution, and the work environment.
11. How does a manager acquire skills in leadership, motivation, and communication?
12. List the major requirements of the controlling function.
13. Compare production and performance, and describe how both are components of quantity control and quality assurance.
14. What factors should be considered in measuring the quantity and quality of work?

REFERENCES

American Medical Record Association. *Professional Practice Standards.* AMRA, 1984.

BENNETT, ADDISON C. *Improving Management Performance in Health Care Institutions.* American Hospital Association. Chicago, Illinois, 1978.

BERMAN, HOWARD J., and WEEKS, LEWIS E. *The Financial Management of Hospitals,* 5th Edition. Ann Arbor, Michigan: Health Administration Press, University of Michigan, 1981.

BLOOMROSEN, MERYL. "The Development of a Quality Control Program: Activity Reporting and Performance Standards." *Journal of the American Medical Record Association.* August, 1980.

CHASE, RICHARD B., and AQUILANO, NICHOLAS J. *Production and Operations Management,* 3rd Edition. Homewood, Illinois: Richard D. Irwin, Inc., 1981.

DEEGAN, ARTHUR X., II. *Management by Objectives for Hospitals.* Germantown, Pennsylvania: Aspen Systems Corp., 1977.

DESSLER, GARY. *Organization Theory – Integrating Structure and Behavior.* Glenview, Illinois: Scott, Foresman and Company, 1982.

DRUCKER, PETER F. *Management: Tasks, Responsibilities, Practices.* New York, New York: Harper & Row, 1974.

ESMOND, TRUMAN H. *Budgeting Procedures for Hospitals, 1982 Edition.* American Hospital Association. Chicago, Illinois, 1982.

HAMPTON, DAVID R., SUMMER, CHARLES E., and WEBBER, ROSS A. *Organizational Behavior and the Practice of Management.* Glenview, Illinois: Scott, Foresman and Company, 1982.

IMBIORSKI, WALTER; FOX, LESLIE ANN; SAMUELS, CAROLYN B.; STEARNS, GERRY; and BREWER, ELEANOR. *Evaluating the Quality of Medical Record Services.* American Medical Record Association, 1979.

KOONTZ, HAROLD, and O'DONNEL, CYRIL. *Principles of Management: An Analysis of Managerial Functions,* 5th Edition. New York, New York: McGraw-Hill Book Company, 1972.

LIEBLER, JOAN G. *Managing Health Records: Administrative Principles.* Germantown, Pennsylvania: Aspen Systems Corp., 1979.

LUTHANS, FRED. *Organizational Behavior,* 3rd Edition. New York, New York: McGraw-Hill Book Company, 1981.

PETERS, ROBERTA L. and FRISCHKORN, ANN E. "The Integration of Quality Assurance and Productivity Monitoring: A Case Study." *Topics in Health Record Management.* December, 1984.

SCHNEIDER, DON, and APPLETON-SCHNEIDER, LINDA. "Development of a Medical Record Management Control System." *Medical Record News.* June, 1980.

STIMSON, DAVID H., and STIMSON, RUTH H. *Operations Research in Hospitals, Diagnosis and Prognosis.* Hospital Research and Educational Trust. Chicago, Illinois, 1972.

TERRY, GEORGE R., and FRANKLIN, STEPHEN G. *Principles of Management,* 8th Edition. Homewood, Illinois: Richard D. Irwin, Inc., 1982.

—— and STALLARD, JOHN J. *Office Management and Control,* 8th Edition. Homewood, Illinois: Richard D. Irwin, Inc., 1980.

WEISS, W. H. *The Management of Hospital Employee Productivity: An Introductory Handbook.* American Hospital Association. Chicago, Illinois, 1973.

chapter *19*

QUALITY ASSURANCE

OVERVIEW

EARLY EFFORTS TO EVALUATE MEDICAL CARE

The evaluation of medical care is as old as medicine itself. There is evidence of public effort to control the quality and cost of medical care throughout history. The code of Hammurabi spelled out a number of conditions which controlled medical practice and specified the fees that could be charged. In the 1600s the legal code of the colony of Virginia stated that a physician could be arrested and compelled to swear to the "true value and worth of the drugs and medicines prescribed." In the 1860s studies were performed which compared hospital size with the probability of surviving an amputation. The larger the hospital, the greater the fatality rate.

In early hospitals, assurance that the medical care provided was of high quality was indirectly controlled through licensure of health care practitioners, the granting of medical staff privileges and peer review mechanisms. One of the byproducts of the American College of Surgeon's hospital standardization program initiated in 1918 was improvement in the quality of patient care. In 1918, only 12.9 percent of hospitals participating in the program were accredited to verify their quality; by 1956, 94.6 percent were accredited.

EARLY INFLUENCE OF JCAH IN QUALITY ASSURANCE

The JCAH was a forerunner in evaluating medical care strictly from a quality standpoint. In 1972, the JCAH established a requirement for medical audits and developed an outcome audit methodology, the Performance Evaluation Procedure (PEP), designed to assist hospitals in objectively reviewing and evaluating patient care. It was during this period the term "audit" became synonymous with patient care evaluation and quality assessment activities. Even today many health care professionals use the terms interchangeably. In 1974, the JCAH specified the number of audits to be performed.

In 1979, the JCAH eliminated the numerical requirements for audits and substantially revised their approach to quality assurance through a new accreditation standard. This standard required hospitals to coordinate all quality of care activities through an individual committee, or group, rather than allowing segmented and individual review activities without any central coordination.

QUALITY ASSURANCE TODAY

Since 1979, quality assurance mechanisms have changed, with the prescriptive requirements giving way to more facility-oriented systems. Today, quality assurance is a process through which the level of desired quality is defined, pursued, achieved, and maintained through the institution of formal mechanisms for detecting and correcting factors which prevent the achievement of desired quality. Quality assurance is a broad term that describes the overall efforts of the hospital to achieve effective care without compromising quality. Quality care is care that does not over- or underutilize available resources (efficiency) but achieves the best outcome possible given the patient's condition (effectiveness).

In overutilization, a patient receives medical care which is not medically necessary for the diagnosis or treatment of the patient's illness or injury. Examples: excessive ancillary services such as respiratory therapy; repeated care because the original test results were not available promptly from another provider or did not appear in the patient's chart on a timely basis; and care provided as an inpatient which could have been provided on an ambulatory basis.

In underutilization, a patient fails to receive all of the care needed for the diagnosis or treatment of an illness or injury. Examples: premature discharge; transfer to a long term care facility lacking the appropriate services; or omission of necessary tests.

Although the JCAH standards currently allow each hospital considerable flexibility in determining the structure and mechanisms it will use to "objectively and systematically monitor and evaluate the quality and appropriateness of patient care, pursue opportunities to improve patient care and resolve identified problems," the standards identify many characteristics a hospital quality assurance program must display. The current *JCAH Accreditation Manual for Hospitals* should be consulted annually to evaluate the adequacy of an institution's quality assurance program.

COMPONENTS OF QUALITY ASSURANCE

Quality assurance includes all assessment activities conducted in the hospital including Utilization Management, Quality Assessment, and Risk Management. Although each of these activities will be discussed individually because each originated as a separate activity, these assessment activities are closely related and may be efficiently conducted in a coordinated program. Integrated data collection may be performed by medical record technicians assigned to the patient care units, quality assurance coordinators or utilization reviewers who review the medical record of all patients every one to three days. Regardless of who performs the review, it should be a comprehensive review including: occurrence screening, necessity for continued stay, medical record completeness, antibiotic and other drug use reviews, and blood use review.

UTILIZATION MANAGEMENT

Utilization management is one of the methods encouraged by federal and private insurers to control health care expenditures. Utilization management includes a review of medical appropriateness and an analysis of the hospital's efficiency in providing necessary services in the most cost-effective manner possible. Utilization management not only looks at continued hospitalization, but also evaluates alternate, lower cost health care options.

Earliest utilization review efforts in hospitals can be traced back to the 1950s when guidelines were developed by the Allegheny County Medical Society. This was the first review plan focusing on both the quality and cost of medical care. From these efforts, the Hospital Utilization Project (HUP) was formed to provide data support and consulting services for utilization review activities in western Pennsylvania. Originally, utilization review was conducted by hospital admissions committees. These committees were assigned the task of allocating scarce hospital beds to patients who could demonstrate the greatest need for hospitalization. Only hospitals with frequent bed shortages regularly conducted utilization review prior to federally mandated review.

MEDICARE

Utilization review first became mandatory in 1965 with the passage of Medicare (Title XVIII of the Social Security Act). The Medicare law required that hospitals and extended care facilities establish a plan for utilization review, and that a standing utilization review committee be maintained. While intended as a physician peer review function, the Medicare law established the fiscal intermediaries as the overseers of appropriate utilization and gave them the power to deny payment where medical care was deemed not necessary.

JOINT COMMISSION ON ACCREDITATION OF HOSPITALS

The Joint Commission on Accreditation of Hospitals has required utilization review since the early 1970s. Physicians were required to periodically review bed utilization and the diagnostic, nursing and therapeutic resources of the hospital, with respect to both the availability of these resources to all patients in accordance with their medical needs and the recognition of the medical practitioner's responsibility for the costs of health care. In 1980, the JCAH separated the utilization review requirements from the overall Quality of Professional Services Standard by developing a Utilization Review Standard which requires the hospital to demonstrate appropriate allocation of its resources through an effective utilization review program.

This new emphasis on utilization review by the JCAH paralleled Medicare and other third-party payer interests in decreasing inappropriate hospital utilization. The Medicare utilization review requirements focused only on Medicare beneficiaries. The JCAH requirements expanded the utilization review concept to all hospital patients, regardless of payment source.

Hospitals are required to implement a utilization review plan, describing the methods for conducting review of the appropriateness and medical necessity of admission, continued stays, and supportive services, and for providing discharge planning. The standard specifies that retrospective monitoring of the hospital's utilization of resources shall be ongoing, and concurrent review shall be focused on those diagnoses, problems, procedures, and/or practitioners with identified or suspected utilization related problems. The JCAH emphasizes discharge planning as a method of ensuring timely discharge at that point in time when an acute level of care is no longer required. The JCAH requires that the hospital's utilization review program including the written plan, criteria and length of stay norms be reviewed and evaluated annually and revised as appropriate to reflect the findings of the hospital's utilization review activities.

PROFESSIONAL STANDARDS REVIEW ORGANIZATIONS

In 1972, the Social Security Act was amended (PL 92-603) which provided for significant expansion of the utilization review process. Under the 1972 amendments, utilization review committees were required to engage in concurrent review of all admissions reimbursed by Medicare, Medicaid, and Maternal and Child Health Programs. These amendments also required extended stay review for covered hospital and long term care patients. Physician review committees were required to establish norms, standards, and criteria for use in evaluating the necessity of admissions and continued stays.

PL 92-603 further provided for the establishment of Professional Standards Review Organizations (PSROs), a nonprofit professional organization composed of licensed physicians, organized to perform professional reviews and evaluations of patient care services. PSROs were regionally located according to the number of beds involved. The purpose of PSROs in utilization review was:

1. To determine if the services provided were medically necessary.
2. To assure that care was provided in the most economical setting consistent with the health needs of the patient.

The PSROs also had some quality objectives.

All hospitals were required to have a written utilization review plan which outlined their involvement in utilization review and the norms and standards by which utilization review was to be performed by the physician utilization review committee. The PSROs monitored hospital utilization review activities to assure compliance with the requirements.

During the 1970s the scope of utilization review activities changed. Review of all admissions was found to be costly and without significant benefit. Some hospitals were allowed to discontinue 100 percent Medicare review and encouraged to focus on known utilization problems only. Other hospitals discontinued concurrent review altogether and participated only in long stay and retrospective reviews. Serious questions were raised about the cost-effectiveness of PSROs as experience with the program accumulated. While isolated instances of cost-savings could be documented, the expenditure of dollars for inpatient health care was dramatically increasing, threatening to bankrupt the Social Security fund. The incentive for stringent utilization control did not exist. Hospitals were paid for the services they provided and the incentive for reducing these services was nonexistent. Many hospitals participated in "paper exercise" utilization review programs which did little to reduce Medicare outlays.

In the early 1980s, the Health Care Financing Administration began to phase out the PSRO program and to increase reliance on fiscal intermediaries to perform utilization review functions. In response to growing concern about the adequacy of utilization review under the Medicare program, a redesigned program was passed as the Peer Review Improvement Act of 1982. This legislation coincided with the Prospective Payment System, which changed the Medicare payment system from a cost-based system to a diagnosis-related group system.

PEER REVIEW ORGANIZATIONS (PROs)

Peer Review Organizations (PROs) review the appropriateness of admissions and discharges; the validity of diagnostic information provided by the hospital; the completeness, accuracy, and quality of care provided; and the appropriateness of care for which additional payments are sought (outliers).

Skilled nursing facilities have been subject to Medicare utilization review since 1972. These requirements include:

1. Admission review – to determine the appropriateness of admission
2. Continued stay review – to determine the need for continued stay

The PROs are involved in monitoring compliance with these requirements but have not assumed the responsibility for review, as they have in hospitals. The same is true for other nonhospital participants in the Medicare program (hospice, psychiatric facilities, alcohol and drug rehabilitation, etc.). As the federal government expands the Medicare Prospective Payment System to nonhospital providers, PRO involvement in utilization review for these facilities will undoubtedly increase.

EXTERNAL PRESSURES FOR EFFICIENCY

Hospitals are experiencing significant changes in payment programs – federal, state, and insurers. These constraints are responses to the rising cost of health care. To reduce health care expenditures, businesses are self-insuring and are forming coalitions to negotiate contracts for services. In the 1980s hospitals are seeing third-party reimbursement controls such as:

1. Preadmission certification for all elective admissions.
2. Second opinion programs, requiring a second surgical opinion prior to elective surgery.
3. Use of outpatient settings for procedures considered appropriate for this less-costly alternative.
4. Capitation payments.
5. Audits on all claims over a specified dollar amount.

Historically, third-party payers and insurance premium payers picked up hospital deficits created by cost-based Medicare reimbursement and charity care. The 11.1 percent inflation in the hospital sector in 1982 caused concern not only from Medicare, but all third-party payers. Mandatory utilization management is the backlash from this statistic. Hospitals are subject to reduced payment or nonpayment for services not considered medically necessary in the acute care environment. The institution is, therefore, motivated to strengthen its internal cost containment efforts to protect its financial resources.

A second pressure to control costs comes from the health care industry itself. In an effort to attract and retain their market share of patients, hospitals are entering into Preferred Provider Organization contracts with industry. These insurance plans provide clients with incentives for using particular health care providers – hospitals and physicians. In exchange for a more stable and "guaranteed" patient population, providers negotiate a fixed rate for their services, usually a rate lower than that charged non-PPO patients. In addition, PPOs have strict utilization management programs, to further reduce health care costs of the PPO's clients. In order to retain their contract with the PPO, providers (hospitals and physicians) must comply with the utilization review requirements and demonstrate an effective use of health care resources. Preferred Provider Organizations, through their utilization management programs and provider-negotiated fixed rates, can reduce the total cost of health insurance premiums for the buyer. If a hospital is both a buyer of PPO health insurance for its employees and a provider of PPO services, the incentive for stringent utilization review and control is doubly strong.

A third external pressure being faced by today's hospitals is the competitive environment. People are demanding and getting a variety of low-cost health care choices. Streamlined, historically hospital-based services, are being developed throughout the U.S. Freestanding emergency or urgent care centers, freestanding surgery centers, birthing centers, diagnostic centers, and home health care services, can potentially provide services at a lower cost because they lack the overhead of the traditional hospital. Other, less traditional services, are also threatening the patient's view of the hospital as the provider for all health-related services. These include occupational and sports medicine centers, freestanding industrial health centers, executive fitness centers, health screening and wellness programs, freestanding cancer centers, substance abuse centers, and other ambitious schemes. The growth of alternate care pro-viders is expected to continue throughout the 1980s. Hospitals are faced with a new utilization management problem: how to provide low cost services competitive with those of the alternate providers. A strong utilization management program, coupled with the hospital's development of health care alternatives within their local marketplace, is one answer to meeting the challenges of the competitive health care environment.

ORGANIZATION AND OPERATION OF A UTILIZATION MANAGEMENT PROGRAM

A hospital's utilization management program is based on its utilization management plan which outlines the purpose; lines of authority; committee organization, responsibilities, and func-tions; reporting mechanisms; administrative support; relation-ship to other quality assurance activities and the procedure for updating the plan.

The utilization management program's administrative sup-port may be a utilization management department, a quality as-surance department, or this function may be assigned to the medical record department. Regardless of the organizational pattern utilized at a particular hospital, the medical record practitioner's expertise in data collection and data analysis is needed to develop an efficient utilization management program. The data requirements of the utilization management program must be integrated with other data requirements to ensure that quality data are maintained and that each data element is col-lected only once.

Utilization Review Process

The utilization review process consists of certain basic proce-dures in all hospitals:

Preestablished objective screening criteria are used for all re-views. The time frames for completing reviews are specified in the utilization management plan. Three types of review are commonly performed:

preadmission review – designed to identify patients who do not qualify for inpatient benefits prior to admission and refer them to the appropriate health care setting.

concurrent review – designed to evaluate the need for continued hospitalization at specified intervals throughout the inpatient stay.

retrospective review – designed to identify trends or utilization related problems such as overutilization, underutilization, inefficient scheduling, and patterns of nonacute days.

Some facilities may require preadmission certification while others may conduct the first review in 24-48 hours.

The reviewer assesses the documentation of care rendered or planned for a patient and the patient's physical condition using the criteria.

The case is approved and the reviewer may assign a length of stay if the level of care being rendered and/or the severity of the patient's illness meets with the criteria.

The physician is contacted for more information if documentation in the medical record under review does not conform to the criteria.

The case is referred to a physician advisor for review in situations where there are no applicable criteria, or the need for admission or continued hospitalization is questionable.

The attending physician is contacted to provide further documentation of the need for admission or continued stay if the physician advisor cannot establish medical necessity for admission or continued stay.

The admission or continued stay is denied if after reviewing the additional information provided by the attending physician, the physician advisor decides that medical necessity does not exist. The reasons for this decision must be documented in the utilization review worksheet.

The physician advisor advises the attending physician of this decision.

A second physician advisor is consulted if the attending physician disagrees with the adverse decision.

The denial process is implemented if the second physician advisor concurs with the adverse decision.

Notification of the denial is provided in writing to the: business office; patient; attending physician; PRO, where applicable; employer/insurer, where applicable.

The patient and attending physician are informed of their right to reconsideration of the decision.

Screening Criteria

Screening criteria form an objective base against which specific performance can be measured. Two types of criteria sets are available to the committee responsible for utilization management activities: (1) diagnostic-specific and (2) severity of illness/intensity of service. Most facilities utilize the latter category because it measures the level of intensity of resources used and is easier to use. Figures 1 and 2 illustrate such criteria.

Information System

The utilization management information system should contain data on admission certifications, initial days certified, physician advisor reviews, continued stays, and denied days. This information, however, must be integrated with quality assessment monitoring data and medical record discharge data to identify utilization review problems requiring further study and action.

Outcomes of Utilization Management

A hospital can be assured of appropriate medically necessary admissions, appropriate lengths of stay and appropriate ancillary utilization when structure and process components of the utilization management program are implemented effectively and coordinated appropriately with other quality assurance activities. Additionally, facilities that participate in the Medicare program benefit financially from an effective utilization management program to reduce unnecessary dollar expenditures for which they may not be reimbursed. If Medicare patients can be cared for efficiently and effectively at a cost below the reimbursement rate, a hospital makes money. If a patient consumes more resources than the average, the hospital loses money. In order to survive and grow, a hospital must render quality care while increasing its efficiency, decreasing its costs, and responding effectively to marketplace pressures.

1. GENERIC

SEVERITY OF ILLNESS

VITAL SIGNS
Temperature above 102° F (38.9° C) with WBC above 15,000/
cu. mm or bacteria by smear
Pulse below 40/minute
Pulse above 140/minute

BLOOD PRESSURE
Systolic below 80 mm Hg
Systolic above 250 mm Hg
Diastolic above 120 mm Hg

LABORATORY – BLOOD
Serum Sodium below 123 mEq/L
Serum Sodium above 156 mEq/L
Serum Potassium below 2.5 mEq/L
Serum Potassium above 6.0 mEq/L
Blood pH below 7.30
Blood pH above 7.45 (newly discovered)
Presence of toxic level of drugs or other chemical substance

FUNCTIONAL IMPAIRMENT (sudden onset)
Sight loss
Hearing loss
Speech loss
Loss of sensation or movement any body part
Extreme weakness without paralysis
Impaired breathing
Unconsciousness
Disorientation

PHYSICAL FINDING
Gross, continuous hemorrhage from any site
Wound disruption (requiring reclosure)
Vomiting/diarrhea with any one of the following:
- Serum Sodium above 150 mEq/L
- Hematocrit above 55%
- Hemoglobin above 16 grams
- Urine specific gravity above 1.026
- BUN above 35
- Creatinine above 2 mg%
- Ileus

OTHER
Incapacitating pain

Reprinted with permission of InterQual from "ISD-A Review System"

FIG. 1 – SCREENING CRITERIA – SEVERITY OF ILLNESS

1. GENERIC

INTENSITY OF SERVICE

MONITORING (at least every two hours)
 Special care unit (refer to CCU/ICU/PCU criteria, pp. 4-6 to 4-11)
 Vital signs (T,P,R)
 Blood pressure
 Orientation to time and place
 Urine output
 Pupil reaction to light
 Central venous pressure
 Electrolytes
 Blood gases

MEDICATIONS
 Intravenous therapy if n.p.o.
 Intravenous medications
 Continuous intravenous chemotherapy or chemotherapy requiring
  parenteral medications for control of nausea and vomiting
 Initial Insulin therapy/Insulin pump regulation
 Parenteral analgesics three or more times daily

TREATMENTS
 Respiratory assistance (e.g., ventilator, Bird, MAI)
 Implantation of radioactive materials in doses greater than 30
  millicuries*
 Plasma phoresis requiring hospitalization

PROCEDURE (scheduled within 24 hours)
 Surgery or procedure not on ambulatory surgery list and requir-
  ing general or regional anesthesia (refer to Ambulatory
  Surgery Guidelines, pp. 3-6 to 3-9)

PROCEDURE (NOT scheduled within 24 hours)
 Surgery or procedure requiring preoperative preparation <u>in the
  hospital</u> (2 days only):
 • Bowel preparation (except colonoscopies and sigmoidoscopies)
 • Nutritional supplementation (refer to TPN criteria, p. 5-12)
 • Medication adjustment (potassium, glucose, etc.)
 • Obtain blood products (cardiac and thoracic admissions)
 • Dialysis for living related renal transplant admissions
*See Nuclear Regulatory Commission Requirements.

DISCHARGE SCREENS

 Temperature below 99° F/37.2° C for last 24 hours without anti-
  pyretic such as aspirin, Tylenol, Bufferin
 Prescribed diet tolerated for 24 hours without nausea or vomiting
 Passing flatus/fecal material
 Voiding or draining urine (at least 800 cc) for last 24 hours
 Type/dosage of major drug unchanged for last two days
 No parenteral analgesics/narcotics for last 24 hours
 Wound(s) healing
 Able to clean and care for drainage tubes

Reprinted with permission of InterQual from "ISD-A Review System"

FIG. 2 – SCREENING CRITERIA – INTENSITY OF SERVICE

QUALITY ASSESSMENT

Quality assessment refers to a system designed to monitor and evaluate quality issues within a health care facility. It includes activities such as infection control, surgical case monitoring, ancillary service review, blood utilization review, pharmacy and therapeutics review. The quality assessment structure has three components:

- various committees, departments, and services engaged in review (assessment)
- medical staff leadership and hospital managers accountable to the board to demonstrate that findings are acted upon and that their actions bring needed changes
- staff support structure responsible for facilitating and coordinating the work of those engaged in assessment and assurance functions

Hospitals may use individual committees for conducting the various reviews or may assign the quality assurance committee responsibility for many activities including: infection control, medical audit, medical records, utilization review, pharmacy and therapeutics, and blood and tissue. Quality assessment support functions may be organized as a division within the medical record department or as a separate department. A JCAH approved quality assessment program begins with a clear definition of departmental and medical staff committee objectives. Once the objectives are clarified and agreed upon, monitors are developed to measure success in meeting these objectives.

MONITORING

Ongoing monitoring should be used to evaluate the quality and appropriateness of patient care. Monitoring is a criteria-based review to ensure that a specified standard of performance is always met. Criteria that might be used for blood utilization review appear in Figure 3.

Medical staff reviews may also focus on known or suspected problems but only after sufficient review of all cases. A problem is a deviation from an expected occurrence that cannot be justified as appropriate under the given circumstances.

CRITERIA	YES	NO	N/A
1. Was patient a candidate for type & screen order rather than type & crossmatch?	☐	☐	☐
2. Did patient meet the following transfusion indications?			
A. Hypovolemia due to acute blood loss shown by any one of the following:			
1) systolic BP <90 mm Hg	☐	☐	☐
2) acute drop systolic BP≥30 mm Hg on movement from supine to upright position (sitting or standing)	☐	☐	☐
3) Hct <30%	☐	☐	☐
4) Hgb <10 gm	☐	☐	☐
5) obvious acute massive hemorrhage - ongoing with signs of shock	☐	☐	☐
B. Estimated intraop. blood loss >500 ml	☐	☐	☐
C. Chronic anemia (not due to acute blood loss) plus either:			
1) Hgb <10 gm	☐	☐	☐
2) Hct <30%	☐	☐	☐
D. Prophylaxis prior to surgery for patients with Hgb <10 gm or Hct <30%	☐	☐	☐
E. Blood given to patient on chemotherapy for malignancy when Hgb <10 gm or Hct <30%	☐	☐	☐
F. Platelets only:			
1) Given when count is <30,000	☐	☐	☐
2) <100,000 when given prophylactically preop. or intraop.	☐	☐	☐
3. Were there any contraindications for transfusion present? If yes, specify:_____	☐	☐	☐
_____			
4. Did the patient have a transfusion reaction? If yes:	☐	☐	☐
a. Was the unit wasted?	☐	☐	☐
b. Could the unit have been continued after administration of an antihistamine and antipyretic?	☐	☐	☐
c. Was the appropriate reaction protocol initiated?	☐	☐	☐
5. Were blood or blood products wasted? If yes:	☐	☐	☐
a. Could the wastage have been prevented?	☐	☐	☐

FIG. 3 – SAMPLE CRITERIA FOR BLOOD UTILIZATION

The JCAH also requires that findings of medical staff monitoring activities be coordinated with the medical staff credentialing function to allow a more objective review of a physician's practice at the time of recredentialing. Figure 4 is an example of how Quality Assurance may be incorporated in a Physician's Credentialing Profile.

PHYSICIAN'S QUALITY ASSURANCE PROFILE

Physician: William Blank, M.D.

EVALUATION CRITERIA		YEARS	
	1983	1984	1985
Adverse result of OP Management	2	1	
Readmission for Complications	6	4	
Transfers to Special Care Unit	10	7	
Unplanned return to OR	2	1	
Neurological deficit on discharge	1	0	
Unplanned injury to organ	0	0	
Other complications	6	8	
Nosocomial infections	4	3	
Normal tissue review	0	1	

FIG. 4 – SAMPLE PAGE FROM PHYSICIAN'S CREDENTIALING FILE

In 1985 the JCAH clarified the quality assessment requirement for hospital clinic support services. A common quality assurance standard was added requiring each hospital clinical support service to monitor and evaluate the quality and appropriateness of the patient care services it renders and to resolve identified problems.

This monitoring and evaluation is accomplished by the routine collection of information about important aspects of care and the periodic reassessment of the collected information in order to identify important problems in patient care and opportunities to improve care. When important problems in patient care and opportunities to improve care are identified, action is taken and its effectiveness is evaluated. Figure 5 is an example of a simple monitoring activity for the respiratory therapy service.

When and if monitoring activities demonstrate a problem in patient care or an opportunity to improve patient care, facilities are required to perform a problem-solving activity. This

---

RESPIRATORY THERAPY MONITOR

Order-Treatment Comparison

Objective:

To determine if the respiratory therapy administered corresponds with the respiratory therapy ordered.

Instruction:

1. The schedule of respiratory treatments log identifies patient records to be reviewed.

2. The respiratory therapy staff should collect the information by applying the screens to a predetermined number of records at a specified time (e.g., screen 20 records each week for 4 weeks).

Demographic Data:

Patient identifier
Respiratory therapist identifier
Therapy ordered
Physician identifier

Screens:

1. Does therapy administered correspond with ordered:
    a. Therapy?
    b. Frequency?
    c. Duration?
    d. Dose?
    e. Concentration?

2. Does the number of treatments administered correspond to the number of treatments ordered?

    If no,
    a. More treatments given than ordered?
       (Record # administered_____; # ordered_____)

    b. Less treatments given than ordered?
       (Record # administered_____; # ordered_____)

Fig. 5 – Monitoring Activity for Respiratory Therapy

problem-solving activity can take any form. It does not have to follow a certain format or contain specific elements like the audit methodology. Problem-solving activities should be designed to eliminate or alleviate the problem and should include some method by which to measure success.

The results of monitoring, evaluating and problem-solving activities must be documented as well as the actions taken to resolve problems and the impact of these actions.

With the establishment of Peer Review Organizations (PROs) came new quality assessment requirements for hospitals. Each PRO was required to develop quality objectives for its region as part of its contract with the Health Care Financing Administration (HCFA). Following the general guidelines for quality assessment outlined by the HCFA, PROs developed quality objectives designed to:

1. Reduce avoidable deaths
2. Reduce avoidable complications
3. Reduce unnecessary surgeries or other invasive procedures
4. Identify omissions of necessary services
5. Reduce unnecessary readmissions

Each PRO developed a plan to meet these objectives, the most common being a series of state-wide or region-wide intensive medical care evaluation studies.

INTERNAL PRESSURES FOR QUALITY

Whereas quality assessment activities in the past were performed, for the most part, to fulfill accreditation requirements and Medicare regulations, hospitals and other health care providers are beginning to develop a new internal incentive for quality evaluation. Economic constraints from various external pressures have placed an increasing emphasis on productivity and cost-efficiency. In connection with productivity monitoring, facilities are developing quality monitors by which to measure successful productivity. Quality services provided without error and within the time frames expected are less costly to the facility and the patient. Services of poor quality, with procedural errors and ineffectual outcomes are nonproductive and result in higher patient care costs. The concept "Quality is Free" stands true in today's health care industry and quality monitoring and evaluation systems can serve to identify those areas where poor quality translates into unnecessary expenditures.

RISK MANAGEMENT

More than 1,600 years before the development of the Oath of Hippocrates (circa 400 B.C.), the Code of Hammurabi made provisions for defining physicians' liability in the case of certain injuries they might inflict upon their patients. This code stated:

> "If a surgeon has made a deep incision in the body of a free man and has caused the man's death or has opened the caruncle in the eye and so destroys the man's eye, they shall cut off his forehand."

From this beginning, the fundamental principle of physician liability and accountability for iatrogenic patient injury became an integral part of each subsequent society's medical practices. As civilization and the practice of medicine evolved, physician liability and accountability expanded to include nonphysicians who provide medical care to patients and later to include health care institutions that deliver patient care. Today, if a patient experiences, or thinks he has experienced, an adverse medical occurrence in a hospital, he may hold both the private physician and the hospital liable. The extension of liability to hospitals occurred in 1965, with the court case of Darling v. Charleston Community Memorial Hospital. In this instance, the court upheld the patient's right to recover damages for malpractice from both the physician and the hospital. This ended the long-standing philosophy that hospitals were exempt from liability because of charitable immunity and established the hospital's duty to supervise the action of independent staff physicians.

Today, hospitals are corporately liable for:

1. Exercising reasonable care in providing proper medical equipment, supplies, medication, and food for their patients.
2. Exercising reasonable care in providing safe physical premises for their patients.
3. Adopting internal policies and procedures reasonably estimated to protect the safety and interests of their patients.
4. Exercising reasonable care in the selection and retention of hospital employees and in the granting of medical staff privileges.
5. Exercising reasonable care to guarantee that adequate patient care is being administered.

HOSPITAL LIABILITY

Most liability carriers reported a 30 to 50 percent rise in claims between 1970 and 1980. For both physicians and hospitals, the 1970s were seen as a malpractice crisis, with the number of claims and the dollar amounts of those claims rising dramatically.

Insurance carriers responded to this situation in one of two ways: sudden and total withdrawal from the malpractice insurance market; or, for those insurers that remained in the market, astronomical premium rate increases for hospitals and physicians. For some practitioners, these increases totaled 100 to 200 percent.

From the malpractice crisis of the 1970s came the development of hospital-based risk management programs, which included risk financing as well as loss prevention and control. The loss prevention and control aspect of risk management was designed to control preventable risks and keep to a minimum the incidents for which the institution might be held liable.

Although utilization management and quality assessment activities focus on patterns of care, risk management activities such as loss prevention, focus on the individual case and the potential for a claim to arise from it. An individual patient care problem may represent an enormous potential loss but represents no concern from a quality assessment perspective because it is truly an isolated event. On the other hand, it may represent one of a series of cases with important quality of care considerations.

An effective risk management program incorporates the identification, analysis, evaluation, and elimination or reduction of possible risks to patients, visitors, and employees.

RISK IDENTIFICATION

The primary tool used in the identification of risk is the incident report. Incident reporting provides early detection of problems or potentially compensable events (PCEs) and provides a foundation for an early investigation of serious incidents. Most health care institutions have some type of incident reporting mechanism, requiring all levels of personnel to report happenings not consistent with the routine care of a particular patient.

The format of the incident report varies with the facility, but all require a narrative description of the incident and the actions taken to prevent or avoid further injury. Incident reporting systems identify risks concurrently, at the time the incident occurs.

Other mechanisms are designed to identify potential risks before an incident has occurred. One such tool is the Hazard Surveillance report. Hazard surveillance is required by the JCAH and must be completed at least semiannually. In many facilities, the Safety Officer or Safety committee is assigned the responsibility of identifying potential hazards through the use of a Hazard Surveillance checklist.

A third mechanism used to identify risks, specifically liabilities resulting from physician-related occurrences, is termed "occurrence screening." Occurrence screening allows for the concurrent or retrospective identification of physician-related adverse patient occurrences whereas most incident reporting systems only identify institutional problems. Occurrence screening is sometimes termed "generic screening" because the criteria used in the screening process may be applied to all patients, regardless of the patient's diagnosis or procedure. Examples of common occurrence screens are:

1. Admission for adverse results of outpatient management (i.e. delayed diagnosis, conditions attributed to outpatient drug therapy, or complications from outpatient management).

2. Admission for a complication resulting from incomplete management on a previous hospital admission.

3. Adverse reaction to medications, transfusions, and anesthetics.

4. Unplanned transfer from a general care to a special care unit.

5. Unplanned return to the operating room on the same admission.

6. Perforation, laceration, tear, or injury of an organ during an invasive procedure.

7. Myocardial infarction during or within 48 hours of a surgical procedure.

Occurrence screens are used to identify specific events that occur during a patient's hospitalization. Liability is assigned only after review of the case by both administration and the medical staff. If the system is used concurrently, health care practitioners, often medical record professionals, are employed to analyze cases and identify the events while patients are still hospitalized. If the review is performed retrospectively, the identification of the events occurs postdischarge and data collection is conducted during medical record discharge analysis.

ANALYSIS AND EVALUATION

In the case of incident reporting, the event is analyzed while the patient is still hospitalized and potential liability is assessed. In some instances, the patient involved is contacted by hospital personnel and arrangements made for amicable resolution. Studies have shown that early patient contact in the event of a potentially compensable occurrence, prevents later court action. Many of the incident reports filed do not require such patient contact, with the analysis limited to an assessment of the appropriateness of the actions taken to prevent further problems.

Occurrence screening data are used in much the same manner as incident report information, although physician involvement is required. If the system is concurrent and the events identified while the patient is still hospitalized, steps are taken at that time to reduce potential liability. If the system is retrospective, cases are reviewed by medical staff committees and inappropriate physician practices are handled within the medical staff peer review structure.

ELIMINATION OR REDUCTION OF POSSIBLE RISKS

The incident report is also used as a tool to eliminate or reduce future adverse occurrences. In many instances, the event is discussed with those involved and serves as an educational device to prevent future problems. The data from incident reports are also collated and analyzed to identify high risk areas which may require more intensive education and/or restructuring to eliminate future risks. By analyzing the most frequent areas of injury or risk, risk control programs can be targeted to the problem area.

The Hazard Surveillance function is used to identify areas of potential environmental risk prior to an adverse occurrence. In this way, liabilities may be prevented entirely.

The physician-related adverse patient occurrences identified through an occurrence screening procedure are usually coordinated with the medical staff peer review and credentialing function. Disciplinary action, including loss of staff privileges, may occur if data indicate a pattern or trend of unacceptable physician practices.

ORGANIZATION AND OPERATION OF A RISK MANAGEMENT PROGRAM

The organizational structure of an institutional risk management program varies. Larger facilities may employ a risk manager with a staff of specialists to maintain an effective program. In other facilities the medical record practitioner may be responsible for the risk management program through a committee. In either structure, the medical record department may perform occurrence screening, analyze and display incident report and occurrence screening data, and assist the risk management or quality assurance committee with follow-up activities.

To be effective, the risk management program should be integrated with the facility's quality assurance program. Without such integration, inadequate communication, duplication of effort, excess costs, and questionable impact of the quality of care can occur. With the quality assurance program moving away from periodic audits of patient care and into quality monitoring and problem-solving, the functions of risk identification and analysis can easily be integrated with those of quality assurance.

THE MEDICAL RECORD PRACTITIONER IN QUALITY ASSURANCE

The medical record practitioner with a knowledge of health care information systems and data systems can provide invaluable leadership in quality assurance functions. This leadership may be manifested by accepting responsibility for directing the hospital-wide quality assurance program, coordinating one aspect of the program – i.e., quality assessment, utilization management or risk management, or a more limited role of managing data for the various aspects of the quality assurance program.

The primary data source for quality assurance monitoring is the medical record. Medical record personnel have the unique opportunity of analyzing each patient record. No other department is so closely involved with the documentation in the record. While others may individually write patient care notes in the medical record, only the medical record professional has the advantage of evaluating the record *in toto*. By evaluating the documentation in the record, medical record professionals can identify unrecorded diagnoses, over- or underutilization of services or resources, complications or other inappropriate patient care, inadequate documentation, medication errors, or other procedural problems. For the risk management component of quality assurance, medical record professionals may identify patient complaints, patient incidents, equipment failures, deficiencies in informed consents, inappropriate record alterations, or other documentation problems which may increase liability.

Many medical record departments are actively involved in identifying patient care problems through the use of a generic screening mechanism or other systematic record monitoring. Through the efficient use of medical record professionals in the problem identification phase of quality assurance, duplicative record review by others is eliminated.

The records management expertise of the medical record professional is invaluable in the problem resolution phase of quality assurance. If documentation is a problem, the medical record professional can suggest methods for improvement. In-service programs on the legalities of record documentation can be prepared by the medical record professional. If new chart forms are proposed, the medical record professional should be involved in format design.

Medical record professionals also play an important role in the follow-up phase of problem resolution. Once a problem in patient care has been identified and steps taken to resolve the problem, the medical record professional can assist in monitoring to assure satisfactory problem resolution. This assistance may take the form of ongoing record review or a one-time collection of patient care information. The data obtained by the medical record department are then shared with the medical staff committee or department interested in resolving the problem.

Medical record professionals play a key role in all aspects of a facility-wide quality assurance program. Intradepartmentally they monitor to insure efficiency and effectiveness of their procedures. More importantly, they assist all other components of the program in the problem identification and problem resolution phases. By virtue of their expertise in data collection, record documentation, and forms design, medical record professionals can enhance the overall effectiveness of the health care quality assurrance effort.

SUMMARY

Quality assurance encompasses Quality Assessment, Utilization Management, and Risk Management Activities. Quality assessment activities are required by JCAH and other accrediting bodies and include a review and evaluation function for both physician and facility-related services. The basis for a quality assessment program is ongoing monitoring of important aspects of patient care. When problems or opportunities to improve care are identified, efforts to reduce or eliminate the problem are undertaken.

Utilization management looks at both overutilization and underutilization of services in an effort to provide the best possible health care at the lowest cost.

Risk management programs grew out of the malpractice crisis of the 1970s. An effective risk management program incorporates the identification, analysis, evaluation, and elimination or reduction of possible risks to the institution's patients, visitors, and employees. Incident reporting, occurrence screening, and hazard surveillance are the three primary data collection methods used in a risk management program.

Whatever the approach to the evaluation of patient care, a data-gathering effort is necessary. Medical records supply much of the data for quality assurance activities, hence medical record practitioners are highly involved in collecting such data. Data display and coordination of data within the institution are another important aspect of a quality assurance program. The medical record professional plays an important role in each of the following steps in quality assurance: gathering of data, analysis of data, acting on the findings, and continuing the monitoring process. Data used for quality assurance activities must be accurate and reliable so the medical staff leadership and hospital manager can confidently utilize quality assurance data as a basis for action.

STUDY QUESTIONS

1. Identify three components of a quality assurance program. How do they differ?
2. What is the purpose of quality assessment activities?
3. What is the purpose of utilization management?
4. Identify the procedures which compromise the utilization review process.
5. What was the impetus for development of risk management programs? What are the factors involved in an effective risk management program?
6. What is the role of the medical record practitioner in each of the three components of a quality assurance program?
7. What external and internal pressures in today's health care environment impact on quality assurance programs?

REFERENCES

CONNER, MELODY; MACK, GLORIA; and HANDELMAN, EUGENE. *Dynamics of Utilization Management.* American Hospital Association, Chicago, Illinois, 1983.

DEMUTH, WILLIAM E. "Health Care Costs: One Surgeon's Perspective," Colloquim, *CPC Communications.* Greenwich, Vol. 2, No. 1, February, 1982.

GLAZIER, DON C. "How to Deal with the Impact of Alternate Providers." *Hospital Forum*, September/October, 1984, pp. 57-59.

GREENSPAN, JACK. *Accountability and Quality Assurance in Health Care*. The Charles Press Publishers, 1980.

Joint Commission on Accreditation of Hospitals, *Accreditation Manual for Hospitals*, Chicago, Illinois, 1985.

Joint Commission on Accreditation of Hospitals, *The QA Guide: A Resource for Hospital Quality Assurance*. Chicago, Illinois, 1980.

LAMPREY, JOANNE. *The ISD-A Review System*. InterQual, Chicago, Illinois, 1984.

Medicare Policy: Peer Review Organizations. Chicago, Illinois: American Hospital Association, Special Briefing, July, 1984.

ORLIKOFF, JAMES E., FIFER, WILLIAM R., and GREELEY, HUGH P. *Malpractice Prevention and Liability Control for Hospitals*. Chicago, Illinois: American Hospital Association, 1981.

Quality Assessment: Action and Accountability: Maximizing the Effort. Chicago, Illinois: InterQual, Inc., 1983.

"Quality Assurance Update," *Topics in Health Record Management*. Gaithersburg, Maryland: Aspen Systems Corporation, Vol. 5, No.2, December, 1984.

SPATH, PATRICE L. *Cost Effective Quality Assurance*. Portland: Brown-Spath & Associates, 1984.

LIST OF ILLUSTRATIONS

LIST OF ILLUSTRATIONS

LIST OF TABLES

LIST OF TABLES

INDEX

INDEX

A

Abbreviations, 73
Abstracting, 425
Abstracts, discharge, 417-420
Accident reports, 198
Accreditation, 54-58
Accreditation Association for Ambulatory Health Care, 57-58, 145
Accreditation Manual for Hospitals, 6
Accreditation of medical record professional, 36-39
Administrative data, 76-80
Admission
    form, 76-78, 80-83
    note, 104-105
    register, 430-431
Admitting
    department, 63-64
    evaluation, 186-189
Allied health practitioners, 17-18, 19
Alphabetic filing, 204-206, 403-405
Ambulatory care, 12-13, 134-153
    classification systems, 389-391
    computerized records, 147-148
    emergency records, 137-140
    free-standing, 142-153
    free-standing facility records, 145-149
    group practice, 143
    health maintenance organizations, 144
    home care, 153-160
    hospice programs, 160-169
    hospital-based, 134-141
    neighborhood health centers, 143
    outpatient records, 136-140
    preferred provider organizations, 144

quality assurance, 149-153
satellite care units, 141
statistical definitions, 152-153
statistics, 495, 497
surgery facilities, 141
uniform data set, 150-151
urgent care, 145
American Academy of Pediatrics, 127-128
American Association of Blood Banks, 110
American College of Obstetrics and Gynecology, 119
American College of Physicians, 21
American College of Surgeons, 3-4, 6, 20-21, 56-57
American Hospital Association, 21-22
American Medical Association, 20
American Medical Record Association (AMRA)
    Board of Directors, 25
    classification systems, 368
    code of ethics, 28-30
    continuing education program, 39
    councils/subcouncils/committees, 25-26
    emblem, 30-33
    executive office, 26-27
    Foundation of Record Education (FORE), 27
    House of Delegates, 25
    independent study program, 36
    membership categories, 24
    mission of, 24
    official colors of, 32
    organization of, 4-6
    pledge, 30-33
    publications, 28